Infant Previewing

Paul V. Trad

Infant Previewing

Predicting and Sharing
Interpersonal Outcome

Springer-Verlag
New York Berlin Heidelberg
London Paris Tokyo Hong Kong

Paul V. Trad
Department of Psychiatry
The New York Hospital-
Cornell Medical Center
White Plains, NY 10605
USA

Library of Congress Cataloging-in-Publication Data
Trad, Paul V.
    Infant previewing : predicting and sharing interpersonal outcome /
Paul V. Trad.
        p.   cm.
    Includes bibliographical references.
    ISBN 0-387-97197-1
    1. Infants—Mental health.   2. Mental illness—Diagnosis.
3. Mother and infant.   4. Infant psychiatry.   I. Title.
RJ502.5.T73   1990
155.42'2—dc20   89-26237

Printed on acid-free paper.

Media Conversion by David E. Seham Associates Inc., Metuchen, New Jersey.
Printed and bound by BookCrafters USA Inc.
Printed in the United States of America.

9 8 7 6 5 4 3 2 1

ISBN 0-387-97197-1 Springer-Verlag New York Berlin Heidelberg
ISBN 3-540-97197-1 Springer-Verlag Berlin Heidelberg New York

Preface

Although a good deal of recent research in the area of infant and early childhood development has probed the nature of the interaction between the caregiver and the infant, few researchers have articulated a comprehensive thesis that captures the full impact of the normative developmental processes of the mother-child relationship. In the past several years, I have devoted myself to articulating a theory of early infant psychopathology. The etiology of such psychopathology appears to lie in deficits that plague the dyadic relationship. These deficits can often be rectified when adaptive behaviors are reintroduced into the primary interaction between mother and child and when the overwhelming potency of the trends of imminent development are appreciated, acknowledged and responded to. Thus, from my work with caregivers and infants who suffer interactional failures, I began to understand that the dyad must align itself with the rhythms of adaptive development if the infant is to mature in a psychologically healthy fashion.

My work in this area also led to the notion of *previewing*. As will be discussed more fully in the following chapters, previewing refers to a unique quality, manifested in varying degrees by virtually every caregiver, which helps propel development forward by introducing the infant to imminent maturational trends. Previewing requires that the caregiver represent or envision the direction of incipient development, convert these representations into behavioral manifestations which may be enacted during interaction with the infant and then, in a supportive fashion, ease the infant slowly back to his previous developmental state. Not only did I discover that adaptive previewing was an integral part of the dyadic relationship between mothers and infants who were interacting in an optimal fashion, but it also became apparent that previewing techniques could be used as an interventive tool by therapists to help realign relationships that had gone awry and to help stimulate infants who had been deprived of adaptive interaction.

Moreover, a review of the recent clinical and experimental literature revealed that certain caregivers appeared highly competent at stimulating their infants appropriately and encouraging the manifestation of maturational skill. The infants of such caregivers tended to be extraordinarily motivated in the sense that they communicated, through gestures and facial expressions, a desire to perpetuate the interaction with the caregiver. Investigators have labeled caregivers who display these characteristics as "intuitive," "empathic," and "responsive." Despite the label, however, on closer examination these caregivers appear to be exhibiting a cluster of behaviors which, taken together, comprise previewing manifestations. Although the overarching concept of previewing has not been introduced before, the normative components of this phenomenon have been associated with adaptive caregivers. Thus, clinical and experimental studies have already provided some substantiation for the concept of previewing.

This book, then, serves to launch the theory of previewing by providing an explanation of the concept, by describing how previewing heightens the maturational processes of the infant, and by offering guidelines for using previewing behaviors in the treatment of caregiver-infant dyads. Because this concept has proven to be such a potent instrument for effecting change within the mother-infant relationship, several other volumes that explore various clinical implications of this phenomenon are in preparation. The fundamental notion of previewing as an all-encompassing concept and its dramatic effect on the early infancy years is described in the following pages.

My understanding of previewing required a good deal of thought and analysis. During this process, I was deeply fortunate to be able to discuss my ideas with Wendy Luftig, whose keen intelligence and encouragement were given consistently and without reservation. My warm thanks also go to Richard H. White for his unflagging support. My appreciation is also extended to Craig C. Berggren who was always willing to discuss my ideas and share his insights. I am grateful to Sharon Yamamoto, James Wtorkowski, Stephanie Hill, and Vernon Bruette who assisted in preparing the manuscript. My warm acknowledgement is extended to Paulina F. Kernberg, M.D. whose critical insight and compassion have guided my career.

Finally, this book is dedicated to Jorge, Pilar, Emilio, Emily, Roberto, Ligia, Alex and Lorena—my brothers and sisters-in-law. They have always made me feel special.

Contents

The Concept of Previewing: Introduction

Just as fairy tales of childhood begin with a predictable "once upon a time" and end with the familiar "they lived happily ever after," so too does this book suggest that infant development is a tale whose beginning and end may be predicted.This book is an adventure story. It concerns two main characters—the mother and the infant, with the father as an occasional third protagonist. The adventure is about growth and change, which in the parlance of modern psychiatry is referred to as *developmental processes*. In particular, though, this book highlights both the phenomenon of growing up during the first two years of life, a period that has been labeled infancy, and introduces a new concept—*previewing*—which facilitates our understanding of how the transformations of maturation that occur during this period modify the relationship between mother and infant.

Unlike other approaches to the study of infant development during the first two years of life, this book strives to offer the reader a new perspective from which to view maturational phenomena. This new perspective comes from numerous clinical observations by the author of mother-infant interaction, as well as from a critical analysis of research data pertaining to the interactions characteristic of parents and infants. As a result of these efforts, the concept of previewing was born. Previewing refers to many aspects of the interpersonal exchange that occurs between caregiver and infant. Distilled to its essence, previewing encompasses all of the processes, enacted by both members of the dyad, that serve to propel development of enhanced skill and mastery of the increasingly complex challenges posed by the interaction between two developing individuals—caregiver and infant. It is the contention of the author that, although maturational progression will occur in any event as a result of the infant's constitutional endowment, this maturation requires an interpersonal component in order for development to evolve in the most adaptive fashion. The infant must be exposed to caregiver-initiated behavior that encourages adaptive interactions. This form of interactive behavior provides the dyad with insight into the contours of imminent developmental acquisition and permits the infant to obtain a full awareness of what lies over the next developmental horizon, as well as a sense of the implications that these changes will have on the interaction. Once the infant is exposed to this form of nurturing response by the caregiver, his own developmental skills are heightened. In this manner, previewing perpetuates the mutually fulfilling relationship. The primary reason why this relationship is so fulfilling is that it offers to both dyadic members a paradigm for deriving an enhanced sense of control and mastery over the myriad of developmental changes.

Previewing as a Parental Manifestation

Given the wealth of knowledge derived from clinical studies, we can begin to predict how a specific mother and infant dyad will undergo the ritual of developmental evolution. But beyond the predictions of the researcher—be he or she a therapist, clinical investigator, or bystander—are the predictions of the two crucial characters in the drama of development—the mother and the infant. From the contours of their representational images, each of these individuals formulates future interactions which allow them to evolve a unique sense of partnership. This developmental pattern will transform two lives, that of the infant and that of the caregiver. The goals of the following chapters are to provide insight into the dynamic processes that occur during this interaction and to reveal how the predictions of both mother and child that emerge in the form of previewing behavior leave an indelible interpersonal imprint on the lives of both.

How can we detect this behavior when studying the caregiver-infant relationship? As discussed in the beginning chapters of this book, the caregiver's interactive skills during the early months appear imbued with *intuitive* qualities. Caregivers who engage in previewing manifest particular behavior that suggests an awareness of the infant's imminent developmental status. These behaviors appear to be spontaneous and yet indicate an awareness of subtle cues being given by the infant. It is almost as if the caregiver possesses a comprehensive image or representation of how the developmental processes will unfold for her individual infant; such representations guide the dyad in the direction of developmental achievement. As explained in detail in the opening chapters, previewing incorporates that caregiver behavior which offers the infant a *prediction* or *foreshadowing* of the social implications of imminent developmental change and achievement.

Broken down into its components, previewing consists of a trio of specific behaviors. First, the caregiver must *anticipate* the trends of upcoming maturational attainment. Once the caregiver has, in a sense, felt the infant's developmental pulse and envisioned future maturation, she can begin helping the infant to predict which imminent milestones will occur in the near future. The attuned caregiver will be able to sense these milestones from their onset because of her exquisite sensitivity to the infant's behavioral cues. Sensitivity to these cues allows the caregiver to anticipate what kind of developmental achievement is imminent. The second stage of previewing requires that the caregiver *transform* her sense of milestones into behavioral manifestations which can be shared with the infant during interactional sequences in order to help him coordinate emerging precursory functions. Exercising the limbs of the infant to simulate crawling patterns or guiding the hand of the infant who is beginning to grasp for utensils are just two examples of how caregivers convert their predictions about imminent developmental change into previewing exercises. Finally, previewing requires that the caregiver be sensitive to cues that the infant wishes to return to an already-mastered developmental level. A caregiver who senses such cues will gradually abate the previewing activity and will slowly ease the infant back to the developmentally mastered status manifested prior to the initiation of the previewing exercise. In order to derive adaptive results from previewing exercises the dyadic members must "cue" one another reciprocally. Such cuing generates predictions about imminent developmental trends and about the implications these trends will have on the relationship between mother and child.

Previewing exercises are also significant in helping the infant develop a sense of self and self-regulation. As will be described in the following chapters, it is my contention that previewing facilitates the evolution of the infant's self-regulatory capacities in two main ways. First, the infant is provided with an interactional arena where his intentions, actions, and feelings can be reflected by the caregiver who reinforces the infant's anticipations of future interpersonal changes. The caregiver who previews adaptively conveys the message that developmental and adaptational changes can not only be predicted, but can also be mastered within the interpersonal arena. In addition, the exposure to previewing enables the infant to reinforce cause-effect relationships. In other words, the infant gradually learns to tailor behavioral responses which convey that he is either ready for yet a new previewing experience or that he wishes to rehearse again a previous previewing experience. The adaptive caregiver understands these cues and pursues the infant's intentions. As a result of these interactions, the dyad masters the flow of interpersonal changes in two ways. First, by learning to coax the caregiver to begin or finish a previewing episode, the infant begins to experience mastery over social interactions. This mastery suffuses the dyad with feelings of security and competence, staving off the debilitating effects that emanate from the incongruity between what is intended and what is experienced. Second, in the infant, previewing fosters the perception that developmental processes can best be anticipated and mastered through social interaction.

As will be discussed in Chapter 1, in some ways the behavior of the caregiver during previewing episodes may actually be a continuation of the kinds of anticipatory reveries or fantasies the caregiver engaged in prior to the birth. Thoughts which occupy the mind of the pregnant woman can offer insight into the ultimate nature of the relationship of the dyad. With the arrival of the infant, however, the caregiver is challenged to transform these representational musings into a palpable reality. In this, most caregivers will be assisted by the infant himself who is poised on the brink, ready and eager to absorb the diverse stimuli that surround him.

As will be discussed in Chapter 2, these intuitive behaviors predominate the interactions of adaptive caregivers and their infants and help to create a fluid and attuned relationship. However, these behaviors are deficient or lacking in those caregivers whose response to the infant is detached or maladaptive. Moreover, it also appears that these intuitive behaviors act as the building blocks of the previewing behavior sensitive caregivers use to introduce their infants to imminent developmental trends. As such, a knowledge of these intuitive behaviors becomes crucial for the therapist engaged in diagnosing and treating mother-infant dyads in which adaptive patterns of interaction have gone awry. A catalog of these behaviors includes: *visual cuing, verbal cuing, tactile stimulation, feeding competence,* and *appropriate holding behavior.* As will be seen in the following chapters, these behaviors not only reinforce the infant's current developmental status and fulfill his immediate needs, but also serve the deeper purpose of fostering predictability as the infant progresses to more sophisticated tiers of development.

Previewing as a Dyadic Manifestation

Although previewing which specifically introduces the infant to imminent developmental acquisition is largely a caregiver initiated activity, the infant also participates actively in this process by anticipating and engaging in behaviors designed to elicit a particular caregiver response. If a specific chain of interactive events occurs, the infant will gradually acquire the skill to convey to the caregiver his eagerness to be introduced to the skills of the next developmental level. In order to be able to engage in this fairly sophisticated means of communication with the caregiver, the infant must first be able to *represent* developmental change. Representation here is defined as a reflective state during which knowledge comes through images of the external world, which are perceived on the stage of active consciousness. Representation, in other words, requires that the infant inculcate himself with various perceptions gleaned from the experiences to which he is repeatedly exposed.

Once the infant solidifies his representational capacities, he can begin making associations between discrete representations. Such associations have been labeled *contingencies,* and refer to stimulus-response sequences involving a recognizable object or event that triggers a distinct behavioral response. For example, the fact that the infant's cry (stimulus) causes the mother to feed the infant (response) is an example of a classic contingency relationship. As the infant begins to recognize various contingencies, he can begin to anticipate or predict them. Eventually, he will begin to manipulate or vary these contingencies in order to experiment with his ability to elicit a new or a different response.

Infant previewing is also bolstered by a trio of developmental skills that motivate the infant to predict and thus control the experiential world surrounding him. One of these developmental skills involves the capacity for *symbolic thought*. Essentially, symbolic thought involves the capacity of the infant to recognize that a particular symbol, such as a word, stands for or represents a particular object.

As explained in Chapter 6, previewing demonstrations engaged in by the dyad involve several kinds of manifestations. These manifestations may be conceptualized on two levels. First, the immediate behavioral gestures the caregiver exhibits convey direct nonverbal messages. In other words, a caregiver who is previewing the act of crawling to the baby by exercising his limbs in a particular way is communicating the message that the concept of crawling consists of that particular combination of neuromuscular alignment and movement. The caregiver's physical manifestations (gestures and nuances) thus serve to communicate a unique and distinctive message. This mode of communication, whereby the content of the message and the means used to convey the message overlap, is referred to as *analogic mode*. However, when the caregiver engages in previewing exercises with the infant she is not only conveying a message about the current activity, but she is also orienting the infant towards the interpersonal implications that will arise from imminent developmental achievement. In the above example, previewing is one way in which the caregiver communicates to the infant the notion of "this is what the sensation of crawling will feel like some day soon when you develop sufficient skill to engage in this behavior on your own." This message, however, is a symbolic one, in the sense that the behavior engaged in contemporaneously actually serves as a metaphor for the future experience the infant will undergo when he articulates the developmental milestone on his own. The mode of conveying symbolic meanings is referred to as the *digital mode,* whereby the means used to represent the message is different from the message itself. The most sophisticated type of digital communication is obviously language, whereby arbitrary symbols can signify or represent objects and concepts entirely distinct from their own intrinsic meaning.

I am not suggesting that the manifestations of previewing resemble the digital mode of communication in the same fashion that words do. However, I am proposing that previewing may signify a unique form of communication for the infant because it combines elements of both the digital and the analogic modes of communication. As such, it is a *hybrid mode* of communication which allows the infant to capture the direct visceral feel of analogic communication while simultaneously experiencing a symbolic or digital component. Because previewing serves as this interim type of communication, it may help the infant evolve the capacity to engage in sophisticated symbolic thought and to use this capacity as the vehicle for beginning to think in symbolic terms. Although researchers have not yet discerned each of the discrete steps involved in acquiring the capacity for symbolic thought, it is not farfetched to suggest that through episodes of repeated previewing the infant eventually comes to develop symbolic representational capacities. Symbolic representations emerge as the infant begins to manipulate and experiment with internal imagery. This activity is stimulated by previewing.

A second developmental skill that reinforces the infant's capacity to engage in predicting the future is *play*. As will be explained in Chapter 5, play activity is essentially defined as consisting of three primary components—a *cognitive component,* which encourages the infant to experiment with already familiar contingency patterns; an *affective component,* which consists of positive emotions that imbue the play activity; and, a *social component,* which involves the fact that, at least during the first year of life, play is primarily an activity that is initiated by the caregiver who provides reciprocal cues to maintain the interaction.

In assessing the effect of play behavior on the infant's development, researchers have been particularly cognizant of the social aspect that characterizes play during the first year of life. It is this social component, comprised of attentive caregiver ministrations designed to stimulate the infant to maintain the interaction, which has been interpreted as being a prerequisite for adaptive cognitive and emotional development. Significantly, both previewing and play share similar characteristics. Both phenomena occur within the context of dyadic exchange and both result in a positive affect that appears to suffuse the entire interaction. Moreover, each of these activities appears vital in engaging the infant in behavioral challenges designed to enhance new skills. Perhaps the main difference between these activities is that play focuses on experimentation with representations and skills which have already been attained whereas previewing is oriented towards the future and those developmental capabilities which lie on the next developmental horizon. Despite this difference, it is clear that both activities are instrumental aspects of the developmental process and warrant exploration and examination. Play enriches cognitive operations by providing the infant with an arena in which he can experiment with his newly discovered skills while interacting with the caregiver in a pleasurable fashion. Through play, the infant varies familiar configurations and restructures new outcomes. It is through play, then, that the infant gives his predictions about the world a dress rehearsal.

Rounding out the trio of developmental skills explored is *multimodal perception.* Multimodal perception refers to the infant's capacity to coordinate and integrate perceptions infringing upon him in various modes. For example, the integration of visual and auditory modes allows the infant to perceive both perceptions simultaneously and to scrutinize the invariant characteristics of a single object. The capacity to integrate all of the varied perceptions emanating from a particular object, as well as the ability to identify the invariant qualities emanating from different objects, represents full-fledged intermodal functioning.

Intermodal capacities are seminal to the infant's development for a variety of reasons, as discussed in Chapter 4. It should be remembered that in order for the infant to make sense of the messages being conveyed through previewing or play activity, he must first comprehend the source of the message in a coherent and integrated fashion. In addition, the evolution of intermodal integration is critical for the infant's capacity to delineate boundaries between himself and the world. By understanding the nature of the perceptual stimulation he is receiving, the infant comes to recognize that there is an "other" participating in his maturational journey. The awareness of the "other" fuels the burgeoning recognition of the "sense of self."

Previewing as a Therapeutic Goal

Given the bold dynamics of previewing, it is logical to inquire whether this interpersonal phenomenon may be used by therapists working to instill more adaptive patterns of interaction between new mothers and infants as the dyadic relationship matures during the early years of life. The answer to this question is definitively positive. Previewing represents a valuable clinical tool for therapists working with new parents as well as for the parents themselves. Individual chapters are dedicated to explaining how previewing can be reinforced through stimulation and play, and how therapists can encourage previewing behavior in caregivers who, because of psychopathology or the birth of a premature or developmentally disabled infant, are not integrating these manifestations into the typical daily experience of the infant and are thereby failing to represent the infant's imminent development.

Caregivers may be taught, for example, that development is a process which is capable of being both predicted and mastered. Through the relationship with the therapist such predictions begin even before the baby is born when the mother formulates expectations about a whole host of phenomena from the infant's temperament to how she herself will undergo a developmental transformation in assuming the role of a nurturing caregiver. Indeed, for many expectant parents a representational reverie of the child is conjured up. The potency of such parental expectations, confirmed in documented interviews with expectant caregivers, prompts researchers to ask how these fantasies are eventually transformed into behavioral manifestations enacted in the caregiver-infant relationship that shapes the infant's developmental course. And, if the actual baby possesses habits and idiosyncracies that diverge from the parental expectations, how do parents cope with these discrepancies and how does their behavior reflect how they have adapted to the infant's unique and individual personality. Moreover, how do such discrepancies between the parental antenatal fantasy of the infant and the actual infant effect the evolution of an attachment between mother and infant during the infancy years? In therapy, caregivers can examine how their predictions and expectations effect the maturing infant and the environment in which his development will unfold. One chapter of this book explores these antenatal fantasies and the way they may be analyzed by the therapist to predict and modify the course of future interaction between mother and child.

Since previewing also addresses the infant's role in the journey of development, it is important that caregivers in treatment recognize that the infant is not merely an amalgam of parental expectations and hopes but is a creature capable of influencing the shape of representations and interactions. As such, the infant can learn to predict future interactions, as the parent can, and can then engage in behavior that indicates genuine mastery and control over his universe. Recent data suggest that the infant is equipped with a broad spectrum of innate skills which help him navigate his way through this new world. Researchers have demonstrated that the wizened and crying creature who emerges at birth possesses remarkable capacities for responding to the diverse stimuli. Beyond these constitutional endowments, however, lies the prolific realm of developmental potential. Within the first three months of life, infants emerge from the cocoon of neonatal status and begin to display such sophisticated skills as contingency awareness and discrepancy awareness. This level of perception indicates that memories are accumulating at a rapid pace, both in terms of the diversity of information that can be stored and subsequently retrieved and in terms of the way in which past images are connected. From manifestations of these abilities researchers have inferred that infants begin to represent the world around themselves at an extraordinarily young age. Representation ultimately facilitates the infant's ability to discern contingencies and to develop predictions about himself and the world around him.

But these predictions will only occur if the infant is exposed to sufficient previewing exercises that help him to understand the developmental changes occurring within his body. If the caregiver fails to provide the infant with sufficient support and stimulation in the form of adequate previewing exercises, the infant may be unable to control or master the developmental changes he is undergoing. This sense of uncontrollability can lead to somatic, affective, and cognitive deficits that hinder adaptive interaction. The emergence of any or all of these deficits leaves the infant trying to master a maladaptive interaction without overcoming the deficit(s); instead, the infant may come to incorporate these deficits into his interpersonal behavior and sense of self. However, if the caregiver's previewing behaviors provide the infant with a means of predicting and coordinating his burgeoning skills, dysphoric feelings will be assuaged. Indeed, the infant will acquire a sense of competence over his own developmental destiny. Therefore, in order to create an optimal relationship with the infant, it becomes vital for the therapist to insure that caregivers are using previewing in an adaptive manner. This book strives to demonstrate how this goal can be accomplished so that previewing becomes a primary vehicle for enhancing the infant's developmental journey.

CHAPTER 1

Prelude to Previewing: The Effects of Prenatal Representations

Introduction

This book delves into the relationship that is forged during the first years of life between the caregiver and infant, and seeks to explore this relationship from a unique perspective. According to this perspective, the most vital characteristic of early interaction concerns how the caregiver prepares the infant for imminent developmental achievement and for effectively surmounting the challenges posed by the environment.

To describe the full implications of such caregiver behavior, the word *previewing* has been coined. Essentially, previewing represents a three-stage process that virtually every caregiver engages in to varying degrees. During the first stage of previewing, the caregiver is called upon to *represent* the contours of development by envisioning the infant's current developmental status and then by anticipating how imminent maturation will unfold in the context of interaction with the infant. This representational phase of previewing may be conscious or unconscious, but it emerges largely from the caregiver's fantasies and imaginings about her relationship with the infant. Moreover, as will be seen in this chapter, the fantasies pertaining to future dyadic interaction between mother and infant first surface during the antenatal period.

The second aspect of previewing requires the caregiver to operationalize these expectations of infant development through behavior aimed at the infant. The caregiver who senses that the infant is on the verge of exhibiting full-fledged crawling behavior will, for example, begin exercising the infant's limbs to simulate crawling motions or the mother who observes that fine motor skills are becoming more apparent will guide the infant in the consolidation of these skills by helping him reach out and grasp objects. These episodes, during which previewing is most evident to the observer, serve several purposes. First, they function to acquaint the infant with the sensation that will actually attend crawling behavior. Such previewing exercises also serve to familiarize the infant with how the milestone will be experienced as an event that will modify subsequent interactions with the caregiver. In other words, the notion that developmental achievement not only emerges, but also modifies the contours of the relationship with the caregiver, is reinforced. Another benefit gained as a result of such previewing exercises is that the infant comes to rely upon the caregiver as a repository of knowledge about future development and as a guide who can help him refine his burgeoning skills to achieve interpersonal and developmental goals.

Finally, the third aspect of previewing involves the caregiver's capacity to sense when the infant has been sufficiently exposed to the new maturational experience and is ready to return to his current developmental status. As a result of this perceptual sensitivity, the caregiver gradually tapers off the previewing exercise and, in a supportive fashion, reacquaints the infant with the developmental level he manifested prior to the initiation of the previewing exercise. This final phase of previewing requires that the caregiver be attuned to the infant's affective and mood state, as well as to his level of cognitive arousal.

As will be seen, the caregiver's role in initiating and sustaining interaction with the infant remains the most vital contribution to the evolution of the infant's ability to predict and subsequently control the challenges posed by internal and external forces. It is only when the infant can predict with some certainty the events in the world that he acquires a sense of mastery that motivates his self-development. Perhaps the most significant way in which the caregiver fosters these predictive capacities is through previewing. Previewing behavior assumes many shapes and forms and yet all previewing behaviors incorporate aspects of prediction about imminent maturational change. This chapter will focus on how previewing actually begins during pregnancy with the caregiver envisioning her relationship with the infant. At that time the caregiver formulates a variety of speculations about the infant, ranging from what the infant will look like to what the infant's characteristical disposition will be like. In addition, the caregiver will often engage in deep and prolonged reveries about what the relationship with the baby will be like and how this relationship will affect her relationship with other significant people. To what extent are these speculations or anticipations about the infant eventually converted into maternal behaviors designed to elicit certain specific responses in the infant? In other words, how does the mother's behavior toward the infant after birth act as a kind of self-fulfilling prophesy, causing the infant to develop in the particular fashion the mother has anticipated? This theme of how prenatal expectations influence the caregiver's eventual previewing behavior is explored in depth in this chapter.

In addition, this chapter focuses on how other maternal experiences and behaviors that trace their origins to pregnancy, such as stress and psychopathology, contribute to the attitude the caregiver conveys to the infant after birth. Once again, previewing plays a key role here because it is from these nuances of maternal behavior that the infant begins to acquire knowledge of himself and the world. A mother who subjects her infant to stress may preclude him from experiencing contingencies in his environment and such an infant may acquire a distorted perception of his ability to interact with others. Moreover, a caregiver who has experienced stress during pregnancy may have special difficulties in later differentiating these representations from the reality of the infant. As a result, the infant may begin to manifest developmental change at a precocious pace as a means of distancing himself and thereby coping with the caregiver's distressing emotional states. Or, the infant may develop somatic, affective, cognitive or motivational deficits, which emerge in the form of behavioral disorganization, because the impaired representations the caregiver conveys to the infant have not permitted representational skills to emerge adaptively. To understand how these phenomena can occur, it is necessary to focus first on the pregnancy period. Thus, in this chapter we explore the concept of previewing from the earliest days of pregnancy and examine how the caregiver's expectations of the future eventually affect the relationship with the infant.

Why, though, are we positing that previewing begins even before the birth of the child? Until quite recently virtually all research concerning the evolution of social interaction between mothers and infants began with the premise that the dyadic relationship commenced at birth. It was assumed that until the infant emerged from the womb no genuine communication or contact could transpire. New investigations, however, have been far more ambitious in delineating the starting point of interactional patterns between mother and child. Indeed, some investigations have posited that the period of gestation itself heralds the onset of the mother's relationship with the infant and the beginning of maternal expectations about the child's psychological make-up, physical characteristics and the type of relationship that will ensue between mother and infant.

Studies of this genre explore both the physical and psychological changes wrought by pregnancy. Some studies focus on how the physiologic changes occurring in the mother's body affect the infant's ultimate physical status at birth and may exert an impact on the mother's psychological attitude towards the infant. These studies indicate, for example, that mothers who experience high levels of daily stress during gestation may be prone to giving birth to low birth weight babies or babies with temperamental dispositions that may be classified as "difficult." In a similar vein, physiologic phenomena like elevated maternal blood pressure and tachycardia may be related not only to such immediate outcomes as prematurity, but also to such long-term conditions as childhood enuresis and hyperactivity, according to some researchers. Essentially, these investigations probe the issue of whether the mother's physiologic status creates a *predictable outcome* in the infant that may color the nature of dyadic interaction during the infancy and early childhood years. This chapter also explores the possibility that caregivers who experience a physically difficult pregnancy may subsequently have difficulty in representing the infant as a healthy and thriving interactive partner. As a result, the caregiver's ability to preview will be impaired.

In addition to such physiologically oriented studies, however, over the past decade researchers have explored how the mother's psychological status, as evaluated by such measures as self-concept and self-esteem, can impact on preconceived notions of the developing fetus. Psychological attitudes are later transformed into behaviors manifested during interaction with the infant. Such inquiries have led to investigations of maternal and paternal prenatal reveries and to the correlation of these fantasies with subsequent patterns of infant interaction. In particular, the way in which these fantasies may affect the caregiver's ability to preview imminent development to the infant is highlighted. These fantasies offer a rich source for discerning the contours of an inchoate relationship between caregivers and infants that first surfaces during the pregnancy.

Material of this type has proven indispensable to researchers for a wide variety of reasons. First, it should be remembered that pregnancy itself is a period of stress for the expectant mother. Just as she undergoes enormous upheaval and dramatic change in her physiologic states, so too is the mother's physical state paralleled by psychological alterations. These psychological alterations provide insight into how the new mother envisions or previews her relationship with the infant. For example, some researchers have suggested that the somatic changes that occur during the first trimester are evocative of changes in body dimension and image that women experience during puberty. By the second trimester, when fetal movement begins to occur, the mother is confronted with the sometimes startling realization that there is, in fact, a creature within her who is dependent upon her for sustenance. Many researchers believe that this period of quickening is the time when expectant mothers first fully comprehend the notion of motherhood and, as a consequence, reassess and reflect upon their relationships with their own mothers. Finally, late pregnancy is a time of preparation for the impending birth. With the approach of this event, the mother experiences yet a third dramatic psychological realization—the notion that separation and feelings of loss are an inevitable part of the developmental process of giving birth.

Thus, the expectant mother will most likely re-experience in the relatively short period of nine months, three of the most critical phases of her own development:

1. The uncertainty and anticipation of attaining womanhood through the physiological changes of puberty;
2. The recall of feelings about her nurturing experience with her own caregiver; and,
3. Earlier life experiences with separation, loss and depression involved in the achievement of independent status.

Depending upon the mother's own life experience with these events, the way in which she ultimately comes to preview developmental experience for the infant may well replicate her own emotional history. As a result, the physical and psychological changes the mother endures during the pregnancy period will be likely to exert an effect on the nature of the relationship she forges with the infant.

Nor are expectant fathers immune from undergoing similar emotional turmoil during the period of their spouse's pregnancy. As recent studies reveal, husbands may experience feelings of isolation because their wives are absorbed in the gestation process and in the anticipation of giving birth. Isolation and alienation may be further exacerbated as the future father becomes aware of the physiologic changes in his wife, which in turn create changes in the sexual patterns between the couple. Moreover, just as an impending birth arouses maternal insecurity at the prospect of caring for a newborn, so too may the expectant father become anxious at the notion of responsibility that the new infant represents. In addition, fathers may feel left out of the birth process because, unlike the expectant mother, they do not experience the visceral changes that attend pregnancy. Because of this, some expectant fathers may feel physically and emotionally separated from their infants and this sense of detachment may later manifest in the form of difficulty in establishing an interactional bond with the infant. Expectant fathers, then, may feel deprivation and loneliness, and in contrast to earlier challenges posed by the marital relationship, they may not be able to share these feelings with their mate; in fact, the expectant mother may actually be viewed as the source of these conflicting and confusing emotions. Lastly, fathers, too, will be forced to view their wives in a new role (that of being a mother) and this changed perception of their mate can lead to a resurrection of a conflict that existed with their own caregivers during childhood. Thus, the psychological alterations the expectant father undergoes during the pregnancy will likely have implications for how he previews development for the infant.

Research into all of these phenomena has resulted in three basic findings that will be explored in depth in this chapter. First, a relationship does in fact exist between the mother and the infant during the gestational period, and this incipient relationship serves as a paradigm for predicting the type of interaction that will transpire between the caregiver and infant after birth and the caregiver's subsequent ability to preview development adaptively to the infant. This relationship is best investigated and defined by examining studies that have elaborated upon both maternal and paternal fantasies during pregnancy. The reader here should not be misled by use of the word *fantasy*. In this instance, fantasy refers not to a pretend or imaginary state of being that is transitory and fleeting, but rather to profoundly felt beliefs and cognitions which will most likely exert an impact on the mother's manifestations towards the infant and are likely to permeate the entire relationship forged during the period of infancy. The practitioner can gain access to these fantasies by asking the expectant mother to report on both her physical status and her emotional perspective. Both of these inquiries will reveal how the caregiver is beginning to represent the infant and her future relationship with the infant. In addition, these fantasies suggest how the caregiver will envision future development and preview how maturational trends will have an impact for the infant.

The second significant theme to emerge from these studies of the perceptions of expectant women is that the antenatal relationship with the infant has *predictive validity*. That is, therapists can interpret the caregiver's fantasies to anticipate future areas of harmonious interaction, as well as domains of potential discord, which will predominate the relationship with the infant after birth. Indeed, researchers have drawn correlations between the mother's antenatal, largely fantasy-oriented relationship with the infant and such postnatal phenomena as infant temperamental traits, behavioral abnormalities (such as enuresis and hyperactivity), and patterns of secure and insecure attachment. Once again, the caregiver's fantasies can be used as predictors for discerning the eventual relationship which emerges after birth. Finally, perhaps the most challenging finding of these research efforts is that antenatal relationship patterns that are indicative of risk and future maladaptation can be modified during the period of pregnancy itself or during early infancy so that a potentially maladaptive relationship with the infant is averted. It is possible, in other words, to apply the research findings gleaned from these studies to reshape and realign the mother's relationship with the infant into an interaction that is more conducive to adaptive development.

In order to accomplish this goal, the practitioner must be able to understand how the caregiver's antenatal perceptions will be converted into a particular attitude towards the infant, as well as into particular kinds of previewing behaviors that convey a specific view of development to the infant. By modifying the content of the caregiver's representations, previewing behaviors themselves will be altered in a more adaptive direction. This last finding signifies a challenge to all therapists who work with dyads.

It is the intent of this chapter to assist such practitioners in honing their diagnostic and treatment skills in order that maladaptive patterns be altered as early in the infant's life as possible. Thus, learning how to detect the caregiver's potential for adaptively previewing development during the pregnancy period, and using this knowledge to help both parents create an atmosphere conducive to optimal development, represents the prime goal of therapists working with expectant and new parents.

Prenatal Representations of the Infant: The Physiologic Repercussions of Pregnancy

Several researchers have suggested that the attachment bond between mother and infant, which becomes palpably evident after birth, actually begins to evolve during the antenatal period.

Relying on studies which focus on the physiologic changes that the caregiver undergoes during the pregnancy, these researchers seek to draw some correlations between these visceral alterations in the expectant mother and the kind of relationship that is eventually forged with the infant. Although the findings of these studies are tentative, we may derive some general theories about the impact of physical changes on the ultimate attachment between mother and infant. In addition, we may hypothesize about how the caregiver's physical status during the pregnancy may affect her capacity to represent developmental change to the infant in an adaptive fashion.

In order to do this, it is necessary to begin with the pregnancy experience itself, which consists in large measure of the objective physical changes the expectant mother undergoes. During this time, the mother's fantasies about the infant will derive, not unexpectedly, from the physiologic changes that she observes and senses in herself as well as from the objective reports provided by her obstetrician. Once fetal movement begins it may be easier to envision the baby. Such medical procedures as sonograms, amniocentesis or simply allowing the mother to listen to the baby's heartbeat provide the caregiver with *objective* perceptions about the infant's status. From such perceptions, the caregiver can fashion representations about what the baby will look, feel, and sound like. Once these basic objective descriptions are obtained, most caregivers will come to acknowledge the infant as a viable being, will endow the infant with a personality and will begin to envision the nature of future interaction with the infant.

It is important to recognize that separation is one of the most significant issues the caregiver must confront during the pregnancy period. Initially, during the first trimester, the infant is perceived as being a physical part of the caregiver's body and during these early weeks many caregivers will have difficulty in envisioning the infant as an other being with a personality and needs separate from those of the mother. Nevertheless, as the pregnancy progresses and the caregiver comes to experience the infant's physical separateness from her through fetal movements, listening to the infant's heartbeat and viewing the infant on a sonogram, the capacity to visualize the infant as a separate creature and to anticipate the separation that will accompany the delivery becomes more real. As a result, by late in the second trimester, most caregivers will begin to relate to the infant as a separate individual in their fantasies and will begin to represent the type of relationship they will forge with the infant as well as the ways in which they will behave to foster the infant's development. Within the span of a few short months, in other words, the caregiver grows to psychologically accept the reality of the infant as a separate *other* with whom a unique and intimate relationship will be forged.

However, in cases where the pregnancy is a difficult one physiologically, the caregiver may have problems in negotiating this degree of psychological separation from the infant. If the caregiver experiences high blood pressure or physical pain or if the infant is born by cesarean, the caregiver may come to attribute her physical injury to the infant in such a way that the gradual process of differentiation is incomplete. For example, as one of the studies discussed below reports, maternal high blood pressure is associated with low-birth-weight babies. Assuming a caregiver manifests hypertension during pregnancy and the infant possesses a low birth weight, the caregiver may interpret the infant's physical status as being due to and somehow connected with her own physical status. She comes to believe, in other words, that she has passed on her physical impairment to the infant and, as a result, it may be more difficult for her to envision the infant as a separate being with an autonomous personality. In addition, the caregiver's capacity to represent the future developmental potential of the infant may be impaired because she may tend to confuse her own physical state with that of the baby. The caregiver's ability to preview imminent development adaptively may thus fail to emerge in an optimal fashion.

This section discusses in greater detail how such physiological phenomena experienced by the caregiver can affect and impair the representational fantasies she subsequently displays. Rubin (1977), for example, has commented that the mother's attachment to the infant begins with the enteroceptive sensations created by fetal movement and that these sensations validate the mother's perception that the infant represents an *other* being within her. This awareness continues throughout pregnancy as the caregiver begins to develop an attachment to the infant growing within her. In order for this attachment to develop, the expectant mother must begin to formulate representations of the infant and to preview upcoming experience with the infant. This form of representation is triggered by the physiologic changes which are experienced by the mother and which facilitate her representations of the infant as a separate individual. Moreover, Rubin adds that all the information the mother receives and processes both cognitively and emotionally about the infant is mediated through her own body image and self-concept. Bibring (1961) offers similar insights on this subject by noting that during pregnancy mothers must progress from a state of narcissistic concern about their own bodies to one of object-love towards the separate life within them, in order for the dyadic relationship to eventually become an adaptive reality. In a similar vein, Brazelton (1975) has observed that, if the antenatal representations of the infant are free of conflict, it is likely that the contours of the mother's subsequent relationship with the infant will be characterized by rhythmicity, reciprocity and overall attunement because she will be able to relate to the infant as a separate personality. The transition from early narcissistic fantasies in which the infant is envisioned, if at all, as being part of the mother to later fantasies in which the infant is represented as an independent, interactive partner is mandatory if adaptive development is to ensue after birth.

What factors affect these antenatal representations of the future dyadic relationship and how can the practitioner draw out the variables that threaten to infringe upon positive interaction? Several insights have been offered by Gaffney (1986) who measured three such variables—maternal self-concept, maternal state (temporary) anxiety, and maternal trait (long-term) anxiety—in an effort to decipher antenatal maternal phenomena that may impair future patterns of harmonious exchange. Gaffney defined the components of adaptive maternal-fetal attachment as consisting of the caregiver's tendency to predict and attribute individual characteristics to the fetus, the ability to engage in role-taking and perspective-taking with respect to the fetus, and a sense of self-differentiation and evidence of forecasting the interaction with the fetus.

In Gaffney's investigation, one hundred primiparous pregnant women were studied during their third trimester. By this point in the pregnancy, it may be assumed that the caregiver has begun to represent the infant as a distinct individual, separate from herself. These future caregivers were administered the Tennessee Self-Concept Scale (Fitts, 1965), which consists of a hundred statements about an individual's perceptions of self to which the subject responds with one of five responses ranging from "completely false" to "completely true." In addition, the dimensions of the anxiety variable (state vs. trait) were given to these women. According to the researcher, *state* anxiety represents the individual's reaction to a perceived threat or danger within a specific time or in response to a specific event, as pregnancy, for example. *Trait anxiety,* in contrast, is viewed as the individual's overall long-term tendency to become aroused in the presence of perceived danger. Each of these anxiety scales consists of twenty statements about feelings of anxiety; the subject selects one of four responses which rate the intensity of anxiety level.

Among the findings of the Gaffney study was that the overall level of the maternal representational skills did not correlate significantly with self-concept, as might have been expected. One possible explanation for this finding lies in Deutsch's (1945) hypothesis that a woman with low self-concept may experience a "vacation" from her ego during her pregnancy. That is, a woman who might ordinarily engage in a self-denigrating assessment of herself views pregnancy as an opportunity to say, "Now I do not have to be anything else; after all, I am pregnant." As a consequence, the representations such a woman harbors about the unborn infant would be relatively positive. Nevertheless, such mothers may be at risk for developing impaired relationships with their infants, because they are superimposing their own psychological status on the infant. After the birth, feelings of low self-esteem may resurface and the caregiver may even blame the infant for the resurgence of her feelings of inferiority. As a consequence, it may subsequently be difficult for such caregivers to engage in adaptive interaction based on previewing with their infants. The study also revealed significant inverse correlations between state or temporary anxiety and overall maternal-fetal attachment.

Other researchers have further probed the nature of maternal anxiety during pregnancy and have attempted to correlate this psychological characteristic with fetal outcome. Lederman (1986), for example, focused on the psychosocial conditions, relationships and developmental conflicts that give rise to maternal anxiety, which in turn may have an adverse physiological effect on the intrauterine environment and on fetal and neonatal health and development. Lederman relied on definitions of anxiety and stress that had been previously operationalized such as Spielberger, Gorsuch and Lushene (1970) for example, who defined state anxiety as a transitory emotional state or condition of the human organism that is characterized by subjective, consciously perceived feelings of tension and apprehension, along with heightened autonomic nervous system activity. Trait anxiety, on the other hand, refers to relatively stable individual differences in overall anxiety proneness or to differences between people in the tendency to respond, with elevations of state anxiety during situations perceived as threatening.

Lederman's review of the literature included a study by Heinicke, Diskin, Ramsey-Klee and Given (1983) which used standardized personality and infant development measures to follow the progress, from the middle of the pregnancy to an infant age of one year, of forty-six births occurring in married couples. Significant predictors of the twelve-month-old infant's endurance on the Bayley Test (Bayley 1969) included the prebirth maternal characteristics of optimistic representations of future interaction (a broadly defined factor of adjustment and problem-solving efficiency), confidence in visualization as a mother, and The Minnesota Multiphasic Personality Index Scale of ego strength. Each of these measures can reveal the nature and degree of anticipatory fantasies the caregiver is engaging in about the infant. By analyzing the nature of these fantasies, researchers can explore how a particular caregiver envisions future interaction with the infant and what kinds of behaviors the caregiver is likely to manifest in previewing development to the infant. Moreover, such fantasies provide insight into the caregiver's ability to differentiate herself from the infant in an adaptive manner and relate to the infant as an individual personality.

Other studies, such as those of Standley, Soule, Copans and Klein (1978) and Blomberg (1980a,b), have revealed similar findings. Standley et al., for instance, revealed that older, more educated, and financially secure couples were at an advantage in that they had a more satisfying pregnancy and predicted more confident outcomes regarding childbirth and the parenting experience than the younger subjects studied. These women also tended to anticipate more positive relationships with the infant after birth and, finally, they expressed more sophisticated representations of how the relationship with the infant would be experienced. This sophistication emerged from the wealth of detail with which caregivers endowed their antenatal representations. The pregnancy and newborn data showed that antenatal parental orientation, age and socioeconomic status also correlated with infant motor maturity scores.

Blomberg followed 1,263 infants of women who were emotionally stressed due to the denial of an abortion request. The incidence of malformations was higher in the abortion-request group than in a control group with similar prenatal care and evaluation and, within this malformation group, older age and lower social class were associated with an increased number of anomalies. Significantly, during the prenatal period these women disclosed relatively few fantasies and representations pertaining to their infants. Indeed, it was not unusual for these mothers to express virtually no anticipation fantasies regarding the infant. This finding suggests that such expectant mothers may fail to represent their infants as autonomous personalities during the pregnancy and this impairment in representation may interfere with the subsequent ability to preview adaptively during infancy. In yet another study, Ottinger and Simmons (1964) found a significant relationship between maternal prenatal anxiety and neonatal crying. In a similar investigation, Farber, Vaughn and Egeland (1981) indicated that anxiety was not a factor in the incidence of pregnancy and delivery complications or infant physiologic anomalies, but, nonetheless, their results showed that the more anxious mothers interacted less skillfully, communicated less, seemed less sensitive to their babies' needs and were less able to adjust their own behaviors to infant responses. Prior to the birth these women had engaged in fewer positive representations about their infants. Here again, the caregiver may inappropriately associate her anxiety with the infant, preventing her from establishing an adaptive relationship.

In two other studies, investigators examined relationships between prenatal maternal blood pressure (a measure assumed to be indicative of maternal stress), and infant irritability (Korner, Gabby & Kraemer, 1980; Woodson, Jones, da Costa-Woodson, Pollack & Evans, 1979). Woodson et al. found that primigravid women who developed a peak blood pressure between twenty and thirty-two weeks had significantly smaller for date newborns than women whose peak blood pressure reading occurred after the thirty-second week. These investigators concluded that fetal growth retardation was associated with the development of peak pregnancy blood pressure from the twentieth to thirty-second week and later with lower intrapartum fetal heart rate. Lower heart rate, in turn, was associated with greater crying and irritability in the newborns. In the Korner et al. study, the researchers replicated these results with a group of Caucasian mothers and infants with normotensive blood pressure during the third trimester and found that maternal blood pressure in the latter part of pregnancy, even within normal limits, is a factor in the emergence of irritability in newborn infants. Although maternal prenatal representation was not investigated in these studies, it would be of interest to see what kinds of fantasies these pregnant women had about their unborn babies and how these anticipatory fantasies correlated with the physiologic measures studied.

From the foregoing studies, it appears that prenatal anxiety can be manifested in a variety of different psychological and physiological responses measurable during pregnancy. Further, these responses, whether resulting solely from the prenatal environment or from the combined prenatal and postnatal environment, may serve as useful guides in predicting the subsequent dyadic relationship and course of development. In many instances, it appears that the emergence of physiologic problems during the pregnancy manifest later in the form of impaired interaction with the infant.

Other investigations have examined the relationship between maternal pregnancy complications and subsequent psychiatric disturbance or maladaptive behavioral syndromes in preschool or school-age children. For example, Nilsson, Almgren, Kohler and Kohler (1973) examined 165 randomly selected women during pregnancy and the post-partum period for adaptation to reproductive functions. Four years later, seventy-one mothers and children from the original sample were reexamined. The results showed that caregivers with conflicts between reproductive function and their status as mothers more frequently reported the presence of enuresis and other adaptational problems in their children. The etiologies of some of these problems are believed to stem from a less-than-optimal primary relationship between the mother and child. Studies by McNeil and associates (McNeil & Wiegerink, 1971; McNeil, Wiegerink & Dozier, 1970), compared data of children under treatment for psychologically related behavioral disturbances with data from control subjects. Seriously disturbed subjects had mothers with slightly higher frequencies of pregnancy and birth complications than did moderately to mildly disturbed subjects. The researchers reported that prematurity and prenatal problems were especially noted in the histories of disturbed children; however, there were no significant relationships between type of behavior patterns and specific pregnancy and birth complications. In another study, Mura (1974) interviewed the mothers of seventy-four children under psychiatric care to obtain pregnancy and delivery histories of the mentally ill children. Significantly more pregnancy and delivery complications were found for emotionally disturbed children than were found for their siblings. The reviewed data suggest that in instances of a difficult pregnancy, the mother's representational abilities may be impaired to the extent that forging an interactional bond with the infant becomes problematic. In particular, expectant women who experience physiologic difficulties during their pregnancies may be unable to fantasize adaptively about what the future relationship with the infant will be like and how the infant will behave as an individual. This inability to anticipate an adaptive interaction with the infant prevents the caregiver from engaging in adaptive previewing behaviors, with the result that the infant is deprived of the experience of imminent development. As a result, such development may be delayed or impaired.

Finally, Lederman reviewed studies concerned with the cumulative effect of perinatal complications on cognitive, language, and hearing development in preschool age children. One such study by Werner, Simonian, Bierman and French (1967) observed that with increasing severity of perinatal stress there was an increase in the proportion of two-year-olds who were below normal in physical status, intellectual, and social development. The researchers also noted that the quality of the home environment had a significant effect on both mental and social development and that these factors tended to be highly negative in cases where perinatal complications were severe. They emphasized the importance of the benefits of a good early home environment in minimizing the disadvantages of severe perinatal complications. Once again, this study indicates that failure of the caregiver to engage in positive anticipatory fantasies during the prenatal period is likely to have a detrimental effect on the caregiver's ability to represent the infant in a positive fashion and to subsequently preview imminent developmental changes for the infant, thereby interfering with the infant's overall developmental progress.

Istvan (1986) made a similar assessment of the role of stress and anxiety during pregnancy and the effect of these variables on birth outcome. This researcher focused on characteristics that had been identified as maternal predictors. One predictor, for example, was a stressful maternal life-situation during pregnancy. Outcome measures like excessive vomiting during the pregnancy, toxemia, and prolonged labor were considered. It was found that life-stress during pregnancy was higher in excessive vomiting and toxemia groups than among the normal pregnancy groups.

This researcher also observed that a woman's response to pregnancy implicates a matrix of social and psychological factors on the one hand, and a series of endocrinological and metabolic changes on the other. The contradictory results reported in a number of studies may reflect a failure to consider each of these complex factors and their implications for pregnancy outcome. The Istvan study illustrates this complexity by seizing upon the example of alcohol abuse. Alcohol consumed during pregnancy, the researcher notes, has a damaging effect on the fetus. One documented effect of alcohol consumption is reduced birth weight (Little, 1977). Marlatt (1983) has pointed out that one potential mechanism for stress may operate via increased alcohol consumption. Conversely, however, it is also true that alcohol use may reduce perceptions of anxiety in nonalcoholic individuals. When alcohol is ingested late in the third trimester of pregnancy, one proximal effect is to suppress the release of both maternal and fetal oxytocin and vasopressin, potentially inhibiting the onset of labor (Fuchs and Fuchs, 1984). Indeed, Istvan reports that alcohol has been used therapeutically for precisely just such a purpose. Thus, alcohol use may result in either greater gestational age (within limits, a positive reproductive outcome) or lower birth weight (often a negative reproductive outcome), depending on the pattern of use. In addition, given recent widespread reports of the effects of alcohol abuse on unborn infants, one may also question the attitude of an expectant mother who consumes alcohol. Is such a caregiver able to represent her infant positively as a differentiated individual with a unique and separate identity, and if so, why is she engaging in behavior known to have a detrimental effect on the infant.

Expectant mothers who have experienced an earlier perinatal loss may also be more susceptible to undergoing intense anxiety during the gestational period. Such expectant mothers may engage in a lower degree of adaptive representations about the infant. Theut, Pedersen, Zaslow, and Rabinovich (1988) reported on twenty-five expectant couples who had experienced a perinatal loss within the previous two years. These couples were compared with thirty-one couples expecting for the first time. The researchers examined the hypothesis that during a subsequent pregnancy, caregivers with a previous loss would exhibit anxiety that was specific to the pregnancy experience, rather than a more generalized anxiety. The results of the study demonstrated that caregivers who have undergone a previous perinatal loss in fact had a proclivity toward heightened anxiety. In these cases therapy may be warranted to encourage these expectant parents; such patients should be encouraged to engage in positive anticipatory representations of the impending birth.

Another study by Tennen, Affleck, and Gershman (1986) found that mothers whose infants experienced perinatal complications tended to manifest a high level of defensive attribution and self-blame, and that both of these patterns interfered with representational capacities with respect to envisioning the infant. The study involved mothers whose infants were born with a full spectrum of heterogenous medical problems including perinatal asphyxia, seizures, intraventricular hemorrhage, bronchopulmonary dysplasia, severe apnea, and were significantly smaller for gestational age at birth. When caregivers of these infants were asked to rate the severity of their child's condition and its causes, these caregivers engaged in a high level of self-blame and defensive self-attribution. The researchers hypothesized that such mothers may experience heightened guilt over their infant's physical condition which triggers increased levels of self-blame and self-castigation. This psychological state may play an indirect role in hindering the development of an adaptive relationship within the dyad, preventing the caregiver from engaging in adaptive representations about the infant's development and conveying these representations while interacting with the infant in the form of previewing.

Thus, therapists should be alert to the repercussions the infant's physiological status may have on the caregiver's overall ability to forge a relationship with the newborn or to represent and subsequently preview development to the infant positively. One useful exercise in these cases is to ask the caregiver to describe how she thinks her infant's physical condition will affect his development.

Another physiological factor that warrants consideration by the therapist is the mother's age and status at the time of the pregnancy. Culp, Appelbaum, Osofsky and Levy (1988), for example, found significant differences between adolescent and older mothers during both the prenatal and postpartum periods. In the study, one hundred thirty adolescent mothers and eighty-six married primiparous nonadolescent mothers were followed longitudinally. Prenatal interviews were performed with all of the women and, following the birth, in-hospital observation of mother-infant interaction during feeding was conducted. All of the expectant women were interviewed in the latter part of their second trimester and the first part of their third trimester.

Among the measures of birth weight, gestational age and one- and five-minute Apgar scores, none revealed differences between the two groups of mothers. Maternal psychosocial characteristics, however, did differ markedly between the two groups. In general, adolescent mothers reported being less happy about being pregnant and had less social support. Moreover, these adolescent women tended to have fewer anticipatory representations pertaining to future interaction with the infant. Adolescent mothers also reported less support from the father of the infant. The most striking differences between the two groups emerged, however, during observations of newborn feeding sequences. For example, the adolescent mothers engaged in fewer instances of vocalization with the infant and when such auditory stimulation did occur, it was less appropriate and of a shorter duration than was the case with the older mothers.

This study suggests that adolescent mothers may be less equipped than older women who are either married or involved in a secure relationship to forge an adaptive relationship with the infant because they have fewer positive expectations about the nature of the long-term interaction with the infant. Eventually, if these representations are not converted into adaptive previewing experiences to be shared with the infant, developmental progress may be hindered. As a consequence, therapists assessing and treating adolescent mothers should evaluate the degree to which these women can represent future infant behaviors. Predictive exercises should be initiated during the pregnancy, whenever possible, in order that the caregiver will develop adaptive interactive skills by the time of the birth.

The results of these studies offer insight into how the caregiver's emotional status can affect her physiological status, and how her physiological status affects such psychological capacities as the ability to differentiate from the infant and envision future development. In turn, both of these factors impact on the fetal outcome and on the nature of the initial relationship that transpires between caregiver and infant. In order to stave off any detrimental effects on the newborn's development, it is vital that during the prenatal period therapists begin to explore the caregiver's physiological and psychological status and strive to devise strategies for ameliorating detrimental phenomena, such as anxiety, which have been demonstrated to exert a negative effect on birth outcome and on the caregiver's ability to interact adaptively with the infant through previewing. In addition, therapists are encouraged to explore the caregiver's capacities for representing future interactions or future developmental changes with the infant and for devising previewing exercises designed to enhance adaptive development (Trad, 1989b). The caregiver's skills in this area will likely provide some profound insights into the nature of the future relationship with the infant.

Prenatal Representations of the Infant: The Psychological Fantasies of Pregnancy

Another group of researchers has focused on the role maternal and paternal psychological fantasies play in helping or hindering the forging of a bond with their infants and the enhancement of adaptive development. Pines (1972), for example, has written that a first pregnancy is a particularly stressful time for the expectant mother in whom the psychological equilibrium required to deal with the ever-present demands of a helpless, dependent human being has often not been thoroughly recognized by researchers. According to Pines, one of the most noteworthy features that emerges during the analytic process of pregnant women is the reemergence of repressed fantasies into preconsciousness and consciousness, and the fate of these fantasies once the reality of the newborn infant and the infant's autonomy have been established. Pines notes that the revival of conflict belonging to earlier developmental stages of the mother is a fundamental aspect of pregnancy and, as a result, the gestational period is a time when the expectant caregiver is in need of both emotional and physical support, so that she can eventually preview imminent development to her infant in a manner that facilitates adaptation.

Pines explains that pregnancy, particularly the first pregnancy, marks a crisis point in the search for a female identity. Pregnancy implies the end of the woman as an independent, single unit and the beginning of the irrevocable caregiver-infant relationship. Pines observes that for the primigravida, pregnancy offers proof of a gender identity, along with the visible emblem to the outside world that the expectant mother has had a sexual relationship. Physiologically, it is the confirmation that she has a sexually mature body capable of reproduction. The hormonal changes which accompany pregnancy produce unaccustomed mood swings and physical discomforts which impose an added burden on the pregnant woman and those around her.

Understandably, then, for the future mother such dramatic changes in both her physical and psychological status represent a critical *transitional phase,* as Rapoport (1963) has described it. Indeed, it is not farfetched to argue that pregnancy is, in and of itself, a developmental phase. As a consequence, this period is inevitably accompanied by a revival of past conflicts and anxieties. Pregnancy also alters the relationships within the family unit, so that each pregnancy and birth is paralleled by a kind of family crisis that culminates with the absorption of a new family member and the realignment of family relationships.

Pregnancy is, in other words, a time of reflection, when representations of previous relationships are reevaluated and predictions about the future relationship with the infant are formulated. Not surprisingly, then, during this period the expectant caregiver's early childhood identifications with her own mother are rekindled and evaluated against the panorama of anticipatory reveries involving the new mother's relationship with her own child. At the same time, the new mother's relationship with her own mother may modify and mature with the expectant woman's enhanced understanding of the tasks demanded of motherhood. Thus, says Pines, a previously ambivalent identification with the caregiver's maternal figure may be resolved during pregnancy, to be replaced by a new and more tranquil relationship.

Nevertheless, while the successful achievement of a feminine sexual and gender identity can be strengthened by the proof and confirmation of pregnancy, the process of making and developing a new kind of object relationship—namely, motherhood—can only begin once the infant emerges from the mother's body into the object world. The infant thus combines features of an extension of the mother's self-representation and of her sexual partner (i.e., the father), but is also perceived as a separate individual.

Caplan (1959) has discussed the conflicts and anticipatory fantasies of the expectant mother in terms of three stages corresponding to the trimesters of pregnancy. Stage one encompasses the time of conception until the fourth month when the baby begins to move in utero. Caplan has written of this period that progestin levels are high, leading to physical lethargy and changes in body image such as the growth of the breasts. These physiological transitions mimic some of the changes of puberty and thus it is natural that during this time adolescent fantasies about body change are revived. Characteristically, there are dramatic mood swings and periods of anxiety which may stem from feelings of uncertainty about the dramatic physiological changes the woman is undergoing. Caplan reports that, from the very beginning of this stage, some women experience a feeling of supreme fulfillment and pleasure, marked by an increased investment in the self and a withdrawal from the object world. For other women, this stage may be a time of mild depression, coupled with an increase in physical activity in an effort to stave off newly felt feelings of passivity.

For some women, from the moment the pregnancy is confirmed the fetus is considered as a baby, a distinct representation of an infant with a unique physical appearance and even a sexual identity is formulated. In contrast, for other expectant mothers, the fetus is a part of their body, which can be dispensed with as easily as an inflamed appendix.

Other common representations which predominate during of this first stage of pregnancy incorporate the fact that there is often a marked regression to earlier developmental stages. Women may also begin to identify with the fetus as envisaged in fantasy at this juncture in the pregnancy. For example, Caplan relates the case of a young woman who brought dream material into treatment. The woman reported that in the dream she experienced herself becoming progressively younger as the pregnancy progressed. Finally, shortly before term, she dreamed that she was a baby herself, sucking at the breast, thus merging the representation of herself as a mother and as a newborn child.

A notable shift occurs during the second of Caplan's stages of pregnancy. With the advent of fetal movements, the mother begins to formulate a more realistic representation of the infant who has begun to exert its own independent presence. Now the caregiver must recognize that, although the infant is still within her body, it is a separate entity with an independent existence that the mother cannot entirely control. This is the juncture at which a recognition of differentiation from the infant is achieved and the caregiver's representational fantasies are likely to incorporate this new realization of the infant's separateness and autonomy. It is at this time that the caregiver may begin to engage in fantasies or predictions about what the relationship with the infant will be like. Moreover, even in the most eagerly anticipated pregnancy there is an accompanying awakening of anxiety during this period. This anxiety stems from the realization that the infant will eventually become part of the external world, and may also reflect the fear evoked by separation that is experienced on the part of the mother. Caplan observes too that during this period vivid regressive fantasies tend to emerge. For example, sexual fantasies may surface in the form of the fetus representing a dirty or shameful object that the mother needs to expel. In other instances, women have reported that the fetus is visualized as a devouring destructive creature within the maternal body.

The third and final trimester of pregnancy is marked by bodily discomfort and fatigue as the future caregiver prepares for labor. Memories of sibling rivalry may often surface if the caregiver perceives herself to be in competition with the infant. This final trimester is often characterized by mood swings from pleasure at the imminent prospect of the baby becoming a reality to an inevitable anxiety that is experienced by virtually every pregnant woman that she might die in childbirth or that her child may be abnormal or damaged during the delivery process.

Fantasies of expulsion from the body are more prominent at this stage, and for some women there is a feeling of exhilaration at being able to exchange the passive role that was enforced during pregnancy for an active role in the delivery process. The reality of the infant as a separate entity only emerges into the mother's consciousness when the child is actually born. It is at this time that the anticipatory fantasies that dominated the pregnancy will be converted into a realistic perception of the infant. From this perception the caregiver will devise previewing behaviors to introduce the infant to upcoming developmental changes.

During the latter portion of the pregnancy, expectant mothers may also come to formulate some anticipatory representations about the infant's temperamental makeup. In a study conducted by Mebert and Kalinowski (1986), it was discovered that the kinds of predictions the expectant mother makes about the infant's disposition can be influenced by such factors as parity and mode of delivery. The study involved forty-one couples, fourteen primiparous and twenty-seven multiparous, who were tested at sixteen weeks of pregnancy. All of the couples received the Infant Characteristic Questionnaire (Lounsburg, 1979) which probed expectations of infant temperamental characteristics and dispositions. It was found that multiparous parents expecting a vaginal delivery had the lowest scores, indicating predictions of more temperamentally optimal infants. These findings were replicated when the same instrument was administered to the same population in both late pregnancy and at three to four months postpartum. The researchers commented that the results indicated that parity and childbirth experience affect the way the caregiver represents the infant's temperament and also influences the kinds of behavior the caregiver eventually manifests during interaction with the infant.

This study has several implications concerning the role of prenatal predictions about what the experience of motherhood will be like. Mothers who were informed by their obstetrician that the delivery was likely to be vaginal, rather than by cesarean, tended to attribute a more positive temperament to their unborn infants, as did the multiparous pregnant women. These findings suggest that when the pregnancy itself is viewed as being routine, uncomplicated and nonproblematic, the expectant woman tends to envision the infant positively and to represent these positive characteristics to the infant. Moreover, if the woman has undergone the experience of childbirth before, as in the case of the multiparous women, anxieties associated with the birth process itself may be alleviated and as a result the woman can devote her energies to representing a positive interactional outcome and to devising previewing exercises that will be conducted during interaction with the infant. Thus, this study indicates that beyond any objective determination of the infant's temperamental status, the caregiver's predictions of what the infant's disposition will be like play a strong role in determining the kinds of behaviors the caregiver subsequently manifests to the infant.

There are, in addition, a variety of other variables that therapists should be alert to during the period of gestation. Numerous expectant caregivers, particularly those who are experiencing an unplanned pregnancy, may express denial, especially during the first trimester. As a result of this denial, representations about the infant will be minimal. In one study that focused on this phenomenon, Shereshefsky and Yarrow (1970) found that the presence of denial during the first trimester was correlated with serious adaptational complications later in the pregnancy. Shainess (1968) reported that denial expressed verbally in the first three months of gestation appeared to undergo transformation into somatic complaints during the second and third trimesters. Moreover, obstetric exams revealed that these physical complaints were often psychosomatic in nature with no discernible physiological etiology. Denial here may function as a defense whereby the caregiver prevents herself from acknowledging the independent status or even the presence of the infant. As a result, there is a dearth of anticipatory fantasy about the impending relationship.

As noted earlier, fantasies of regression (generally in the form of a revival of images associated with suppressed developmental conflicts) are another frequent event during pregnancy that therapists should explore. Most commonly, such regressive phenomena pertain to the caregiver's relationship with her own mother, as has been reported by Raphael-Leff (1986), Leifer (1980) and Benedek (1970). While these resurrected fantasies are often beneficial in helping the expectant caregiver prepare for her new status as a mother, in instances where the caregiver's relationship with her mother has been troubled or disturbed, a revival of such memories can pose a threat to the future relationship between caregiver and infant. In such cases, the caregiver may be representing maladaptive interaction which may eventually affect her capacity to forge a positive relationship and may interfere with her ability to preview the infant adaptively. In other instances, the caregiver may regress to the period of her adolescence when feelings of uncontrollability about her body predominated. It is imperative, then, that therapists working with pregnant mothers ascertain the woman's attitudes toward their own caregivers and their adolescent experience. This information will be of use if regressive behavior and/or fantasy material surfaces.

Also vital for the therapist treating expectant mothers is familiarity with the changes that occur during each trimester. Rubin (1975) has reported, for example, that the first trimester represents a period of evaluation, during which the caregiver deals with the issue of acceptance. Acceptance in this sense refers to an ability to acknowledge the physiological state of pregnancy, the psychological awareness of the fetus as a separate, autonomous being and the corresponding recognition of oneself as a mother-to-be. The first trimester, then, is accompanied by a reexamination of the status of the self and self-image and, as Shereshefsky and Yarrow (1970) note, an emphasis on the importance of the immediate reality of the pregnancy itself.

In contrast, during the second trimester quickening marks a shift in focus from the caregiver to the infant, its well-being and care, acceptance by family members, anticipatory fantasies of interaction and a growing sense of psychological attachment on the part of the caregiver, according to such researchers as Ballou (1978), Rubin (1975), and Shereshefsky and Yarrow (1970). This is a time when the caregiver begins to represent her future relationship with the infant and to devise previewing strategies for interacting with the baby. Shereshefsky and Yarrow (1970) have observed that the transition from the third to the seventh month of pregnancy is marked by less overtly expressed anxiety about the infant, a clearer, more descriptive visualization of oneself as a mother, increased feelings of physical and psychological well-being, heightened husband-wife adjustment, validation of both prospective parents as a couple, and an overall diminishment of the anxiety that prevailed during the beginning of the pregnancy. Thus, the second trimester appears to signify a period of adjustment with relative equilibrium for the majority of expectant caregivers. It is at this juncture that the expectant mother begins to consolidate an image or representation of what the infant as an individual will actually be like. For some expectant mothers, this representation is quite sophisticated, as specific personality traits are attributed to the infant; for other expectant mothers, the image of the infant is far more primitive and crude. Nevertheless, in virtually all expectant mothers representation becomes evident at this time, as a kind of exercise in anticipation of the birth and the future dyadic relationship that will ensue.

But with the onset of the third trimester, vulnerability and uncertainty assert themselves once again, as the caregiver becomes increasingly aware of the danger posed by delivery. This new wave of anxiety is tempered by the acceptance of and preparation for separation from the fetus and a readiness to receive the child. Two prospective studies using third trimester interviews revealed that most of the mothers' trepidations during the immediate delivery period were concentrated on fetal well-being and the impending twin events of labor and delivery itself (Areskog, Uddenberg, & Kjessler, 1981; Standley, Soule & Copans, 1979). At this juncture, the caregiver is beginning to envision the nature of future interaction with the infant and to represent specific sequences of exchange. In many cases caregivers will be able to describe their expectations about the infant's future development.

The postpartum period marks the advent of yet another time of uncertainty for the new mother during which common fantasy material may surface. For example, following delivery there is a period of adjustment to the physiological sensation of emptiness in the abdominal region. Now the mother's body image must change once again, in order for her to experience a feeling of wholeness and bodily integrity. Unless this feeling of bodily wholeness is reestablished, there cannot be a reconciliation with the actual birth and an acceptance of the infant's status as a separate individual. Mothers will also begin producing milk, another change that may awaken fantasies associated with their own nurturing experience. Therapists should, therefore, inquire as to body image and perception during the immediate postpartum period in order to gauge whether the caregiver has the psychological capacity to perceive of the infant realistically.

Other researchers, such as Strang and Sullivan (1984), have reported that the caregiver's perceptions of body image, particularly during the pregnancy and postpartum period, can have a negative impact on the caregiver's sense of self-esteem and hence, can intrude upon the incipient relationship being forged between caregiver and infant. By studying pregnant and postpartum body attitudes, these researchers found that primiparas in particular may require support and counseling to more fully understand the dramatic changes their bodies have undergone and to accept that only gradually will their prepregnancy physiological status reassert itself. It is particularly important for therapists working with new caregivers to investigate the caregiver's attitude toward her body image because if a negative image lingers the caregiver may either inadvertently or intentionally represent and transfer hostility to the infant as the cause of her changed body image. These negative emotions must be dissipated before the caregiver can begin to represent and enact positive previewing experiences to the infant.

The pediatrician plays an indispensable role in helping the new mother adjust to the postpartum period. Both the physiological and psychological changes the mother experiences after the birth can trigger representations tinged with positive, negative or ambivalent moods about the impending birth. Such phenomenon can be conveyed to the infant during the first few months after birth by the way the caregiver represents the infant's upcoming maturation and previews future development. Perhaps no health care professional is in a better position than the pediatrician to assess the nature of the caregiver's feeling towards the pregnancy experience and the new infant. Moreover, the pediatrician is in a unique position to promote adaptive behaviors in the caregiver. Thus, pediatricians should familiarize themselves with the caregiver's psychological status and to any changes or fluctuations which occurred during the pregnancy and postpartum period that may yield insight into the unique psychological and physiological condition of each caregiver in treatment.

Another commonly reported response during the postpartum period, reported by both Pines and Caplan, is one of maternal bewilderment at not experiencing an overwhelming emotional response upon first viewing the neonate. In cases where this phenomenon occurs, the caregiver may lapse into depression because of this unanticipated nonresponsiveness. This unsettling lack of enthusiasm for the infant is usually only temporary and with reassurance from medical personnel, caregivers will in most instances begin to represent the future relationship positively, initiating an interactive and nurturing relationship with the infant within a few weeks after birth (Mehra and Pines, 1972). If, however, the caregiver displays minimal curiosity about initiating contact with the infant after one week has elapsed, it is advisable to have a mental status exam performed upon the caregiver in order to determine the source of her apathy and to evaluate the nature of her representations of the infant and of the future relationship with the infant.

Maternal adjustment during pregnancy and immediately after delivery may also be assessed by virtue of various questionnaires that seek to ascertain the caregiver's perceptions of her body, of somatic symptoms, of the marital relationship, of attitudes toward sex, of the pregnancy itself and of how the newborn is represented during separation intervals. One such questionnaire was administered by Kumar, Robson, and Smith (1984), who studied ninety-nine women in late pregnancy and repeated the assessment during the postpartum period in the obstetric service setting. The questionnaire covered a broad spectrum of topics and included such inquiries as: "Have you gotten out of breath recently?" "Do you feel attractive?" and "Have you worried that you might not be a good mother?" These questions probed a diversity of areas, including the caregiver's physiological status, and her psychological attitude towards herself, her husband and the infant.

Use of a comprehensive questionnaire of this type can be of assistance to therapists who wish to formulate an overall impression of the caregiver in order to focus on areas of potential conflict with the infant. Does the caregiver blame her pregnancy and by extension, the infant, for a troublesome weight gain or is the caregiver using the infant as a scapegoat to disguise difficulties that have arisen in the context of the marital relationship? How is the caregiver representing and previewing upcoming development in her daydreams and reveries? Since it is important for the therapist to determine any sources of conflict relatively early in the therapeutic milieu, such questions should be asked of the new mother, who should be encouraged to describe both her individual feelings now that the experience of pregnancy is over and her perceptions of the interactive relationship she is forging with her infant.

The psychological demarcations between trimesters have, therefore, been established in numerous investigations that have been able to pinpoint the specific types of anticipatory fantasies most commonly experienced by expectant mothers. It becomes crucial for therapists to familiarize themselves with the typical attitudes that emerge in adaptive caregivers. This pattern of attitudes may be expressed in the following terms. The first trimester is defined by an almost exaggerated emphasis on the self, which may initially appear to be out of proportion or even narcissistic to the outward observer. In fact, this period is striking for its egocentrism and self-absorption on the part of the caregiver. But this psychological attitude, which might be characterized as being mildly abnormal in nonpregnant women, is in actuality an adaptive reaction on the part of the expectant caregiver. These unusual fantasies may be attributed to the dramatic physical and psychological changes the woman is experiencing, as well as to her complex evaluation of her desire to become a mother. Representations about the infant are minimal and often unrealistic during this period, and if the infant is represented at all, it is often as an extension of the caregiver's body. If these doubts about motherhood are resolved, the period of the second trimester is one of relative socioemotional balance. However, therapists should not confuse balance and the acceptance of one's future role as mother as the equivalent of mental inactivity. In fact, this period is one of rich and profound fantasy as the caregiver comes to accept the relatively autonomous status of the infant. During this period therapists should verify that the expectant mothers they are treating are evincing the myriad of detailed representational fantasies that predominate as the caregiver comes to acknowledge the infant's autonomous status.

The most commonly reported fantasies of this time involve episodes of pretended interaction between the caregiver and newborn, with the caregiver holding conversations with the infant and providing a vivid description of the infant's physical features and behavioral disposition. Such behavior signifies, in part, a desire to anticipate or predict how interaction with the infant will actually be experienced. In essence, during these imaginary sequences the caregiver is experimenting with how she will preview upcoming development to the infant. Practitioners should encourage as much of this type of mental representation as possible, because it will offer parameters for predicting the contours of future interaction within this particular dyad. Finally, it is important that the therapist recognize that the resurgence of anxiety during the third trimester is both normal and expectable given the imminence of the birth and consequent maternal separation of the fetus. In fact, if such trepidations are absent in the weeks immediately preceding delivery, it is worth encouraging the expectant mother to voice her emotional perceptions.

Beyond these patterns other factors also exert influence on the caregiver's mental attitude during pregnancy. Anxiety, for example, appears to be influenced by such variables as age, education, parity, gravidity, socioeconomic status, previous obstetrical experience, current and previous physiological history, marital status and relationship, the expectant mother's personal resilience and history of coping with critical life events and social support. Clinicians should also give careful consideration to each of these factors in evaluating individual patients while planning therapeutic protocols.

Yet another variable that affects the caregiver's mental status during pregnancy and may impinge upon future interaction within the dyad is the caregiver's degree of acceptance or rejection of the pregnancy itself. It is vital for the therapist to explore the caregiver's feelings here, since they will likely have predictive value for anticipating the nature of the relationship that is eventually forged between infant and caregiver. Caplan (1959) reported that eighty-five percent of one study group he investigated revealed some initial rejection of the pregnancy, but by the end of the first trimester eighty five to ninety percent of the mothers interviewed had come to accept and even welcome their new status. This notable shift is characteristic of the psychological upheaval that corresponds to maternal egocentrism in the first months of pregnancy and should not alarm therapists unless the caregiver remains adamantly resistant to the pregnancy. A shift in representational fantasies is also noted during this period as the caregiver engages in an increased number of reveries about future interactions with her infant.

Whether or not the pregnancy is planned is a further variable which can affect maternal attitude. Shereshefsky and Yarrow (1970) reported that seventy-three percent of their primigravid sample had planned the pregnancy. Two-thirds of a sample population investigated by Entwisle and Doering (1981) reported that the pregnancy was entirely planned, while thirty-four percent commented that it was planned to some degree, meaning that the couple had anticipated having children in the near future, but had not specifically anticipated and prepared for that particular pregnancy. Planning in general, however, was found to be unrelated to the expectant caregiver's attitude toward being pregnant in the Entwisle and Doering study, and was not correlated with adaptation to pregnancy in the Shereshefsky and Yarrow study. Thus, it appears that the practitioner working with pregnant women needs to closely scrutinize both the planning of the pregnancy and the separate issue of the acceptance of the infant which generally arises towards the end of the first trimester. Moreover, from early knowledge of pregnancy to the end of the first trimester, there is a significant increase in acceptance. In the Shereshefsky and Yarrow study it was found that unplanned pregnancies correlated with youthfulness of the couple, shorter marriage, the husband's dissatisfaction with his job, his lack of enthusiastic response to the pregnancy, a less positive maternal mood at the three-month prenatal demarcation point and a lower incidence of positive maternal representational fantasies about the infant or predictions about future interaction with the infant.

Altman (1968), who conducted several studies focusing on the factor of birth planning, advised caution when interpreting rejection or acceptance of the pregnancy. For sociocultural reasons planning of pregnancy may not be associated with acceptance of the baby and of parenthood. Primigravidas who find themselves pregnant before they are ready may actually be more amenable to acceptance if social and financial circumstances are deemed adequate. Multiparas, on the other hand, who feel they have more children than they want may not be able to stave off the feelings of rejection that are aroused by another pregnancy. Acceptance for such women might be termed resignation, a mental attitude achieved by rationalization. Moreover, Pohlman (1968) has suggested that there is some degree of stability in parental attitude regarding acceptance over the course of the pregnancy. It is important, therefore, to explore the caregiver's genuine feelings about the pregnancy and this is often best accomplished by examining representational reveries relating to the infant's upcoming development and the future interaction between mother and child.

Lederman, Lederman, Work, and McCann (1979), who also assessed the acceptance of pregnancy on the part of expectant mothers, discovered that the variable of acceptance correlated with other personality dimensions as well as with the presence of state anxiety and progress during labor. Primigravidas, who had difficulty in accepting the pregnancy and whose pregnancy was unplanned, voiced a greater degree of anxiety with respect to their relationship with their own caregivers and with regard to their identification with the role of motherhood. These women conveyed heightened trepidation about labor which caused them to experience a more prolonged period of labor.

Other data which may be used to predict the expectant caregiver's future patterns of interaction with the newborn can be gleaned by assessing the mother's representation of her relationship with her own mother (Lederman et al. 1981; Main, Kaplan and Cassidy, 1985). To test this hypothesis, Bibring (1961, 1966) followed primigravidas in each trimester of pregnancy, labor and delivery and during the postpartum period for up to one year, with interviews and projective psychological evaluations. Bibring's analysis revealed that these caregivers formed a new identification and alliance with their own caregiver during the pregnancy, demonstrated a new respect, and experienced a resurgence of affection for their caregivers who were now perceived as adult equals. Moreover, Bibring reported that the pregnant daughters also displayed greater tolerance and acceptance of their own mothers. The more positive view of their relationship with their mothers was transformed into an adaptive relationship with their infants.

Ballou (1978), who conducted interviews and psychological evaluations with twelve primigravidas through pregnancy and up to three months postpartum, placed stronger emphasis on the significance of *reconciliation* between the expectant mother and her own caregiver. Reconciliation was described as a gradual progressive process wherein by the third trimester women pleasurably envisioned their own childhoods, perceived of their caregivers in an altruistic fashion and remembered the mother-child relationship as being a gratifying one. Ballou's work confirmed and built upon Benedek's (1970) findings, whose study had emphasized that expectant mothers acquire a renewed sense of kinship with their own mothers and of being mothered as a prerequisite to attaining a adaptive sense of one's identity and of the role of mother. As important as reconciliation was, when the relationship with the mother was marked with hostility, Ballou found that a nurturing husband could reassure a doubting wife and thereby assuage and attenuate the negative influence of a poor mother-daughter relationship.

Other researchers have examined the relationship of expectant women with their own mothers and its influence on labor, delivery and postpartum adaptation in forging an adaptive relationship with the infant. Levy and McGee (1975) reported that sixty primigravidas who received no information from their own mothers concerning the mother's childbirth experience were relatively unprepared for the experience themselves, were less able to predict what the birth experience would be like, had a poorer evaluation of labor and delivery than women who received such information, and engaged in fewer representations of future interaction with the infant. This study suggests the importance of the caregiver's own repository of representations in anticipating the contours of the future interaction with the infant. Women who received extreme evaluations from their mothers, whether positive or negative, had a poorer opinion of childbirth than women who received only moderately negative or positive evaluations from their mothers. Extreme impressions conveyed to the expectant caregiver, creating too high a level of confidence or anxiety, tended to preclude the necessary preparation by the caregiver for the impending birth and interfered with the expectant caregiver's ability to envision development realistically. By examining these patterns in detail, Levy and McGee were able to glean and interpret complex information pertaining to the relationship with the mother and the labor experience. Once again, the capacity to predict or represent outcome was crucial to the woman's capacity to adjust adaptively to the situation.

Each of these studies highlights the fact that the mother-infant relationship does indeed commence during the pregnancy period as the caregiver engages in a series of rich and detailed representations in preparation for giving birth. Fantasies that dominate during the first trimester may reflect self-absorption and the caregiver's preoccupation with her changing physiological status. Fantasies evoked during this period tend to signify revivals of memories from earlier periods of developmental change such as puberty. For example, the woman's weight gain and swelling of her breasts are reminiscent of the physiological changes that occurred during adolescence and, hence, developmental issues from that period of her life may be rearoused. Moreover, fantasies during this period may be somewhat narcissistic, since the caregiver has not yet acknowledged the independent status of the infant.

By the second trimester, however, the physiological changes that accompany the pregnancy, such as the movement of the fetus in utero, the caregiver's expanding abdomen, and medical procedures performed by the obstetrician, all create a growing recognition on the part of the caregiver that the fetus is a separate, autonomous being who is only occupying the caregiver's abdomen temporarily. With this realization a new and different type of fantasy emerges. Now the caregiver is challenged to represent the infant as being separate from herself and to endow the infant with certain subjective characteristics beyond the objective features she has become aware of as a result of the physiological changes in her body. For the first time, the infant begins to acquire a distinct personality, often temperamental qualities are attributed and, most significantly, the caregiver begins to envision what future interactions with the infant will be like. From such representations, it is possible to determine how a particular caregiver will represent the imminent development of her infant and subsequently use these representations to formulate and structure previewing exercises for her infant. Such previewing exercises will acquaint the infant with imminent developmental achievement, as well as help the caregiver work through separation issues and enhance the intimacy of the relationship between mother and infant.

As was pointed out in this section, in some instances the caregiver will have difficulty representing the infant and will not manifest these types of adaptive fantasies about future interaction even until late in the second trimester. Such caregivers may still harbor ambivalent feelings about the infant. They may be engaging in denial or may themselves possess a representational deficit that impairs their capacity to differentiate from others. As the studies discussed suggest, failure to engage in these kinds of antenatal representations and fantasies appears to result in an impaired relationship between the mother and infant after the birth. Indeed, unless the caregiver can engage in antenatal fantasies pertaining to the infant as an autonomous being, it may be virtually impossible for her to envision future interaction with the infant and to develop an adaptive relationship that is characterized by an optimal level of previewing experiences. As a consequence, the infant's development will suffer because he will lack an interactional partner with whom he can share the challenges of imminent development.

The Representations of the Expectant Father

Recently researchers focusing on the numerous psychological transitions undergone by expectant mothers have also begun to recognize that the expectant father undergoes emotional upheaval during the period of his wife's pregnancy as well (Boehm, 1930; Freeman, 1951; Jaffe, 1968; Coley & James, 1976). Moreover, unlike his mate, the husband is not the focus of attention during this time and may in fact experience feelings of isolation and loneliness. These negative emotions can become exacerbated if the father is not involved in anticipating and planning the birth. Such feelings may be acted out overtly in the form of resentment toward the expectant mother, and ultimately, through subtle rejection of the infant.

Understanding why expectant fathers may sometimes feel alienated from the pregnancy experience is not difficult. For the mother, the experience of pregnancy is a palpable reality because she undergoes continual physiological change which serves to remind her of the infant developing within her. In contrast, for the father pregnancy is, in a fundamental sense, almost a vicarious experience (Rose, 1961; Jarvis, 1962; Bogren, 1983). Although the expectant father will observe his wife's growing abdomen and be able to touch her stomach to feel the infant moving within her, he is not privy to the visceral sensations associated with development. In essence, the infant's movements and the discomfort of carrying the infant remain alien sensations to the father.

Thus, for the expectant father, pregnancy is less of an *objective* experience than it is for the expectant mother. Indeed, the father will be forced to rely more on his psychological capacity both to envision the infant *subjectively* through representation and to predict what the future relationship with the infant will be like. The difficulty that future fathers experience can lead to problems in their subsequent ability to establish a harmonious relationship with the infant and to engage in previewing exercises.

Although certainly not all expectant fathers experience such a sense of distance from the objective experience of their wives' pregnancies, enough fathers do experience a range of negative emotions. Among the most commonly reported affects in expectant fathers are a rearousal of intense dependency needs, rage towards unresponsive parents, sibling rivalry, and competition with the child for the wife's attention. Issues such as these not only evoke fears of damaging their wives or the fetus, but also evoke guilt for not providing nurture and support. As a result, therapists working with new parents need to particularly encourage the representational capacities of the father. The father must come to understand that his role in promoting adaptive development through previewing is as significant as that of the mother.

The following studies describe recent findings with respect to expectant fathers. Given the risk factors and the detrimental repercussions the father's attitude may exert on the infant's future development, it becomes important to delineate the typical physical and emotional responses endured by expectant fathers during the pregnancy and postpartum period. One attempt to chart these paternal transitions was performed by Clinton (1987). This researcher compared physiological and psychological status in eighty-one expectant fathers and sixty-six married nonexpectant husbands over the course of a year at monthly intervals. A total of 877 monthly data collection episodes were compiled. It was found that compared to nonexpectant men, expectant fathers experienced relatively similar episodes of both physical and psychological symptomatology throughout the three trimesters of pregnancy. For example, during the first trimester, expectant fathers experienced a higher incidence of colds and irritability. Symptomology of expectant fathers was indistinguishable from that of nonexpectant men. However, by the third trimester, unintentional weight gain, restlessness and insomnia were bound to be more prevalent among expectant fathers. The health of the expectant fathers was found to differ significantly from that of nonexpectant men during the immediate postpartum period. Evaluations performed during this time revealed a greater incidence of emotional discomfort, as well as a dramatic upsurge in psychosomatic symptomatology in both its duration and perceived seriousness. Such factors as the father's affective involvement with the expectant mother during pregnancy, the number of children the couple has, the family income, ethnic identity, perceived levels of stress and recent health were all key predictors of how the father would respond to the pregnancy and postpartum period.

Similar data also appeared in a study conducted by Gerzi and Berman (1981) who focused on a sample group of fifty-one expectant fathers with wives in the final trimester of pregnancy. A control group of fifty-one married men without children was evaluated for the purposes of obtaining comparison measures. This study disclosed that expectant fathers scored significantly higher on tests of overall anxiety, both overt and covert, as well as on scales measuring tension and apprehensiveness. Such anxiety may be traced to the expectant father's uncertain representations about how the arrival of the infant may interfere with his relationship with his wife. Administration of a picture apperception test demonstrated heightened oedipal dynamics, a resurgence of previously suppressed sibling rivalry and the presence of guilt feelings in the expectant fathers. Clinical interviews with several of the subjects indicated the presence of considerable ambivalence about assuming the role of father, rearousal of infantile fantasies, feminine identifications, castration fears and oedipal themes, as well as a strong attempt to defend against these ambivalent feelings by engaging in such defense operations as repression, denial, negation, intellectualization, reaction-formation, and isolation. The researchers noted that, while the higher levels of anxiety would be interpreted as a reaction to a real stress situation, the picture apperception results and interview material pointed to more specific dynamic factors. Such men often discover that their wives' physical condition has aroused previously suppressed conflicts pertaining to their male status. These studies suggest that pregnancy may be a time of psychological, as well as physical, upheaval for expectant fathers. In fact, the changes experienced by the expectant fathers in many respects paralleled the kinds of changes their wives were undergoing.

The expectant father's relationship with his wife is also likely to undergo a significant alteration during pregnancy, as was confirmed in a study conducted by Assor and Assor (1985). These researchers examined the emotional involvement of twenty-seven husbands and their wives in their marital relationship during the stressful period of the last trimester of the first pregnancy. Four behavioral measures indicated a high state of emotional involvement in the marriage. These included: a) a striving to gratify interpersonal needs primarily through the marital relationship; b) the need to receive affection and a corresponding desire for support; c) the desire to satisfy these needs in a mutually gratifying fashion; and d) the degree to which irritation and hostility erupted in the marital relationship when one partner felt that these needs were not being fulfilled. These researchers reported that husbands were less emotionally involved and invested in the marital relationship than were their wives. However, on the measure evaluating desire to support one's spouse, husbands consistently received high scores.

This study is revealing because it may inadvertently suggest ways in which husbands can become more emotionally isolated from their wives during the period of pregnancy. If, as Assor and Assor suggest, expectant fathers are, in general, less emotionally invested in the marital relationship than are expectant mothers, this may be because wives provide the additional emotional glue that on a daily basis sustains mutually fulfilling interaction. However, with the onset of pregnancy, the wife's emotional energies come to be invested first in herself and her uncertainties about the pregnancy during the earlier trimesters and only second in the evolving representational relationship that transpires with the fetus from the second trimester onwards. These findings strongly indicate that, in fact, the father may remove or withdraw emotional involvement from the wife since he feels left out or abandoned because of the impending birth and the generally strong emotional fusion that occurs between caregiver and infant shortly after birth as demonstrated during interaction episodes. Feelings of isolation may increase if the father continues to feel he will be excluded from the relationship between mother and infant.

These studies focusing on the physical and psychological alterations experienced by new fathers indicate that by ignoring the paternal role during the pregnancy and postpartum period, researchers may have been omitting one crucial source of dysfunction in both the marital relationship itself and in the parental response to the neonate. Moreover, the father's capacity to preview development to the infant may play a vital role in the infant's maturation and should not be ignored. Further investigations of this type are, therefore, warranted and therapists are urged to explore the representations and emotions of expectant fathers in their evaluations of dyadic interaction.

Conclusion

This chapter has posited the notion that the caregiver-infant relationship actually commences during pregnancy, when the expectant parents re-evaluate their status through representational fantasies concerning the infant and their future relationship with the infant. These psychological assessments, coupled with the dramatic physiological changes that attend pregnancy, create an atmosphere within which the contours of the incipient dyadic relationship are formed. Representations of the infant first emerge during this period, as does the caregivers' capacity to envision the future dyadic relationship and to begin devising previewing exercises. In addition, it is during this formative period that the expectant parents begin to create a relationship with the infant which is comprised of representational images of what personality and disposition of the infant will be like and of what caring for the infant will consist of. These representations may ultimately fuel previewing behaviors which are manifested during the interaction with the infant and which stimulate the infant's development. As a result, an evaluation of such prenatal maternal and paternal representations offers invaluable insight into how parents will actually preview development to the infant after birth.

It is imperative, then, that the therapist ascertain how the periods of pregnancy and postpartum are affecting the caregiver. In addition, recent studies focusing on expectant fathers and their perceptions have opened a new vista of exploration for therapists. How the expectant father will respond to the pregnancy and to the presence of the newborn may also have dramatic repercussions for the infant's development, for the nature of the relationship each caregiver forges with the newborn, and for the ability of each parent to preview development adaptively to the infant. The therapist thus must approach two avenues of investigation when dealing with expectant caregivers. First, the mother's prenatal history, encompassing both physiological and psychological status as well as her representations, need to be evaluated. Second, the attitudes of the expectant father need also to be assessed. By considering each of these variables, practitioners can obtain a more accurate prediction of what the dimensions of interaction within the dyad will be like, can isolate and diagnose problem areas in which adaptive exchange may go awry, and can predict the type of adaptive or maladaptive patterns that will ultimately exert an overwhelming impact on the infant's development.

CHAPTER 2

Previewing: A Means of Fostering the Infant's Predictive Abilities

Introduction

The recent application of microanalytic techniques to the study of human development has allowed researchers to observe a myriad of previously imperceptible events that occur during the maturational process of living organisms. In particular, sophisticated time-escalated sequences captured on videotape have permitted examination of the most intimate of events: the in utero alteration of human gametes from diffuse cell clusters into differentiated systems with unique functions. As the tape advances, we see how clusters of cells form an incipient spinal cord and we wonder what mysterious force impels this movement toward growth. From such sequences a distinctive impression emerges. It appears that the processes of nature move relentlessly toward development, by means of rapid change, increased control, and the acquisition of specialization.

At no time is this inexorable spasm of development more evident than during the first two years of life. Indeed, development proceeds at such a feverish pace during this interval that researchers have conveniently demarcated the period and given it the special label of "infancy". During these early years the infant begins to manifest the impressive array of developmental capacities that constitute his maturational endowment. Fine motor skills emerge as the infant's gestures become increasingly more refined. Some degree of autonomous control over physiological functions becomes apparent as feeding, sleeping, and elimination cycles acquire patterns of regularity. The infant begins to recognize familiar faces and objects in the environment and even formative language abilities surface. These developmental transformations generally depend on basic maturational growth which takes place on a physiological level and may be *objectively* observed and measured by the caregiver, a pediatrician and even by the infant himself to the extent that he is conscious of his burgeoning skills. As the infant matures, the caregiver's skill in validating this form of objective maturational change through previewing becomes vital. In essence, previewing exercises which rely on already mastered skills to introduce the infant to imminent developmental achievements help reinforce for the infant the sense of mastery and control over the transformations of his body.

Beyond these acquisitions, however, another type of developmental transformation surfaces during infancy. This category of developmental attainment involves the evolution of affective and cognitive capacities, both of which are fueled by the interaction that transpires with the caregiver. Such developmental progression may be deemed *subjective* in nature because it emerges from the intimacy and trust embedded in the relationship forged with the caregiver, and is experienced on a uniquely individual level. This is not to say that developmental skills of this type cannot be objectively measured. Nevertheless, unlike the infant's more objective attainments, subjective maturational achievements are best evaluated by assessing the quality of interaction within the dyad and by investigating the degree to which both infant and caregiver can predict one another's behavior, as well as the infant's imminent developmental milestones.

Foremost among the infant's subjective developmental achievements are the capacity to formulate predictions about upcoming events, the capacity to engage in behavior designed to elicit a particular response from the environment, and the capacity to maintain a coherent and stable representation of the outcome of interactive sequences with the caregiver. Underlying each of these developmental attainments is the ability to somehow formulate anticipations about the future, whether it be the future course of interaction with the caregiver or future maturational skills such as walking, and to behave in a fashion intended to provoke the kind of experience the infant has anticipated. Each of these developmental skills fosters and enhances the infant's *predictive abilities*. It is from the formulation of such predictions that the infant develops a sense of mastery and control over his environment. In turn, the adaptive caregiver engages in attuned ministrations which validate the infant's predictions, leading to a more enriched and heightened sense of control, and stimulating the infant to strive for even greater degrees of mastery over both the objective physiological changes occurring in his body and the more subjective alterations he is experiencing internally.

From this description it is clear that the caregiver plays a vital role in fostering the infant's predictive capacities. Indeed, it may be argued that it is because of the continual nurturing the caregiver provides that the infant is motivated to hone his affective and cognitive skills. Once he becomes adept at these skills, he can perpetuate the relationship with the caregiver. Although caregiver behavior may be characterized in diverse ways, one quality that permeates virtually all adaptive caregiver-infant interaction involves the orientation toward prospective development. In other words, it has been observed that caregivers who behave in an optimal fashion appear to orient the infant towards the future, towards the next developmental horizon and the skills that await. Such caregivers seem to possess an internal representation of the general contours of imminent development and are able to guide the infant in the direction of these maturational attainments at an appropriate pace. To capture the full implications of this predominant feature of dyadic interaction, I have coined the term *previewing*.

At its core, previewing represents an organizing principle that helps to explain an overriding feature of the infant's development: the fact that both infant and caregiver devote themselves to enhancing maturational skills and achieving ever more sophisticated techniques for mastering the challenges posed both by the environment, and by the physiological and psychological waves of development the infant is undergoing. Moreover, the concept of previewing also provides insight into how such mastery is painstakingly achieved by the infant and how the caregiver plays an indispensable role in shaping the infant's developmental destiny.

At the beginning of the caregiver-infant relationship, it is the caregiver who serves as the prime initiator of behaviors. Because of the caregiver's representational capacities, she can, unlike the infant, envision what developmental skill lies on the next horizon. By this statement I don't necessarily mean that the caregiver will possess a comprehensive roadmap of how development will progress and precisely when a maturational achievement will surface. Rather, most caregivers will display what is best described as an acute sensitivity to the moods and general trends of development being demonstrated by their infants. By sensing the infant's status on several levels simultaneously, the caregiver can begin to form *representations* of behaviors and developmental skills that are on the verge of consolidating. For example, a sensitive caregiver will be attuned to the infant's temperature, will notice patterns of eye movement and will be alert to the implications of the infant's gestures. Such a caregiver will be able to gauge when the infant's neck needs support and when support of this type can be withdrawn, if only momentarily, to enable the infant to experience the sensation of holding his head up by himself. From these representations, which apply to both small gestures and major developmental milestones, the caregiver begins to devise behavioral strategies for gradually introducing the infant to an imminent developmental achievement. During periods when the caregiver attends to the infant's needs, she will be able to distinguish between those changes that are more objective in nature and those that affect the infant's subjective perceptions.

The kinds of caregiver-initiated behaviors referred to above are examples of previewing that may be observed and assessed. For example, a caregiver who has sensed that the infant's kicking gestures are precursory to full-fledged crawling motions will begin to exercise the infant's limbs in an effort to both stimulate actual crawling and to gradually acquaint the infant with what the sensation of crawling will be like. Similarly, the caregiver who echoes the infant's vocalizations with carefully devised "baby talk" sequences is introducing the infant to the rhythms of human speech and preparing the infant for dialogues which will occur at a later date. In addition, by engaging in these previewing behaviors, the caregiver is helping the infant to predict not only how these new skills will be experienced, but also how these skills will influence the relationship being forged within the dyad itself. That is, such previewing behaviors convey to the infant how he will change autonomously with the advent of new developmental acquisitions and also how the relationship with the caregiver will be modified as a result of these new skills. *Indeed, it may be suggested that, by reinforcing the continuity of the primary dyadic relationship through previewing behaviors, the caregiver stimulates the infant to strive for even greater degrees of control and mastery over his body and the environment through developmental skill.* This is because mastery enhances both the intimacy of the infant's primary relationship with the caregiver and the autonomy he derives from control over his developmental capacities.

Another aspect of previewing should be mentioned at this juncture. Just as the sensitive caregiver is able to anticipate or represent imminent developmental achievement and to devise behaviors to introduce the infant to such skills so too will she be able to sense when the infant is ready to cease engaging in the previewing exercises and return to his previous developmental status. In other words, an adaptive caregiver will not overtax or exhaust the infant through previewing but will instead gradually integrate these behaviors into the infant's repertoire and then, with equal sensitivity, guide the infant back to his current developmental plateau.

This chapter attempts to analyze in detail the kinds of behaviors manifested by adaptive caregivers who engage in previewing exercises with their infants. It has been observed, for example, that such caregivers tend to exhibit a specific cluster of behaviors, referred to by several researchers as *intuitive responses,* that appear to promote the infant's capacities to predict events in the world around him and facilitate the subsequent introduction of the infant to imminent developmental achievement. In this cluster of behaviors are specific types of *visual cuing, vocal communication, and holding and feeding behaviors* which reinforces the infant's awareness of being ministered to by a responsive caregiver. Over the past two decades, technological advances in the area of video recording have enabled researchers to study these behavioral clusters. It is now possible to observe the universe of miniature, micromomentary interaction between infant and caregiver. From such investigations, researchers have codified the behaviors that occur beyond the awareness of visible perception. These intuitive behaviors, which appear to play an indispensible role in helping both infant and caregiver to predict one another's actions, will be considered in depth in the first part of this chapter.

The second part of the chapter is devoted to examining certain phenomena which further stimulate the infant's predictive capacities, making him receptive to the introduction of previewing exercises. In this section discussion will focus on how the caregiver's behaviors facilitate the infant's recognition of *discrepancies* and *contingencies* in his environment, eventually enabling him to devise predictable sequences of interaction and to formulate *expectancies* about what future development and future interactional patterns will be like. A brief discussion of play is also included in this section because it is through such playful behaviors with the caregiver during the first years of life that the infant is provided with an unparalleled opportunity to experiment with his burgeoning skills in recognizing discrepancies and contingencies. As will be seen, the emphatic caregiver is one who is acutely sensitive to the infant's perceptions and who responds to these perceptions in an appropriate fashion. The infant will seek to match the caregiver's sensitivity by attuning himself to her perspective. As a consequence, an awareness of self and of others will gradually emerge, allowing the infant to recognize that genuine communication requires consideration of one's own, as well as the other's, point of view.

Finally, the chapter delves into the notion of *meaning attribution*. This phrase refers to the caregiver's tendency to imbue the infant's behaviors with meaning and significance thereby enabling the caregiver to respond to the infant in a manner that creates purpose and order and provides the infant with some insight about the future direction of development. It is from the contours of meaning attribution that the infant begins to realize that emerging developmental skills are not chaotic and disorganized, but are instead capacities that can be controlled in order to master challenges in the environment and to fulfill physiological and psychological needs.

This chapter, then, outlines the basic interactional phenomena during the first two years of life that serve to enhance the infant's developmental skill and encourage him to master and control this skill through the primary interaction with the caregiver. The realization of these goals is attained through previewing interactions and, as will be seen in the following pages, the intuitive behaviors the caregiver engages in to promote the infant's predictive capacities and the stimulation she provides to reinforce these predictive capacities serve as preludes to the experience of previewing. By actively exposing the infant to these behaviors, the caregiver instills in the infant a sense of the predictability of his own physiological and psychological development and of his environment.

Maternal Intuitive Behaviors That Foster Infant Predictive Capacities

Careful examination of studies involving maternal behavior during the early years of infant life reveals two identifiable patterns of manifestations of dyadic interaction. According to such researchers as Papousek and Papousek (1987), the first pattern is dominated by behaviors that occur on the level of *intuitive response*. Papousek and Papousek explain that on a scale distinguishing *reflexive action* from deliberative *rational action*, an intuitive response is more closely akin to a reflex. In other words, the response is of such a fleeting nature that it appears to surface spontaneously and unconsciously. Microanalytic studies of caregivers and their infants have revealed that specific behaviors fall into the realm of intuitive responses. The most prominent examples of these intuitive behaviors include *visual cuing*, various forms of *vocal communication*, such aspects of close *bodily contact* as holding or cuddling behavior and *feeding competence*. This is not to suggest that other behaviors are not typical of mothers interacting intuitively with infants. Nevertheless, one reason why these four behaviors have captured the attention of researchers is that each manifestation appears to promote the infant's ability to predict upcoming events, as well as to anticipate the type of interaction that will occur with the caregiver. In addition, these behaviors are instrumental in introducing the infant to imminent developmental achievement during previewing exercises. As such, visual cuing, vocal communication, holding behaviors and feeding competence may be considered the building blocks from which the caregiver eventually sculpts and designs previewing interactions.

Visual Cuing

Even novices in the area of infant research are able to identify a crude form of visual exchange between caregiver and infant beginning immediately in the postnatal period. Papousek and Papousek (1987) refer to such optical manipulation on the part of the parent as *visual cuing*. In measuring this behavior, researchers have relied on naturalistic observations of face-to-face interaction and the seemingly orchestrated regulation of direct eye contact between the dyadic members during episodes of normal exchange. Visual cuing on the part of the caregiver evokes a distinctive greeting response from the infant and appears to be contingent upon presentation of the caregiver's face (Haekel, 1985). In fact, maternal visual cuing followed by a reciprocal infant gaze appears to be one of the first contingent sequences experienced by the infant. Repetition of this sequence may eventually help the infant formulate an internal representation of the caregiver's features which can later be used to predict a particular caregiver response or to elicit a desired behavior from the caregiver. It is also likely that visual cuing enables the infant to develop an internal representation of optical patterns which can later be manipulated through play, as with the game of peek-a-boo during the latter portion of the first year.

In addition to naturalistic observation of the gross patterns of visual cuing, researchers have also dissected the precise dimensions of maternal visual cuing. Microanalytic studies enable us to describe minute responses manifested during a sequence of visual cuing. Papousek and Papousek comment, for example, that caregivers characteristically gravitate to the middle of the neonate's visual field and strive to achieve direct eye-to-eye contact. When such contact is achieved, the caregiver typically displays an exaggerated greeting response, which these researchers have labeled "rhythmic noise." Moreover, it has been noted that mothers respond to the motor responses of the infant (limb gestures, clenched fists) with heightened attention to the infant's face, particularly the eyes. Thus, visual cuing in response to virtually any notable infant behavior appears to be assigned a preeminent position in the caregiver's responsive repertoire.

Blehar, Lieberman and Ainsworth (1977) have also recognized the primary role of visual cuing during their observations of interactions between caregivers and infants of six to fifteen weeks of age. In dyads where mothers coordinated visual cuing with playful behavior, it was found that infants were more frequently labeled as "happy," as demonstrated by joyful bouncing, smiling, and vocalizing. Mothers who relied on visual cuing were also rated as more skilled in terms of pacing and modifying behavioral initiations to infant signals. Infants who experienced harmonious interaction with caregivers were capable of differentiating their behavior significantly when confronted with a stranger. This study suggests, then, that early visual cuing fuels a host of other infant developmental skills in a proliferative fashion.

To explore the ramifications of such early infant differentiation, the researchers also observed dyads in which maternal visual response was muted. In such pairs, the mother initiated face-to-face contact less frequently and visual cuing as manifested by direct eye-to-eye contact was significantly less apparent, with a virtual absence of vocalization and emotional displays directed at the infant. It was noted that among such dyads, infants seldom sought maternal gaze, and rarely vocalized or bounced rhythmically. Interactive sequences were brief, often ending abruptly before any playful sequences emerged. Interestingly enough, infants in these latter dyads failed to evince any signs of discrimination between mothers and strangers during taped trials of face-to-face interaction. These findings indicate that unless the infant receives an adequate amount of responsive visual cuing from the caregiver, representational processes may become impaired and the infant's ability to distinguish among stimuli, to make predictions about the world around him and to express preferences through previewing may be delayed. In addition, Blehar et al.'s data reveal that infants who are not exposed to sufficient visual cuing will not establish a strong bond with the caregiver and, consequently, will lack support for their developmental journey. The lack of visual cuing between caregiver and infant during the first months of life, therefore, may be evidence of a maladaptive interaction and may be used as one indicator for predicting subsequent developmental deficits.

In a related investigation conducted by Tronick, Cohn and Shea (1986), it was found that, during the latter portion of the first year, infants who ordinarily experienced an abundance of visual cuing during interaction exhibited notable distress when such a response was withheld by mothers who had been instructed to feign a nonreactive, depressed mood and to avert their gaze. In accord with the work of Blehar et al., it was also found that among dyads where visual cuing and other forms of playful interaction were *not* ordinarily in evidence, infants were relatively indifferent when caregivers simulated depression. Thus, visual cuing may stimulate the infant's capacity to understand and discriminate among affective signals emitted by the caregiver, and, in particular, infants who are not exposed to a diversity of emotional expressions shared by the caregiver may exhibit deficits in their own affective functioning.

Field (1978) has emphasized that the caregiver's capacity for engaging in visual cuing with the infant during the first few months of life has a significant impact on whether interaction in the dyad will be harmonious and rhythmic. This researcher cautions that if the caregiver fails to use visual cuing to elicit alertness in the infant, a disturbed or asynchronic exchange can ensue, a finding also supported by Brazelton, Koslowski and Main (1974). Field maintains that the caregiver's role during early episodes of visual cuing is especially vital because this form of behavior stimulates the infant during periods of interaction and fosters continuation of the interaction. In addition, the caregiver's visual cuing behavior must be attuned to the visual manifestations emitted by the infant in order for a rhythmic exchange to occur. As Robson (1967) has pointed out, the infant's visual behavior, including gazing, looking away, eye closing and head turning, represents the fundamental motor system over which the infant has substantially *voluntary control* during the first months of life. In order for adaptive interaction to occur, it is essential not only that the caregiver display visual cuing but also that the caregiver take the lead in responding visually to infant cues. The caregiver should encourage the infant to exercise this form of interactional skill so that more sophisticated controlling experiences can evolve.

Because visual cuing appears to play such a crucial role in the early development of the infant's predictive abilities, a key issue is raised when the infant is either congenitally blind or possesses a visual handicap. In such cases, does the caregiver abandon visual cuing entirely, relying on other adaptive modes of interaction to substitute for direct eye-to-eye contact or does visual cuing remain a part of the mother's intuitive repertoire? Moreover, if visual cuing is an essential characteristic of early interaction that serves as both an immediate model and as a guide for future behavioral exchanges, how does the visually impaired infant cope in the absence of visual stimulation?

Answers to some of these inquiries have been provided by Als (1985) who traced the progress of a congenitally blind infant and her sighted mother from birth through eighteen months. During the first few days of life the infant displayed more difficulty than would a sighted neonate in controlling her states and recovering from crying, although she was gradually consoled when her mother spontaneously administered soft tactile input coupled with quelling vocalizations. The caregiver had developed after ten days a distinct method of communicating with the infant, involving gentle tactile stimulation administered with a series of melodic vocalizations. These behavioral patterns elicited a distinct response from the infant: his facial contours suggested pleasure and responsiveness and he turned his head toward the sound of the caregiver's voice.

By two months of age, however, this mode of interaction changed. The infant became restless, was easily upset, and difficult to console. His mother, in turn, became depressed at this unexpected regression in the infant's development and required psychological support to continue her efforts. By three and a half months, the infant's disorganization remitted rapidly and she emerged at a new, more sophisticated level of stability which endured through follow-up. Interaction with the mother was rhythmic and the infant demonstrated a unique attunement to the touch and voice of his mother.

Als' study is instructive for several reasons. First, this case history indicates that when either the caregiver or infant is deprived of one means of controlling the dyadic interaction (here, visual ability) other modes of control will be heavily relied upon to compensate for the infant's inability to transform phenomena into predictable events that can be controlled and mastered through specific responses. In this case, the infant seized upon caregiver's vocal communication and tactile contact to navigate toward harmonious interaction. Second, although the caregiver knew the infant was blind, she nevertheless engaged in visual cuing (holding the infant face-to-face, establishing direct eye contact, and modulating visual distance) suggesting that this form of interactional behavior is intuitive to the caregiver who is eager for interaction with the infant. Finally, the period of disorganization briefly observed in this infant may indicate that even if other adaptive modes of behavior can be used as substitutes, the absence of visual cuing itself may interrupt the forging of the interpersonal relationship between the mother and child. In fact, the period of disorganization observed in this infant highlights the significant role visual cuing plays as a fundamental intuitive behavior used by the caregiver to orient the infant to interaction and to the predictive nature of dyadic exchange.

All these studies suggest several general conclusions about the phenomenon of visual cuing. First, such maternal responsiveness is predictively valid. Infants deprived of visual cuing during the months immediately following birth will likely interact in a distinctively muted fashion which endures through later infancy. Their skills in discerning discrepancies and contingencies appear impaired (such infants are less adept at discerning discrepancies between the caregiver and an adult stranger, for example.) and they seem less adept at engaging in behaviors designed to exert control and mastery over physiological and psychological development. In contrast, early maternal visual cuing correlates with subsequent infant response both in the neonatal period and the later months of infancy. Visual cuing appears to enhance the infant's ability to predict interaction with the caregiver and consequently to exert control over the interaction. The predictive quality associated with visual cuing may stem from the fact that such behavior stimulates the infant to begin representing the caregiver's facial expressions and the meaning implicit in particular expressions. As a result, affective development is stimulated as the infant comes to associate specific expressions of the caregiver with internal feelings.

Visual cuing also appears to play an integral role in the formation of ever more complex modes of adaptation. These investigations reveal that the repeated pattern of visual cuing leads to some form of incipient awareness or recognition on the part of the infant which is acknowledged by a greeting response at three months and evidence of distress when the cuing is absent by six months.

Ultimately, as Papousek and Papousek point out, visual cuing serves a didactic purpose, enabling the infant to learn in the most profound sense of that word. Learning here involves the acquisition of representations which can be duplicated, modified, and subsequently used to communicate with the caregiver and to encourage more interaction. Through visual cuing the child acquires the capacity to identify discrepancies and contingencies in the environment, to represent behavioral patterns of the caregiver and to predict future sequences of exchange. Thus, visual cuing permits the infant to develop cumulative skills which compound in hierarchical fashion. Indeed, visual cuing may be a prime mechanism whereby the infant orients himself to the caregiver, eventually learning how to predict and thus control the world around him. By understanding that events in the external world can be controlled, the infant also comes to realize that he can exert a degree of mastery over the objective and subjective maturational changes occurring within himself. In addition, visual cuing reinforces and perpetuates the intimate relationship between the caregiver and the infant who relies on the caregiver as a source of information about the world. As a result, visual cuing is an indispensable aspect of early infant development, which captures the empathic communications parents share with their newborn.

Vocal Communication

Linked to visual cuing is another form of behavior exhibited by caregivers beginning during the immediate postnatal period and persisting throughout infancy. This behavior has been labeled *vocal communication*. Although the caregiver emits vocalizations immediately after the birth, a distinctive pattern can be identified at approximately six to eight weeks of age (Papousek and Papousek, 1987).

As with investigations of visual cuing, studies measuring vocal interaction have utilized observational techniques and microanalytic methods to highlight the distinct features of this behavior. During observations of interactive sequences between mother and infant researchers have evaluated changes in voice pitch, voice contour, quality of voice, vocal matching to infant repertoire, naming explanations and onomatopoeic sounds. It has been suggested that caregivers first evaluate the infant's state— whether it is one of arousal, discomfort or quiescence—and then use vocal cues to facilitate transition to another state. In other words, the caregiver evaluates the infant's current status and uses vocal cues to preview an upcoming mood.

When describing vocal communication, researchers have distinguished between two alternating forms of phonetic utterance. Initially, the caregiver verbalizes a reference appropriate to the interactional context. This reference is generally in the form of a question or answer. While maintaining direct eye-to-eye contact with the infant, the mother might comment, "You're not alone. Mommy's here." Almost immediately afterwards this reference statement will be followed by a complementary utterance in the form of nonsense speech, but incorporating melodic contours, rhythmicity, tempo, pauses and dynamics of voice pitch and quality. A typical sequence, when dissected, might sound like, "Yo, yo, ho, ho, heee." The caregiver will often coordinate the articulation of elongated vowels with the simultaneous stroking of the infant's face and an enhanced facial expression. To the outward observer, it might appear that the caregiver intuitively recognizes the need to translate *symbolic* language into a physical *analogue* which can be readily understood by the infant. Field (1978) has reported that during interaction in the first months of life maternal speech is generally slowed and exaggerated, while the range of pitch is expanded. Ferguson (1964) found that maternal "baby talk" is characterized by fluctuations in the range of loudness, contour of pitch, rhythms and stress, with vowel durations being prominently elongated.

The Blehar et al. (1977) study previously cited found that vocal communication during face-to-face interaction correlated with infant responsiveness. By three months of age the infant appears to understand that vocal communication contains a symbolic component, in the sense that the words are conveying a distinct message perhaps having to do with an emotional state such as affection or with the fulfillment of a physiological need such as hunger. Not only will vocal communication by the caregiver evoke reciprocal vocal communication but it will also elicit other forms of response. Infant crying, for example, becomes a way of communicating a desire to receive nourishment, to have discomfort alleviated (by a change of a diaper) or to engage in play with the mother. Parke and Sawin (1975) reported that parents touch and watch the infant closely following vocalization in order to determine which behavioral response will be most appropriate. Gradually the infant comes to understand that particular vocalizations have specific meanings and becomes more discriminating in both attending to caregiver vocalizations and replying with vocalizations and gestures of his own. We see here the evolution of an incipient communications systems designed to help the infant exert control and mastery.

Vocalization has also been examined from the perspective of the infant by Harding and Golinkoff (1979) who sought to ascertain the developmental stage at which infants begin using vocalizations to communicate with the caregiver. The study videotaped infants ranging in age from eight to fourteen months with their caregivers during naturalistic episodes. Two frustration episodes were introduced during the sequence in order to encourage infant vocalization. The researchers relied on Austin's (1962) classification of utterances, which posits that the responses following verbalizations can be of two types. *Perlocutionary responses* usually involve the infant's earliest utterances, when the caregiver reacts to infant sounds as if they were communicative even though there is no indication that the infant is intentionally using the sounds for communication. In contrast, an *illocutionary response* is recognized by both the speaker and listener as being communicative. According to Harding and Golinkoff, the point at which the infant uses vocalizations to signal the listener can be viewed as the illocutionary stage of communicative development.

The researchers found that a greater percentage of the younger infants they examined were perlocutionary, as demonstrated by the fact that these infants seldom channeled vocalizations directly at the mother and appeared oblivious to the fact that their caregivers could act as agents in obtaining desired objects. When such infants did direct vocalizations at the mother, they generally looked at her hands, as if believing that such gazing would set the hands in motion. These infants also tended to bang toys during frustration episodes and rarely gestured to their caregivers as a means of obtaining assistance. In contrast, the older illocutionary infants directed vocalizations not only at their mothers' hands but far more frequently at their mothers' eyes, suggesting that they recognized the caregiver as a separate object from whom they could obtain aid. Such infants used vocalizations to contact their caregivers, to direct attention and to coordinate eye contact a significant amount of the time. As this study reveals, by the end of the first year the majority of infants have acquired the capacity to use vocalization as an *intentional* form of communication with the caregiver. This finding indicates that vocalization aids the infant in formulating predictions about how the world operates and also suggests that the transition from perlocutionary to illocutionary responses are facilitated by an interactive partner who engages the infant with vocalizations even from the first days of life. Such vocalizations can be labeled a form of previewing since the caregiver is using verbal sequences to acquaint the infant with what the experience of linguistic communication will be like. Eventually, the infant participates in these vocalizations to enhance communication with the caregiver and to perpetuate the interaction. Thus, the infant has learned that the unique vocalizations emitted by the caregiver represent "language," a vehicle for expressing one's intentions.

These studies suggest that, like visual cuing, vocal communication acts to help the infant predict upcoming events. On a very basic level, the caregiver vocalizes intuitively to stimulate interaction with the infant. But the caregiver's purpose is also designed to assist the infant in smoothing the transition between emotional states and to encourage communication of needs to the parent who, in turn, will attempt to translate infant signals into meaningful requests. As communicative sequences increase in complexity, the infant begins to grasp the dimensions of symbolic or abstract thought. An internal connection will eventually be forged as the infant begins to formulate representations and to make predictions about a particular stimulus (e.g., cry) and patterns of caregiver response. As these patterns increase, so too will the infant's capacity to refine vocalizations, and from a continual series of caregiver-initiated vocalizations and infant responses, the rudiments of language emerge.

The intricacies of this process can be more fully appreciated if we analyze them in terms of the infant's specific developmental stage. For instance, during the first few months of life the infant's responses to environmental stimuli occur spontaneously without the infant making any particular predictions about these interactions; such responses are perlocutionary. By approximately the third month of life, the infant begins to develop sophisticated skills; he gains a heightened awareness of the meaning of his responses and he begins to comprehend that a particular vocalization will evoke a specific response. At this point, a rudimentary realization of the communicative nature of vocalization occurs. Significantly, this is also the period when contingency awareness (i.e., an understanding of the interdependence of stimulus and response) becomes consolidated. Bimodal perception (i.e., the ability to discern invariant features of a stimulus via different perceptual avenues, such as sound and sight) also becomes evident during this period. It is, then, between the third and ninth month that the infant becomes truly illocutionary. From this development, the infant strives to use vocalization as a means of predicting events and exerting control over interactions with the external world as well as over the developmental transformations occurring within his own body.

By the end of the first year, the infant comes to understand the significance of refining vocal messages to predict and elicit precise responses from the caregiver. The meaning attributed to the infant responses can be now mutually agreed upon or *validated* by both members of the dyad. Such development allows the infant to grasp the fact that a particular vocal response can have a multiplicity of meanings, some of which are symbolic. This process of cumulative acquisition provides insight into the infant's capacity to hierarchically organize interdependent developmental skills into more and more sophisticated responses. Once the infant begins to simulate speech, he is striving to practice full-fledged communication with the caregiver and to elicit further previewing vocalizations from the caregiver.

Holding Behavior

Among the most intuitive or deeply ingrained behaviors the parent engages in with the infant is *holding behavior*. The nuances of this phenomenon can be observed during the first months of life. This caregiver response represents a potent signal from mother to infant communicating that interaction and intimacy is desired. Moreover, holding behavior also provides the infant with the secure sense of an interactive partner, who will guide him in exerting control over the developmental changes of his body.

A distinct pattern of holding behavior has been discerned in dyads where interaction is fluid and reciprocal. Main and Weston (1982) report that within such dyads mothers display tender and gentle gestures when picking up their infants. The caregiver's arms are positioned in such a way as to create a natural cradle, supporting the child's head and body. This position facilitates face-to-face contact and enables the caregiver to engage effectively in visual cuing and vocal communication. Main and Weston observed that infants who were held in this position were touched, caressed and rocked more frequently. The infant displayed a pleasurable response to these gestures, as demonstrated by passing to a quiescent state or by gurgling contentedly. This experience—coordinating visual, vocal and tactile dimensions—fosters the infant's incipient representational capacities. From such experiences, sequences of contingency are represented which the infant uses to formulate predictions about the external world and about his own developmental course.

In contrast to the above dyads in which the caregiver appeared skilled in molding the infant to her body, Main and Weston also identified a group of dyads in which the caregiver was inept at providing a core of pleasurable holding experiences for the infant. These mothers tended to hold the infant in a stiff and awkward fashion and often failed to manifest the cradling gestures necessary to promote adaptive face-to-face exchanges. They generally did not attribute any special significance to the infant's face, nor did they seem aware of the fact that the baby's neck and upper body needed support during periods of holding. It was common for such mothers to express a physical dislike and occasionally a repulsion for bodily contact with the infant, and contact was often limited to such necessary behaviors as diapering and feeding. Main and Weston's findings are reminiscent of the observations documented by Spitz (1946) involving institutionalized infants. Spitz found that infants who had been deprived of consistent bodily contact during the early months of life because of an absent caregiver or who received only sporadic contact with a nurse tended to demonstrate an apathetic attitude when subsequent physical interaction by an adult was attempted.

By holding and caressing the infant gently the caregiver gradually conveys to the infant that his body has a particular form, shape, and temperature. This dynamic exchange of information eventually enables the infant to represent his own physical boundaries in relation to the body of the caregiver and to represent himself with others. These interactions also permit the infant to recognize and subsequently predict events that will affect him. It is likely that the infants described in Spitz' original study were deprived of such stimulation, and therefore failed to learn contingency sequences or to develop flexible representations. As a result, these infants ultimately lacked the ability to communicate their needs, to predict the boundaries of their own bodies and to develop capacities designed to control their developmental skills.

In sum, holding behavior may represent yet another mode of maternal response geared to coax the infant's incipient predictive capacities. By means of holding behaviors the caregiver provides the infant with a "bird's-eye" view of the caregiver's eyes and facial expression and allows the infant to experience at close range the nuances of concurrent vocal communication. By establishing bodily contact, the caregiver both literally and figuratively introduces the infant to didactic patterns of interaction which are vital to the fostering of the infant's predictive capacities. Moreover, appropriate holding behaviors convey a sense of emotional security to the infant. As the infant begins to develop representations and experiment with his developmental skills, further awareness of a supportive partner will foster the emergence of more sophisticated predictive capacities.

Feeding Behavior

The ability of the caregiver to competently satiate infant hunger has captured the attention of numerous researchers. According to Pedersen (1975), this behavior becomes evident immediately after birth and crystallizes into an observable pattern at approximately four weeks. Pedersen states that during an optimal interaction the infant is fed according to a well-paced rhythm. Adaptive caregivers appear sensitive to the infant's needs for either stimulation or brief rest periods. This rhythmic sequence of interspersed activity and rest occurs in a fluid fashion, with the caregiver displaying the skill to burp and soothe the infant in a nondisruptive manner.

Ainsworth and Bell (1969, 1979) offer a similar portrait of the parameters of maternal feeding competence, reporting that competence is demonstrated by a smooth cooperation between the dyadic members. Competent caregivers feed the infant promptly, stave off feedings tactfully, coax the infant to the nipple gently and are relatively comfortable in permitting the infant to initiate sucking manifestations. As in their other studies, Ainsworth and Bell also identified dyads in which a predictable caregiver-infant feeding interaction did not occur. The research team identified mothers who did not adjust their pacing to their infants' cues or who enlarged the nipples of bottles too much and who forced their infants to take solid foods despite protests. These caregivers appeared indifferent and ill-equipped to cope with infants who struggled to move away from the bottle or who choked and spat up. Feeding periods often became a time of battle for these dyads. Other insensitive feeding behaviors included teasing a hungry baby by putting a finger in its mouth and coaxing the infant to continue nursing until it gagged. It is not difficult to discern how such behaviors hinder the infant's capacity to develop representations of contingent experience, and hence, impede the development of predictive capacities.

The Mother-Infant Sensitivity Scale developed by Price (1983) measures the quality of early mother-infant interactions in a feeding context within the first few months after birth. Among the items evaluated are: the spatial distance the caregiver maintains from the infant during feeding; the holding style, including rhythmic or awkward holding; maternal mood displayed during feeding; maternal vocalization and visual behavior. This scale is helpful for practitioners just beginning to engage in dyadic evaluations, because it highlights the types of discrete behaviors to which the therapist should be alert.

Although each type of intuitive behavior displayed by the caregiver plays a distinctive role in the infant's development, *feeding competence* is perhaps unique in that its main purpose is to gratify an immediate physiological need. In fact, the caregiver's skill in staving off the infant's hunger by rapidly offering nourishment may create, on a very rudimentary level, one of the first representations of a contingent sequence of stimulus and response for the infant. This sequence, in turn, leads to the infant's initial predictions about the world and to initial attempts to convey his intentions to the caregiver through previewing exercises. The way in which such abilities emerge may be described as follows. The discomfort experienced by hunger is expressed through movements and the vocalization of a cry to which the caregiver responds. If the caregiver's pattern of response is consistent, these interactions serve as a prototypical model for the infant. These complex associations are gradually represented by the infant and used to formulate predictions about future interpersonal exchanges. Feeding competence is, therefore, a noteworthy behavior because it may signify an adaptive interaction from which other, more complex representations are derived and may provide the infant with a model for predicting future sequences. The caregiver's competence while engaging in this behavior may be equally significant because it creates and reinforces the mood or attitude that both partners will experience in future interactions. As a consequence, feeding sequences, like other intuitive behaviors, have validity for predicting the quality of future interaction within the dyad.

Feeding competence may serve yet another adaptive purpose by providing the infant with an additional opportunity to experience the boundaries between himself and the external world. This occurs as the infant gains increased awareness that the source of nourishment, either the bottle or the nipple, represents a stimulus from the external world. If the caregiver is attuned to the infant's needs and responds to feeding cries in a rhythmic and sensitive fashion, the infant will be able to repeatedly validate and strengthen evolving predictions about the differences between his inner psychological and physiological perceptions and the reality of the external world.Sensitive feeding promotes the realization of separateness in the infant, while at the same time the nurturing presence of the caregiver allays any concomitant anxiety that accompanies this realization. The fears associated with separation are quelled and the infant is motivated to perpetuate interaction with the caregiver, who is perceived as a responsive partner capable of predicting the infant's needs and ministering to them.

Maternal Stimulation That Enhances Predictive Capacities

While the modes of adaptation discussed above rely heavily on precise behavioral manifestations that may be quantitatively measured, such as visual and vocal cuing, the caregiver behavior described in this section are more qualitative in nature. When we refer to the caregiver's ability to *provide adequate stimulation* for the infant, we are speaking of a qualitative mood which permeates early interaction, fostering the infant's predictive abilities and capacity to exert mastery and control. The contours of this mood are not often clearly discernible until the infant is approximately three months of age. Although measuring the level of stimulation presents difficulties—because rather than focusing on specific, discrete manifestations, the researcher seeks to evaluate the overall nature of interaction—this area of maternal competence provides vital insights into how the infant eventually learns to predict events in the world around himself.

Papousek and Papousek (1977, 1987) have evaluated the caregiver's ability to provide adequate stimulation for the infant by assessing various criteria during isolated sequences of interaction. They have focused on several areas: the amount of vocal communication the caregiver directs toward the infant, the ability to regulate intensity of speech to match the infant's integrative engagement, the reduction of linguistic complexity coupled with an elongated rate of articulation, segmenting and repetition of prose patterns, the degree of bodily contact and tactile stimulation, modulation of eye-to-eye contact, and differential responsivity to infant signals. They have also observed the caregiver's capacity to coordinate visual cuing, vocal communication and tactile skills in harmony with the responsive rhythms of the infant. Adequate stimulation was obtained when fluid interactive sequences of relatively long duration were identified; mother and infant appeared to reciprocally attend to one another's cues. Such sequences began gradually, moved to a level of sustained moderate activity and then gradually abated. Temporal divisions between periods of adequate stimulation and periods of quiescence were smooth and fluid.

Papousek and Papousek have stressed that interactive behaviors occur gradually rather than abruptly and that caregiver gestures appear to be acutely mediated by interactional cues. Stern (1985) has labeled this quality of interaction *affect attunement,* although he documents evidence of its appearance at the slightly later date of nine months. One implication of this kind of interaction is that the infant has learned to predict sequences of interaction with the caregiver, enabling him to formulate variations on the patterns of contingency he has come to learn and represent. From such variations the infant begins to initiate his own responses and to manifest them to the caregiver in an effort to communicate what the infant anticipates will happen. These manifestations are predictions to which the adaptive caregiver will respond by continuing to stimulate the infant.

Four particular types of caregiver's stimulation will be discussed here. These are:

1. The caregiver's support of the infant's integrative processes through the introduction of discrepant stimuli, sequences of contingent interaction and the fulfillment of mutually understood expectations;
2. The caregiver's use of play to encourage the infant to experiment with emerging developmental capacities;
3. The caregiver's use of empathy as a means of promoting the infant's realizations of the perspective of the other; and
4. The caregiver's tendency to engage in meaning attribution to imbue the interaction with purpose and direction and to help the infant organize burgeoning developmental skills.

At the outset it is important to note that, as with the intuitive maternal behaviors discussed earlier, the manifestations described in this section tend to arise spontaneously. Researchers who have reported on how caregivers introduce infants to discrepancy and contingency note that these caregiver skills emerge automatically and are integrated imperceptibly into the contours of adaptive interaction. Similarly, play behaviors and maternal empathy share this natural and fluid quality. Caregivers who display these tendencies appear to be exquisitely sensitive to the behavioral cues emitted by their infants and respond to these cues in a highly appropriate fashion (Tronick & Cohn, 1989).

The first capacity implicates evolving cognitive capacities. Discrepancy awareness, a phrase coined by McCall and McGee (1977), refers to the cognitive skill of distinguishing between two stimuli that are somewhat similar but divergent enough to evoke a recognition of difference. According to these researchers, extreme discrepancy causes distress (perhaps because the individual cannot process a stimulus that is completely unfamiliar) while minimal discrepancy fails to arouse interest (perhaps because the individual does not discern a sufficient difference). Thus, caregivers who expose their infants to moderate levels of discrepancy foster the infant's capacities to recognize subtle distinctions in environmental objects and in the behaviors of those surrounding him. If the infant is exposed to these kinds of discrepancies among stimuli, his incipient capacity to make predictions about stimuli in the environment and about his own burgeoning developmental skills will be encouraged.

Contingency awareness functions in a similar fashion (Watson, 1966; Watson and Ramey, 1972). Essentially, contingency awareness refers to the capacity to represent a stimulus-response sequence. In order for the infant to attain contingency awareness, he must be exposed to a connected stimulus-response sequence that has come to be recognized as a predictable pattern. Eventually, the infant comes to understand that a particular cue or stimulus (e.g., his cry) evokes a particular response (e.g., being fed). When repeated enough times, this contingent sequence becomes familiar and the infant begins to formulate an internal perception of the stimulus-response pattern. This pattern is then represented or envisioned by the infant and becomes a kind of blueprint for his behaviors. Once a sufficient number of such representations have been internalized, the infant can begin making predictions about the kinds of behaviors the caregiver is likely to engage in, as well as predictions about how the caregiver will respond if the infant engages in a particular behavior. Thus from the nuances of contingency awareness, expectancies emerge. As a result, the infant is able to anticipate how the caregiver is likely to behave and eventually, how he himself will behave. In turn, these expectations enable the infant to exert a degree of control and mastery over his environment and over burgeoning developmental skills.

Play behavior and experimentation is also discussed in this section. As will be seen, although play behaviors serve the purpose of reinforcing the infant's developmental capacities, in and of themselves these behaviors serve no pragmatic purpose. Instead, play enables the infant to enjoy a respite from the challenges of the environment while experimenting with developmental capacities. It is through play that the infant can experiment with various contingent sequences and learn to master his predictions about the world. The caregiver who engages in play with the infant, in essence, is permitting an exhilarating shift in the expected roles of the dyadic relationship. The infant is permitted to be the initiator in the dyadic interaction by originating behaviors to which the caregiver will be expected to respond. Adaptive caregivers will display a willingness to engage in this type of play behavior and to be the recipient of interaction during these sequences. Not only does such play activity facilitate the infant's capacity to exercise his predictive capacities by experimenting with various behavioral sequences, but it also encourages the infant to adopt the perspective of the other.

Maternal empathy is yet a further quality that permeates the interaction of adaptive dyads. Empathy has been defined by Hoffman (1975, 1984) as the capacity of one individual to experience the emotional perspective of another. The caregiver who is empathic to the infant is thus capable of sensing the infant's affective state and responding to it appropriately. In effect, empathy requires the individual to be aware of another who is distinct from him, to be cognizant of the emotions experienced by this other and to respond to these feelings in a sensitive manner. When defined in this fashion it can be seen how empathy promotes an understanding of self-other boundaries and an appreciation for affective sharing. When a caregiver has responded empathically to the infant, the infant's ability to negotiate these self-other distinctions is facilitated. The recognition that the caregiver represents another who is separate from the infant begins once the infant recognizes that he can experience and share feelings with the other.

Finally, some discussion is devoted to the phenomenon of meaning attribution, whereby the caregiver conveys the notion that the infant's actions are imbued with meaning and responds to infant behaviors as if such meaning is being communicated. As will be seen, if meaning attribution is appropriate and adaptive, it will eventually help the infant organize his perceptions about both the caregiver and the environment.

Support of Infant Integrative Processes

One aspect of the caregiver's ability to provide adequate stimulation is *supporting the infant's integrative processes*. Researchers have generally focused on the period from three through twelve months as a time when integrative processes, such as discrepancy awareness and contingency awareness, become evident during interaction. The purpose of this caregiver mode of adaptation is—as with the provision of adequate stimulation—to *orient* the infant toward making accurate predictions about upcoming developmental and interpersonal maturation, to assuage discomfort and to sustain a pleasurable level of arousal. This type of response is an example of caregiver previewing. Here the caregiver is attempting to create a mood that will help the infant to integrate his own perceptions independently.

Parke and Sawin (1975) examined caregiver responsiveness as a means of tapping maternal support of the infant's integrative processes. They referred to this kind of responsiveness as a disposition that permeates the entire interactive atmosphere. They focused as well on paternal sensitivity to auditory distress during feeding periods. Sosa, Kennell, Klaus, Robertson and Urrutia (1980) also studied caregiver ability to distinguish or "read" the predictive cues from the infant by asking adults to indicate whether the baby was requesting a bottle, a pacifier or a toy.

Although different infant behaviors have been studied, these investigations essentially raise the issue of the caregiver's skills in responding to the infant predictions that emerge in the form of behavioral cues. How well does the caregiver supply an appropriate stimulus based on the infant's predictive signals? When matching sequences or patterns of behavior have been repeated over time, the infant acquires a fixed representation or image of the signal and response, such that a typical response becomes predictable. If this expected response is not forthcoming or if a somewhat discrepant response is presented, the infant will display signs of distress, a reaction that is first evident at approximately three months of age, according to McCall and Kagan (1970). Exhibitions of distress due to a discrepant caregiver response have led theorists to offer a variety of explanations. It is now generally believed that infant-caregiver exchange generates an *expectancy* or *prediction* about the direction of the interactive episode from which the infant derives an internal representation of an anticipated response (Stern and Gibbon, 1978). This sequence signifies a contingency, in that the infant maintains cognitive awareness concerning the connection between his signal and caregiver's response. Underlying these phenomena is the notion that the infant has begun to coordinate cognitive and emotional processes in an effort to experience control over a sequence of predictable interpersonal events. This sense of control can later be analogized to the sense of control the infant will attempt to display over his own developmental processes.

Imitative behavior reveals how internal integration is occurring in the infant. While responsiveness takes place when the caregiver responds to an infant cue, imitation involves the infant's response to a parentally initiated behavior. In harmonious dyads infant imitation is encouraged, gradually proliferating into game-playing behaviors. Imitation may also signify a way in which the infant verifies his prediction about what behavior the caregiver will manifest. Sosa, Kennell, Klaus, Robertson and Urrutia (1980) observed that nine- to twelve-month-old infants engaged in an elaborate form of imitation by projecting their own feeding behaviors onto other objects, such as dolls. Imitation here involved complex clusters of interactions including mouth opening, lip movement and sucking, suggesting that by this age the infant is able to incorporate a variety of discrete manifestations into one behavior.

Infants as young as three and a half months have been shown to have the ability to formulate specific expectations and to predict visual events. In a study performed by Haith, Hazan, and Goodman (1988), a group of twelve infants of this age were exposed to a sequence of projections that appeared to the left or right of a visual center. One of the infant's eyes was videotaped during periods while the infant watched a series of slides that were presented as being noncontingent upon behavior. Subsequently, the infants were exposed to slides at spaced intervals. Based on an analysis of the infants' reaction times, it was determined that the infants developed an anticipatory response or expectation to the regularly spaced slide presentation. The researchers reported that the findings of the study suggest that three and a half-month-olds can discern regularity in a spatiotemporal series, will develop expectancies or predictions about events in the series and will act on these expectancies.

Among the key behaviors such researchers have sought to dissect is the manifestation of anticipation, which has been described as an infant action or behavioral cue that is initiated prior to an event and is adaptive for that event. One explanation of anticipatory capacity provided by this study involves the element of prediction. It was found that the infants displayed increased reaction times and anticipatory fixations when exposed to the noncontingent or nonpredictable slides. As Haith et al. note, this finding suggests that infants respond to regular rhythms of behavior in the environment and are aware of disruptions in that rhythm.

This study reinforces the notion that an adaptive caregiver who attunes her rhythm to that of the infant may be providing the infant with enhanced exposure to a consistent and contingent environment. In turn, this rhythm facilitates the infant's burgeoning capacities to engage in predictions about his environment. Predictions generate expectations which, if fulfilled, reinforce internalized contingency relationships and result in positive affect. If the infant is exposed to sufficient contingency relationships, he will eventually begin generating predictions and experimenting with these predictions during interactive sequences in which the caregiver previews imminent development for the infant. Thus, two factors, the caregiver's tendency to provide the infant with rhythmic behavioral sequences and the infant's attraction to these interludes, enhance the infant's capacity to control the environment.

These studies are significant not merely because they demonstrate caregiver and infant ability to duplicate one another's actions, but also because they indicate the potential of both dyadic members to progressively coordinate responses into more sophisticated representational and interactive configurations. When this duet of modulation is occurring, the caregiver may be said to be adequately supporting the infant's integrative processes, helping him to better represent predictable patterns of contingency encountered in the environment.

It should be noted that the kinds of maternal behaviors discussed above have also been found to be predictive of the infant's ease in achieving developmental milestones. In a study investigating the origins of mother-infant attachment behavior, for example, Isabella, Belsky and von Eye (1989) found that maternal synchronic behavior tended to promote secure attachment patterns in infants of one year, while the absence of such displays of synchronic interaction tended to result in insecure attachment patterns of avoidance and resistance when infants were tested at one year of age. In defining synchronic behavior, Isabella et al. focused on a group of fourteen behaviors, many of which have been mentioned earlier in this chapter as intuitive behaviors. Among these behaviors were: maternal vocalization, maternal soothing through vocalization and body contact, face-to-face gazing patterns, contingent exchange and appropriate stimulation.

The findings of this study indicate that such maternal behaviors, which are often used during previewing episodes, facilitate the acquisition of developmental milestones. This investigation demonstrates that an attachment relationship with the caregiver was promoted as a result of such behaviors, while the acquisition of the milestone of attachment was thwarted in infants who were not exposed to this kind of stimulation by their caregivers. In a related study, Lewis and Feiring (1989) also found that maternal behavior during the mother-child interaction facilitated the eventual attainment for a secure and adaptive attachment bond.

These investigations, therefore, highlight the value of previewing and previewing behaviors as catalysts for promoting optimal developmental change. As a result, the degree to which the caregiver manifests these behaviors individually and in clusters during previewing episodes during the first year of life may be viewed as a valid and reliable predictor of the ease with which the infant will be able to attain and master developmental milestones. One reason for this may be that previewing provides the infant with a sense that development is a process that can be mastered and shared with the caregiver. The more this message is reinforced, the greater will be the infant's motivation to seek such stimulation from the caregiver.

Play as the Arena for Creativity and Experimentation

The conceptual difference between caregiver support for the infant's integrative capacities and caregiver playfulness is not so much a matter of substance as it is one of degree. *Playfulness*, which generally becomes apparent as a distinctive form of interaction late in the first year, may be identified by the ease and willingness with which the dyad engages in variations of interactive behavior along with the pleasurable affect that permeates such interaction. Because genuine play relies upon the ability to vary representations into new patterns, it encourages the infant to devise and manifest new patterns while interacting with the caregiver during previewing exercises. In fact, play may be the ultimate paradigm for explaining how the infant comes to engage in previewing interactions.

The implications of play behavior for both caregiver and infant are numerous. For the infant, the capacity to vary behaviors rapidly and responsively, as in play, indicates that a hierarchical form of adaptation has occurred, enabling him to coordinate and sustain multiple internal representations of interactional sequences. Integrative capacities crystallize as the infant uses his newly acquired skills to mediate both familiar and new interactions with the environment. But the implications of play behavior for the caregiver are equally as significant. By engaging in sustained periods of play with the infant, the caregiver demonstrates a capacity to serve as a steadfast and secure base from which developmental innovations will proliferate. Play, then, reinforces the caregiver's role as the infant's goal-correcting partner and stimulates the infant to experiment by varying patterns of contingency with which he is already familiar. Through play sequences, the caregiver not only previews upcoming development, but also encourages the exercise of the infant's adaptational skills to their fullest developmental potential.

Maternal Empathy

Another phenomenon related to previewing that stimulates the infant's predictive capacities involves the manner in which the caregiver successfully communicates affective experience to the infant. This form of sharing experience whereby the infant is eventually able to perceive the feeling state of the caregiver is called *empathy*. Empathy is the act of adopting the perspective of the other, putting oneself in the other's place or entering into another's state of mind (Demos, 1984). In the caregiver-infant relationship two types of empathic exchanges are evident. First, as Demos explains, in order for interaction to be harmonious, it is incumbent upon the caregiver to be aware of and attuned to the infant's perceptions and to respond in a fashion that supports and encourages the infant's explorations of the world. Second, the infant must eventually be able to discern the caregiver's empathic responses and to distinguish these responses from his own.

Demos conducted a study, involving twelve mother-infant pairs, that sought to assess how these two aspects of empathic response operate within the dyad. Empathy involves not only perceiving the nature of the affective tone of behaviors produced by the other, but also requires attaching a meaning to these behaviors that is consonant with the meaning being experienced by the other. Three types of phenomena were the focus of the researcher's attention: 1) the triggering of events; 2) the affective experience; and, 3) the response of the organism to the affective experience.

From observations of these phenomena several distinct patterns of affective awareness were recognized. In one scenario, the caregiver accurately perceived and understood the infant's affective state and the intention represented by the infant through manifestations. Such caregivers responded by communicating back to the infant in an empathic way, facilitating and prolonging the infant's positive states of interest and joy, and reducing the infant's negative states of distress, fear, shame, or anger. A variant upon this type of optimal empathic response is demonstrated by caregivers who correctly perceive and understand the infant's negative affective state and intent, but whose response does not prevent or end the negative experience for the infant. One example may be in the case of an inoculation. In such situations, the mother may act to help the infant endure the negative experience, although the overall unpleasant affect will still be felt by the infant. Other caregivers studied by Demos were able to demonstrate a perception of the child's positive experiences, but were unable to enhance or prolong these experiences, thus failing to support the child's incipient capacity to regulate affective states. A fourth type of infant-caregiver response reported by Demos involved caregivers who, although aware of the child's experience, tended to heighten the negative experience. This may or may not have been done with hostile intent.

Two other kinds of responses that were clearly maladaptive were also reported. In the first such example, the caregiver misperceives or misunderstands all or some of the components of the infant's affective experience, and acts according to this misperception. In the second such example, the caregiver does not seem to notice or respond to the child, although the child is in her presence. From Demos's observations, then, it is clear that empathy facilitates both the caregiver's ability to predict infant response and the infant's skill in anticipating the caregiver's reaction.

The relationship between empathy and caregiver previewing also needs to be underscored. In order to preview adaptively to the infant, the caregiver must be able to perceive and interpret the infant's affective expression. Indeed, since the infant's primary means of communication prior to the advent of language is through affective cues, it is vital that the caregiver be able to "read" these cues before fashioning adaptive previewing exercises. Empathy, in other words, serves as a key prerequisite that must be present before the caregiver can preview adaptively and appropriately.

Meaning Attribution by the Caregiver

Meaning attribution refers to the caregiver's ability to interpret and attribute a specific meaning the infant's behavior (Cramer, 1987). This proclivity on the part of the caregiver first manifests during pregnancy and continues to exert influence well into the late childhood years. Meaning attribution is not merely the verbal labeling of infant action and expression, but is a highly personalized *interpretation* of the implications of the behavior. According to Cramer, parents score infant behavior according to their own private set of expectations, which in turn, influence the timing and manner of the baby's response. Cramer observed that the symptomatic behavior displayed by an infant often symbolizes the projected anxieties and fantasies of the caregiver that have been attributed to the infant. In a mode of communication thus far not fully understood, caregivers can convey emotional data to the infant who manifests such information by engaging in aberrant behavioral patterns. In infants who exhibited difficulties during feeding sequences, for example, Cramer frequently found that the caregiver attributed idiosyncratic meaning to aspects of nourishment. Some of these caregivers expressed the fear that their infants would wither or fail to thrive if excessive nourishment was not provided. This belief persisted despite the fact that infants turned away or attempted to thrust their bodies when fed.

As the above example demonstrates, caregiver attributions are communicated to the infant and may interfere with the normal development of predictive processes occurring within the dyad. By assigning a special, private meaning to the significance of feeding periods, the caregiver may become less attuned or even oblivious to the actual cues emitted by the infant. But meaning attribution may also function in a more positive manner, causing the caregiver to imbue infant behavior with specific positive cognitive and emotional meaning. A caregiver who is particularly sensitive to the infant's vocalizations, for instance, may claim to "hear" fully pronounced words which to the ordinary observer sound like gibberish. Precisely because the caregiver attributes meaning to the infant's sounds and previews this meaning through intuitive behaviors, she may be more motivated to devote time and attention to the interaction, patiently eliciting responses, via trial and error, which must occur prior to genuine speech.

Cramer devised a four-step procedure for ascertaining the kinds of parental attributions that occur within any given dyad.

1. He recommends that caregiver-infant interaction be observed carefully in a naturalistic setting.
2. Such interactions need to be formally recorded, while investigators describe their own impressions of the dyadic exchange.
3. An in-depth parental interview is advised during which the caregiver

is queried, with particular emphasis on how the affective behaviors of the child are interpreted.

4. Correlations must be drawn between various themes that emerge from caregiver attributional statements and forms of behavior exhibited during interaction.

In this fashion, the types of predictions the caregiver is attributing to the infant may be ascertained.

It is appropriate to conclude this section on caregiver behaviors that stimulate the infant's predictive capacities with the discussion of meaning attribution because, perhaps more than any other phenomenon displayed by the caregiver, attribution colors all exchanges with the infant. Indeed, as was discussed in Chapter 1, caregiver attributions begin during the pregnancy period as the caregiver begins to engage in anticipatory fantasies involving the infant. (The implications of such fantasies on infant development were discussed there). The parent who predicts a receptive and thriving infant will endow each communicative exchange with sufficient rhythm and intensity to encourage the fruition of these or any other developmental capacities of the infant. By communicating such an attitude to the infant, the caregiver creates an optimal atmosphere in which such developmental predictions can unfold productively.

Conclusion

In essence, each of the intuitive caregiver behaviors described above that is indicative of an adaptive orientation towards development may be characterized as a form of *previewing*. The concept of previewing is based upon observations of caregiver-infant interaction, with particular emphasis on a comparison between dyads in which developmentally enhancing manifestations are present and dyads in which interaction is maladaptive.

From such observations, I have discerned a distinct pattern that appears to be emblematic of adaptive caregivers. This pattern involves the caregiver's capacity to be acutely sensitive to imminent developmental changes in the infant. Such sensitivity is converted into a specific kind of behavior whereby the caregiver gradually introduces the infant not only to the manifestations that will be involved in the upcoming developmental achievement but also the caregiver acquaints the infant with an upcoming social milieu helping the infant to better predict changes in the interaction. Such previewing also encourages expectations about how these changes will influence both members of the dyad. For example, a caregiver who anticipates that the infant will soon begin walking, might begin to gently exercise the infant's legs to simulate walking. Similarly, caregivers who intuitively sense the infant's developing manual dexterity will assist the infant in grasping small objects and will begin devising ways to encourage this behavior in the infant. Through such behaviors the caregiver introduces and acquaints the infant to the myriad of implications that the new developmental milestone brings for exerting mastery and control over the environment. Once acquainted with this feeling of mastery, the infant's predictive capacities are stimulated and encouraged.

Another aspect of previewing involves the caregiver's ability to function as an auxiliary partner to the infant while practicing previewing exercises. To this end, the caregiver will be alert to any indications on the part of the infant that the new behavior being previewed could be exhausting for the infant. When the infant exhibits such cues, the adaptive caregiver begins to gradually withdraw from previewing, returning the infant incrementally to the status experienced when the previewing behavior was initiated. Functioning as an empathic partner requires that the caregiver engage in a form of vicarious enthusiasm over the infant's accomplishments. For example, such caregivers will mingle such intuitive manifestations as vocalizations, significant eye contact and appropriate body gestures in order to moderate their previewing interactions. As a result, the infant receives sufficient positive encouragement and comes to perceive that developmental achievement is a pleasurable experience. This realization spurs the infant on to exercise his predictive capacities and maturational skills to their full potential.

A convenient method for identifying those caregivers with a proclivity toward using intuitive behaviors for previewing has been outlined above. One such method involves observing the degree to which the caregiver engages in the catalogue of intuitive behaviors described in this chapter. Another technique involves asking the caregiver to describe her perceptions of the infant's developmental status. Caregivers who possess a tendency to preview adaptively will generally provide a comprehensive and enthusiastic response to this question, because they are so empathically attuned to the nuances of the infant's development. In sharp contrast, maladaptive caregivers will often be unable to describe the infant's developmental status at all. Previewing, then, is a significant caregiver skill that serves as a key indicator for assessing how the caregiver represents the infant and devises appropriate responsive behaviors ranging from the intuitive behaviors discussed earlier in the chapter to the more complex skills of meaning attribution.

Investigative efforts underscoring the caregiver's empathic abilities highlight the importance of assessing the caregiver skill in engaging in previewing exercises with the child. Indeed, it may be argued that the ability to detect the infant's perceptions empathically and to respond appropriately is one aspect of the overall previewing process. Practitioners assessing and treating dyads, therefore, are provided with yet a further reason for ascertaining the degree to which the caregiver is able to predict the infant's responses: such predictive abilities reveal not only the degree to which the caregiver is responding empathically to the infant, but also the degree to which the caregiver is predicting infant needs and responding to these needs in a manner that will foster the infant's own developmental skills and predictive tendencies. In sum, then, during the first year of life the caregiver engages in a series of distinct behavioral manifestations, referred to by some as "intuitive," which serve to enhance developmental skills and to reinforce the degree of interpersonal relatedness that imbues the dyad. Beyond these effects, intuitive behaviors also appear to foster the infant's predictive capacities, underscoring the concept that the interactive domain is a contingent one which may eventually be mastered and controlled. These feelings of mastery extend to the infant's perceptions about his own physiological and psychological developments as well. As the infant's predictive skills become more sophisticated, he will begin expressing his own urges and desires to the caregiver in the form of symbolic behaviors and the caregiver will reciprocate by gradually previewing imminent developmental trends for the infant.

CHAPTER 3

Previewing: A Catalyst for Differentiating Developmental Function

Introduction

Unlike the first two chapters which focused on the way in which the caregiver enhances the infant's development through the use of intuitive behaviors which emerge in the form of previewing, this chapter describes a myriad of developmental skills manifested by the infant during the first two years of life. It is the contention of this chapter that the emergence of these milestones and their corresponding mastery is facilitated by caregiver previewing, the organizing principle which enables the infant to begin predicting upcoming developmental changes and interactional behaviors. Previewing in this context refers to an inexorable process during which all of the behaviors the caregiver manifests spark the emergence and subsequent organization of imminent maturational skills.

While we have already discussed some of the caregiver's contributions to dyadic exchange, our attention now shifts to the other participant in the dyadic relationship, the infant. This chapter raises the issue of whether it is possible to isolate discrete behaviors of the infant which propel development forward. The answer to this question is complex. In some respects, it is relatively easy to catalog infant behaviors because a diverse array of responses has been thoroughly documented by researchers. In other respects, however, the intricacies of infant behavior do not lend themselves to systematic compartmentalization because development sometimes occurs in spurts rather than in evenly spaced sequences, and because certain developmental phenomena tend to surface as discrete events which later proliferate into complex developmental skills. This chapter will strive to describe all of the primary developmental skills the infant manifests that are believed to be essential in the development of predictive capacities.

Although the centerpiece of this chapter is the infant and his evolving developmental capacities, the infant will not be viewed as a creature developing in isolation. Instead, the discussion will rely upon some of the issues raised in earlier chapters. In particular, the role played by the caregiver in previewing development to the infant, as well as the all-encompassing interactional relationship the caregiver establishes with the infant, will be examined. These two phenomena, the relationship itself and the caregiver's predilection to preview imminent development to the infant, serve as primary catalysts to propel the infant in the direction of maturational attainment. As a result of such maturational attainment the infant gradually moves towards mastery over his developmental endowment.

Essentially, the material in this chapter is derived from a compilation of the major infant developmental capacities that emerge during the first years of life. It begins with a discussion of the most primitive sensory responses the infant manifests when the Brazelton Neonatal Assessment is administered and moves on to examine phenomena such as imitation, duetting, social referencing and the infant's differential response to strangers.

Also discussed are such constitutional factors as the infant's temperament, which contributes a distinct quality to the kind of interaction that will transpire within the dyad. As this developmental repertoire was being compiled, however, it became evident that something was missing: a vital component that provides organization to the dyadic interaction was not being described. What was lacking was a description of how the relationship with the caregiver serves to activate the infant's capacities, motivating him to attain ever more sophisticated developmental abilities. In this vein, the way in which the caregiver previews to reinforce the skills the infant already possesses and to encourage the manifestation of new skills is also crucial for understanding how the infant's developmental capacities progress during the first two years of life.

While previous chapters have already explored the dyadic relationship and the capacity to preview from the caregiver's point of view, this chapter strives to elucidate how these interactional phenomena are perceived from the infant's perspective. Although it is one thing to assert that previewing bolsters the infant's developmental capacities by acquainting him with imminent developmental milestones, it is quite another to attempt to describe the way in which the infant experiences the caregiver's urging toward future maturation. In addition, the infant's perspective on the overall relationship with the caregiver is a further aspect of early life that needs to be assessed in order to understand the underlying impetus spurring on the infant's efforts to achieve heightened developmental skill.

In offering insight into these issues, this chapter proposes that the main ingredient supplied to the infant during previewing exercises is the germination of the capacity to *represent* somatic, affective, cognitive and motivational experiences more comprehensively, and in particular, to evolve *representations* about the implications that these developmental achievements will have on future interaction with the caregiver. Representation in this context refers to the infant's capacity to envision sequences of interaction and to maintain these sequences in active memory. As these representational abilities proliferate, the infant begins to evolve elaborate schemas that enable him to better predict his interaction with the caregiver and to better use his current developmental skills in facilitating the interaction. But representational skills serve yet a further function that enhances the infant's imminent maturation and fosters the emergence of new developmental capacities. Since caregiver previewing results in the formation of discrete representational schemas that capture the experiences and sensations of what future development will be like, these schemas can subsequently be used by the infant to recall the memory of previous previewing episodes and to communicate to the caregiver that he wishes to experience new previewing sequences.

These representations also provide the infant with a core of behaviors which he can use in the future either to initiate new previewing sequences or simply to exercise his burgeoning skills. Moreover, representational capacities help the infant to synthesize the repertoire of developmental skills he already possesses, as well as to organize new capacities that have been previewed. In other words, then, through previewing the infant attains a perspective on his overall development and on how diverse categories of skills become inextricably connected, in order to achieve specific adaptational goals.

Developmental capacities manifested by the infant during the first two years of life also serve the diagnostic purpose of enabling the practitioner or other observer to evaluate the degree to which appropriate previewing behaviors are being used in any particular context. This is because certain developmental milestones are known to serve as indicia of the rapport between mother and infant. Indeed, unless the infant and caregiver share an adaptive relationship, it is unlikely the infant will use the caregiver as a model which he can use as a reference for future behavior. Thus, consideration of these developmental phenomena is valuable not only for tracking the infant's maturational course, but also for acquiring insight into the nature of the relationship between caregiver and infant.

The Emergence of Fundamental Representational Skills

Most new parents confirm the findings of researchers that the first few months of life represent a period of remarkable transformation in the infant. Although the infant possesses a fine-tuned capacity to respond to external stimuli during the first few days of life, this sensitivity dramatically proliferates as the infant begins to display a diverse array of other skills.

The developmental capacities of the first few months of life are referred to here as *fundamental representational skills*. This is because each developmental capacity manifested promotes the tendency to develop images of behavioral sequences that can be retained in memory and later used by the infant to assess and assert new manifestations which rely on formerly acquired skills, combinations of formerly acquired skills or combinations of old and new skills. In other words, development here is not to be evaluated as a series of discrete and separate events which may be subjected to objective measurement; instead, each incremental level of maturational achievement nurtures the tendency to use behaviors in a proliferative fashion to further promote the dyadic exchange between mother and infant.

This section then enumerates the fundamental development skills manifested by the infant during the first few months of life and attempts to demonstrate how these skills are promoted by the caregiver through episodes of previewing.

Brazelton's Neonatal Behavioral Assessment Scale (1973) offers perhaps one of the most cogent and systematic tools for understanding the kinds of skills inherent in the neonate. The assessment is generally performed at approximately several days after birth. Among the key findings that can be obtained from this assessment are the presence of the infant's capacity to decrease responses to repeated disturbing stimuli and to virtually shut out disturbance by changing his state of alertness. The Brazelton Assessment, therefore provides insight into the neonates' ability to regulate. For example, a response decrement to an intrusive light, a bell and a pinprick indicate that neonates possess rudimentary capacities for *self-regulation*. This self-regulatory proclivity is also evident when the neonate exhibits the ability to orient to visual and auditory stimuli, as well as when the infant exhibits a self-quieting activity that appears designed to facilitate and ease the transition between states of alertness and quiescence. In addition to these self-regulating responses, the Brazelton Assessment reveals also that neonates possess a repertoire of responsiveness that primes them for interaction with the world. This distinctive responsiveness is observable during periods of alertness when a visual or auditory stimulus is introduced and is also demonstrated by cuddling reactions the neonate displays upon being held. The Brazelton Scale also highlights neonatal responses that fall into the realm of *constitutional* or *temperamental* dimensions. Within this category, we find an identifiable constellation of discrete manifestations which, taken together, qualify the neonate's ability to react. When the infant is excited by a frightening stimulus, for example, he characteristically intensifies motor and crying activity and displays an acute startle response at a rapid rate. The lability of skin color and the facility with which he shifts between states of quiescence and excitement can be also measured. Reactivity can be documented by the neonate's general muscle tone, motor maturity and ability to manipulate his head upon being pulled to sit up.

Although the Brazelton Assessment does not specifically evaluate the infant's temperament, it is necessary to discuss this aspect of infant endowment in this context. This is because temperament is an aspect of the infant's endowment believed to be present at birth. Temperament has been defined as the individual's overall dispositional tendencies and proclivities, those constellations of behaviors that enable researchers to label and individual as being "easy", "difficult" or "slow to warm up." Thomas and Chess, pioneers in temperament research has identified nine temperament dimensions or traits that may be used to evaluate the dispositional status of a given individual. Included among these dimensions are degree of irritability, degree of responsivity, and the individuals proclivity to avoid or withdraw from new stimuli.

In their historic Longitudinal Study which tracked young children longitudinally for over a decade, Thomas and Chess (1986) reported some unusual characteristics associated with temperamental disposition. First, according to these researchers, the infant's temperament can be assessed at an astonishingly early age, since qualities such as irritability and regularity tend to be present and measurable even shortly after birth. Second, the initial characterization of the infant's temperament tends to have statistical reliability in the sense that these traits do not change over time. In this respect, temperament is analogous to a kind of indelible stamp that is imprinted onto the infant's constitution. Third, early temperamental assessments performed during infancy appear to possess a high degree of statistical validity in the sense that a "difficult" attribution during early infancy may predict particular kinds of interactional and behavioral difficulties in later childhood, whereas an individual labeled "easy" will be likely to demonstrate a relatively stable developmental course.

The seemingly irrevocable nature of the infant's temperament has implications for both caregiver previewing and for the infant's own capacity to begin exercising his developmental and predictive skills. If, for example, the infant possesses a difficult temperament, the caregiver may be reluctant to engage in active exchange for fear that the infant will become upset and irritable. A similar situation may exist in the case of a "slow-to-warm-up" infant whose caregiver becomes frustrated by the lethargic response of the infant. Moreover, even if the infant himself possesses an "easy" temperament, if the caregiver's temperament is "difficult" or "slow-to-warm-up", she may have difficulty establishing a reciprocal pattern of interaction with the infant. Failure of the dyad to evolve a mutually rewarding relationship, whereby the cues of each member of the dyad are responded to, can diminish developmental achievement for the infant. Without exposure to a sufficient degree of such previewing, the infant's predictive capacities will not be stimulated and the likelihood that deficits will be created is increased.

The Brazelton Scale discloses that although neonates are, to a certain extent, creatures governed by their natural constitutional endowments, they also possess rudimentary skills in the domains of self-regulation and reactivity, and are, in essence, primed to begin responding to the diverse stimuli of the environment. How then does the infant begin to use the seemingly autonomous qualities of his constitutional endowment to enhance his predictive abilities and eventually master and control the social and physical world around him, as well as the pace of his own developmental transformations?

The answer to this question is complex. As the following studies demonstrate, some of the infant's developmental potential begins to manifest spontaneously, while other skills are best promoted as a result of interaction with the caregiver. For example, Hopkins and van Wulfften Palthe (1985) concluded from their observations of two-month-old infants that autonomous functions are, almost from their first manifestation, coordinated by the infant into an integrated pattern. When presented with an intrusive stimulus, these infants tended to escalate their mobility, heart and respiration rates, knitted their brows, manifested frowns, closed their fists, and exhibited body stiffness and crying. When the aversive stimulus was removed, facial and vocal expressions decreased in reverse order until smiles and other vocal signs of pleasure reasserted themselves. Observation of these responses demonstrated that they were not haphazard and disorganized but instead adhered to an organized pattern.

Brazelton and Yogman (1986) have labeled this capacity for responsiveness during the first months of life as *regulation,* commenting that the infant initially attains homeostatic control over input and output systems by either shutting out or conversely reaching for stimuli. The infant eventually begins to exercise this system of rudimentary control to attend and respond to social cues the caregiver provides by prolonging states of attention to more complex messages from the environment. The emergence of discrete patterns of response to environmental cues or *feedback loops* are another means of explaining how interactive phenomena foster representational mechanisms for predicting upcoming events. Indeed, such feedback loops signify an early form of representation engaged in by the infant. However, it appears that unless the infant is exposed to an adequate degree of stimulation by the caregiver, such feedback loops will either not develop or will be delayed.

Lewis and Feiring (1989) have emphasized that the infant's capacity to attain developmental milestones is also contingent upon certain constitutional qualities and proclivities manifested by the infant early in life. For example, these researchers refer to such infant qualities as irritability, sociability, and pleasure derived from proximal contact with another as being predictive of the ease with which the infant will subsequently attain developmental milestones. These dimensions are reminiscent of the temperament traits identified by Thomas and Chess. It should be emphasized, however, that these researchers also found that the caregiver's behavior during interactive sequences played a seminal role in predicting the degree to which infant development proceeded adaptively. Thus, in designing strategies for introducing the infant to imminent developmental acquisition, a caregiver who is previewing adaptively to the infant will also be aware of the infant's unique temperamental disposition.

When discussing the more advanced forms of regulation that occur from three months onward, Brazelton and Yogman posit that mutually reciprocal feedback loops slowly evolve within the dyad. These loops develop because infants and parents begin to press the limits of the infant's capacity to absorb and respond to information and to withdraw from information for the purpose of recovering homeostasis. The rhythmic nature of adaptive interaction emerges from this description. The caregiver learns to pace her responses to the reactions of the infant so that a sufficient degree of stimulation is provided. For Beebe and Stern (1977) the quality of *engagement/disengagement* represents the infant's capacity to modulate stimulation, particularly when confronted with overstimulation. By four months of age, they report, the infant can regulate his own arousal of environmental stimulation. Using frame-by-frame microanalysis, they studied the infant's visual perception, orientation to the caregiver, and facial expression. Because of the high level of engagement these four-month-olds displayed, Beebe and Stern hypothesized that some composites of early interaction with the caregiver are internalized to form a representation of common behavioral sequences which occurs during dyadic interaction. Because they are recognizable, these sequences help the infant predict the contours of future dyadic interaction. Once again, responsiveness here is intricately tied to the caregiver's interaction with the infant and the degree to which the caregiver strives to supportively elicit differential responses from the infant. By approximately five months of age, the multiplicity of such feedback loops enables the infant to experience a sense of autonomy. Feelings of competence are generated because the infant begins to experience his voluntary control over the environment as he predicts various behaviors and responses. This sense of control over external responses is paralleled by feelings of competence concerning his own maturational skill. Indeed, by this juncture the infant may be able to predict prolonged sequences of interaction with the caregiver.

In addition to signifying a cognitive achievement, Brazelton and Yogman have suggested that the development of feedback loops heralds an emotional maturation as well, because the infant derives a sense of mastery as a consequence of recognizing interactive patterns. Mastery for these authors is associated with an emotional state of well-being. Reissland (1988), Field, Goldstein, Vega-Lahr and Porter (1986), Field, Woodson, Greenburg, and Cohen (1982), and Meltzoff and Moore (1977, 1983 a & b) have identified specific patterns of infant imitation demonstrated by tongue protrusion, mouth opening and emotional expression as early as one hour after birth, suggesting that complex mental representations take place. Mental representations are, therefore, reinforced by a responsive caregiver whose reinforcement propels the infant to perpetuate the interaction.

As the infant develops, however, pure imitative responses appear to decline gradually and are replaced by a new kind of response in which the original imitation sequences are varied or modified in order to create a genuine interactional dialogue. This shift from pure imitation to variations on patterns of imitation suggests that the infant is increasing control and can manipulate and direct internal representations more discretely in order to elicit a predictable response from the caregiver. Early imitation can be more accurately referred to as a *mirroring* reaction during which the infant strives to simply duplicate the caregiver cues. Field (1978) commented that caregivers often imitate their infant's behaviors in an effort to enhance communication and reinforce the interaction, while Piaget (1953) believed that mothers intuitively mimic infant manifestations in order to facilitate the infant's processing of social stimulation. Eventually, however, imitative behavior grows more refined and sophisticated as the infant becomes adept at modifying responses to elicit new signals from the caregiver. At times, the infant appears to experiment with the caregiver, attempting to elicit a varied range of responses designed to identify and communicate his needs. This process is referred to by Kaye and Fogel (1980) and Papousek and Papousek (1987) as *duetting,* and can be seen most clearly during episodes in which members of the dyad take turns in exchanging facial expressions.

Duetting may signify some of the first manifestations of the infant's exercise of his evolving predictive capacities. Kaye and Fogel noted that prior to the advent of duetting at approximately six months of age infant facial expression, though varied, is often random; by six months, a nonvocal dialogue becomes evident as the infant manipulates his own facial behavior to engender a response in the caregiver. At this juncture, then, the infant has come to understand the reciprocal nature of the relationship with the caregiver. Brazelton, Yogman, Als and Tronick (1979) also allude to the phenomenon of duetting in six-month-old infants. They note that the matching or imitation of facial expressions not only indicates the infant's capacity to demonstrate the burgeoning of motor skills, but also suggests that the partners in dyadic interaction are sharing intentionality through affective expression. This is yet another example of how emotional expression serves as the prime vehicle for communication in early infancy. When this form of *emotional synchronization* occurs, the observer characterizes the interaction as reciprocal and harmonious; in contrast, when affective matching is lacking, the interactive sequence assumes a disjointed and dysrhythmic quality. Thus, duetting requires not only infant capacity to modify internal representations, but also a cooperative partner (Tronick and Cohn, 1989).

It should be emphasized that, although duetting indicates the presence of adaptive interaction, it is not observable in all dyads. Papousek and Papousek have occasionally encountered mother-infant pairs in which the caregiver was so talkative and inattentive to infant signals that the resulting communication represented a maternal monologue, with virtually no turn-taking behavior, during which infants fussed or cried. In other instances the caregiver's apathy and failure to respond to the infant precluded infant responsiveness. It is likely that caregiver behavior in these cases interfered with the infant's representational capacities precluding the infant from developing internal patterns of predictable response.

What motivates or propels the infant in the direction of formulating such representations? Trevarthen (1980, 1985) claims that the neonate is born with a readiness to know another human being. This innate proclivity to familiarize oneself with the world is labeled *subjectivity,* while the motivation to communicate with others is referred to as *intersubjectivity.* Such proclivities can be demonstrated during face-to-face exchanges and feeding sequences. Other researchers who have also focused on the rapid unfolding of interactional proclivities that manifest during the first three months of life (Emde, Gaensbauer and Harmon, 1976) have isolated such discrete behaviors as eye contact, cooing and the enhanced frequency for visual scanning.

As such behaviors increase in both quality and quantity, the infant begins to experience a sense of *core-self*. Stern (1985) suggests that the core-self emerges from the infant's capacity to coordinate volition with subsequent motor, verbal and visual outcomes and, as Rovee-Collier and Fagan (1981) note, from the infant's ability to predict the consequences of a given act. It is, then, not merely the external manifestation of coordinated signals that distinguishes infant development during the first three months of life, but also the suggestion that a pattern of representation involving somatic, affective, cognitive, predictive and motivational skills is evolving. Moreover, the role the caregiver plays in encouraging these responses appears to be the vital ingredient catalyzing this form of developmental change.

Further evidence of what is transpiring in the infant's interior landscape during this developmental period has been provided by Legerstee, Pomerleau, Malcuit and Feider (1987), who observed eight infants biweekly from three to twenty-five weeks of age. During observation sequences, infants were studied interacting with the mother, with a female stranger and with a doll. By the age of one to two months, it was observed that the proportion of time that the infants looked, smiled, vocalized, and moved their arms toward people differed significantly from their responses to dolls; similarly, the response to the caregiver was more marked than stranger response. The researchers concluded that this capacity to engage in a differential response indicated that some form of internal mechanism for distinguishing animate and inanimate objects was already in operation. Moreover, the significant role played by the caregiver in promoting and initiating change was highlighted by this study.

In another study, Emde, Kligman, Reich and Wade (1978) devoted their attention to emphasizing the *emotional spectrum* of newborns during the first three months of life. They isolated a trio of emotional responses which were manifested based on appropriate maternal cue. These responses included a hedonic reaction, characterized as encompassing the emotive displays of happy, unhappy, upset and frustrated states; the activation response, described to include startle and excitement states; and the external-internal range of affects which enabled the infant to orient himself to the stimuli of the external world. Within this latter category such manifestations as curiosity, interest and sleepiness were included.

Several other forms of early infant response manifest in the first few months after birth and eventually progress to more complex modes of interaction. *Social referencing* falls into this category and is perhaps the most significant occurrence with respect to the infant's reliance on the caregiver as an interactive partner who catalyzes his development. Social referencing is the active search by the infant for emotional information from the caregiver and the subsequent use of that information to assist in the appraisal of uncertain situations. Klinnert, Campos, Sorce, Emde, and Svejda (1983); Campos and Stenberg, 1981 have traced the origins of social referencing as they emerge during infancy. They have noted that neonates generally don't appear to perceive whole faces. Instead, newborns tend to scan the edges or contours of objects with little tendency to scan the interior of the face. This observation has been confirmed by Haith, Bergman and Moore (1977). However even at this early age, the neonate seems able to discriminate emotional expressions such as happy, sad and surprised (Field et al., 1982). This form of emotional discrimination is the first sign evinced by the infant of socially referencing to the caregiver. During the second stage of social referencing, which occurs between two and five months of age, representations of full faces have developed. By six months the advent of the third stage of social referencing takes place. During this stage the infant's full range of emotional resonance emerges. A clear association between the caregiver's emotional expressiveness and the infant's capacity to visually organize different regions of the face becomes evident.

Walden and Ogan (1988) conducted a comprehensive study of social referencing in forty infants aged six to nine, ten to thirteen and fourteen to twenty-two months of age to investigate how this developmental phenomenon progresses with age and, significantly, how other developmental phenomena contribute to the infant's burgeoning capacity to direct attention to and reference a specific significant other. In this study, social referencing was defined broadly to include the infants' gazes toward parents, their affective expressions and other neuromotor behaviors directed toward parents. An important finding of the study was that the infants' looks at their parents were more selective with increasing age, with older infants preferring not only to look directly at their parent's faces but also to detect their emotional cues. Younger infants, in contrast, displayed minimal preference for facial gazing over looking elsewhere in the vicinity of the parent.

Noticeably younger infants looked most often when parents displayed or expressed positive affect, whereas older infants looked most often when parents evinced fear to a stimulus. Only infants older than fourteen months of age refrained from touching the toy until after referencing the parent. Results indicated that the looking behavior of younger infants may function differently than that of older infants, and significantly, that social referencing involves a number of interrelated skills that develop during the end of the first year and the beginning of the second year of life. Thus, increases in cognitive sophistication and representational abilities along with the growth in social interactions with the caregiver, provide a stronger context for the interpretation of parental behavior. Moreover, the infant's increasing skills in inhibiting, and redirecting his behavior, as well as in regulating his affect, combine to create transformations in the form and function of social referencing during this period. In essence, then, full-fledged social referencing requires the infant's use of the caregiver's expression, gestures and other behaviors in order to predict future interactions with the environment.

Another study examining the contours of social referencing behavior was conducted by Hornik and Gunnar (1988). These researchers observed thirty-two infants, half of whom were thirteen months old and half of whom were eighteen months old. The infants were observed exploring a caged rabbit while their mothers were present. Referencing was operationalized as "looks directed to the mother following a look to the rabbit, accompanied by a quizzical facial or vocal expression." Based upon their initial reaction to the rabbit, the infants were classified manifesting either wary or bold expressions. Wary infants were more likely to reference their mothers when the rabbit was first presented. As the exploration period progressed, however, bold and wary infants referenced equally often. Moreover, although referencing occurred less often than affective sharing, it increased in frequency when the mother was instructed to actively offer information and the infant no longer needed to solicit information by looking at her. Mothers directed both affective and instrumental information to their infants by providing affective information through facial expressions and tone of voice, as well as by emphasizing instrumental information in the semantic content of their vocalizations. The caregiver's expression, then, may signify the first example of how the infant discerns the interaction and then makes predictions about upcoming events and orients his behaviors accordingly. Later, other manifestations of the caregiver, including vocalizations, are further integrated into the infant's referencing scheme.

The adaptive capacity of the infant to integrate associations between external stimuli and a self-generated response, and to organize these perceptions into a coherent internal pattern of representations, appears to stem from a distinct integrative ability. This ability involves the capacity to formulate sequential *expectancies* about the occurrence of particular events in the environment, the capacity to recognize and remember *contingent associations* and the capacity to discern *discrepancies* between an anticipated and the real pattern that ultimately transpires.

Mast, Fagen, Rovee-Collier and Sullivan (1980) investigated how infants acquire expectancies. In their study three-month-olds were pretrained to move crib mobiles containing six to ten objects using foot kicking. After the infants were habituated to the stimulus, the researchers exposed these same infants, as well as a group of controls, to a crib containing two objects. Compared to the controls, the infants who had been pretrained exhibited higher kick rates, their visual attention decreased, and they engaged in negative vocalizations. This behavioral cluster persisted for more than twenty-four hours, indicating that the infants had developed an internal representation of a particular outcome and were distressed at being presented with another outcome that violated their already represented anticipation. Such internal representations may be labeled *expectancies*.

Stern and Gibbon (1978) have noted that by three months of age when the infant can discern temporal sequences an expectation of an anticipated event evolves. For example, as the caregiver repeats various words and phrases, the infant becomes habituated to the rhythms of speech. Once habituation occurs, the infant becomes attuned to deviations of caregiver speech and subsequently habituates to such variations. With time, the caregiver introduces greater and greater amounts of variability and each new pattern becomes gradually internalized by the infant facilitating responses to the environment.

Allen, Walker, Symonds and Marcell (1977) investigated this capacity in a group of infants ranging in age from five to eight months. Two groups of these infant subjects were presented with a standard visual or auditory sequence until habituation was achieved. The infants then were divided into groups in which some subjects were presented with the same sequence while others were exposed to a different sequence. Infants exposed to temporal sequences that were varied from the ones to which they had been habituated displayed significantly more emotive responses than did those infants who were subjected to the same temporal sequence. This finding indicated that infants as young as seven months are capable of perceiving both equivalencies and differences in temporal information. Moreover, this study suggests that infants crave variations of already inculcated expectancies. The stimulation derived from such variations may enable the infant to experiment with internal representational schemes, further enhancing his capacity to predict upcoming events more discretely.

As these studies suggest, the role of the caregiver in fostering expectancy awareness is vital. Not only does the caregiver enable the infant to formulate initial expectancies based upon the stimuli she presents, but she also plays a key role in responding to the pace with which the infant learns information about expected, and hence predictable, sequences of interaction. One distinctive way in which the caregiver stimulates the infant's expectancy awareness is by engaging in previewing behaviors. Previewing operates to expose the infant to a wide variety of experiences that represent future or imminent developmental potential. From such experiences, the infant generates representations about what future maturational skill will be like and about the implications that the new skills will bring into the relationship with the caregiver once these developmental capacities are achieved. As a consequence, previewing facilitates the infant's ability to anticipate not only future development but also the nature of the upcoming relationship with the caregiver.

Contingency awareness is closely related to expectancy awareness as a cognitive developmental achievement. Contingency awareness refers to the capacity of the infant to maintain an interior representation of a stimulus-response association. It has primarily been described as a cognitive capacity, but also incorporates an affective component since the infant experiences pleasure upon being exposed to contingencies. Contingency awareness has been explored by Lewis, Wolan-Sullivan and Brooks-Gunn (1985), who investigated infants at two-and-a-half, four and six months of age. They attempted to habituate the infants to an audiovisual stimulus contingent on arm movement. Measurements were taken of the amount of visual fixation, fussing and smiling. Overall, it was found that at two-and-a-half months the infants did not learn the contingent response and displayed a minimal affective response to the task. Among the four month olds, however, there was evidence of learning both the contingency and an accompanying emotional response: smiling and less fussing manifested at the recognition of the contingent sequence. By six months of age, the contingency task was rapidly learned. Such rapid learning correlated with a full spectrum of emotional display.

Contingent responses on the part of the caregiver can be viewed as behaviors designed to enhance response, to reinforce the infant's predictive capacities and to promote developmental skill. Field (1978) has observed that, if the caregiver's response is appropriate and occurs within a few seconds of the infant's behavior, it is more likely to be perceived by the infant as a direct response to his own behavior. Responsiveness between infant and caregiver also tends to assume a cumulative dimension, as when such infant behaviors as smiling, cooing and eye contact are perceived by caregivers to be contingent responses and stimulate the caregiver to repeat and vary behaviors in order to elicit further response. Pawlby (1977) has identified common caregiver behavior that enhances the infant's contingency awareness and refers to the behavior as "high-lighting," noting that caregivers commonly provide a simultaneous commentary describing behaviors to the infant as they occur. This form of intervention further reinforces the contingent pattern for the infant. Here again, the caregiver's role as a stimulator of the infant's burgeoning skills becomes apparent. As exposure to contingency experiences increases, so too does the infant's ability to predict events. The most contingent experience to which the caregiver can expose the infant is, however, previewing. Through previewing the infant represents in a continuous fashion the notion that manifestations of developmental capacities in their incipient form (stimulus) evoke the behavioral ministrations of the caregiver which help the infant to achieve the full-fledged developmental milestone (response). Once the milestone is fully achieved the interactions with the caregiver and or the environment correspond to what was previously experimented with during the previewing experience.

McCall and Kagan (1970) have charted the appearance of *discrepancy awareness* in infants extensively and have found that as early as seventy two hours after birth a familiar stimulus evoked a stronger response than a novel or discrepant one. A decided shift was observed after three months of age, however, when responses to discrepant events became more pronounced and tended to predominate. Response to a discrepancy was inferred from such behaviors as heightened fixation, increased smiling, vocalization and heart rate.

At what age is the infant capable of coordinating such diverse perceptual dimensions? Lyons-Ruth (1977) investigated this issue in fifteen- to sixteen-week-old infants subjected to audiovisual incongruities. The experimental group was habituated to a sounding object and subsequently introduced to a familiar sound paired with either the familiar or a novel object. A control group was subjected to the same presentation with no auditory component. Infants in the experimental group who were exposed to a mismatched sound and object averted their gaze from the object more frequently and failed to orient to the object more often than when presented with the matched sound and object. Since the control group infants did not display these differences, the researcher concluded that the infant's discrimination of matched and mismatched audiovisual stimuli is compelling evidence that by four months of age infants are capable of constructing bimodal schemata. Bimodal refers here to the capacity to integrate sensory messages emanating from different perceptual domains such as sight and hearing. These findings suggest that infants are attracted to orderly sequences, which can be represented and subsequently recognized as guides in their efforts to elicit new experiences from the caregiver. The infant's development of full-fledged intermodal functioning is described in greater depth in Chapter 4.

All these studies indicate that during the first three months of life numerous capacities evolve in the infant, all of which are designed to heighten the infant's ability to predict upcoming events in the environment. Some of these capacities appear to date from the first days after birth and embody a temperamental dimension, as with the infant's innate tendency to respond to or shut out a stimulus. Other capacities emerge later and ostensibly coordinate several skills derived from an earlier phase of development, as with contingency awareness. The common theme shared by all the phenomena referred to above is that these capacities orient the infant in the direction of enhanced control over the external dyadic interaction and over internal physiological and psychological maturational trends. Moreover, each of these developmental milestones provides continuity of experience as a result of the caregiver's exposing the infant to previewing experiences. Not only do infant capacities for regulation, imitation and social referencing emerge as a consequence of interaction within the dyad, but fluid and supportive interaction initiated by the caregiver serves to stimulate rudimentary skills to differentiate and manifest in more complex forms. Repeated previewing on the part of the caregiver leads to the evolution of feedback loops, which in turn lead to the experience of intersubjectivity. Intersubjectivity is related to the phenomenon of social referencing, whereby the caregiver becomes a pivotal figure to whom the infant orients to obtain perceptual cues. Responses to contingency relationships and discrepant stimuli suggest that the infant by three months of age has schematic representations of the external world that can be used to predict future interaction and to devise infant-initiated behaviors in anticipation of eliciting a particular response.

The acquisition and manifestation of these skills during the first few months of life occurs rapidly and without apparent effort, if a nurturing atmosphere that is filled with sufficient previewing experiences is created by the caregiver. The studies listed above permit us to analyze and segment these burgeoning predictive skills and to chart the contours of developmental trends.

The Consolidation of Representational Skills

Infant development during the first two years of life and well beyond may be said to be designed to enhance interactional skills and predictive abilities, and to provide continuity in the relationship between caregiver and infant. In other words, as a result of maturational advancement, the infant is exposed to increased previewing experiences from which he derives a means of evolving more complex capacities for maintaining and continually arousing interaction between the caregiver and the infant.

The infant is gradually coming to represent his physical and psychological self as being more clearly delineated and existing apart from that of the caregiver. Stranger anxiety, which surfaces at approximately seven months and is evidenced by the infant's distress upon being confronted with a new or different adult, is further evidence that the infant has grown acutely aware of the differentiation between the caregiver and others. Realization of his separate status can, in certain circumstances, be traumatic for the infant. However, the caregiver's adaptive previewing behaviors which provide the infant with the sense of security about the presence of a supportive partner in his developmental experiences tend to assuage any anxiety aroused with the infant's realization of his autonomy. The independent locomotion manifested by the infant at this time is referred to as *practicing,* which Mahler, Pine, and Bergman (1975) suggest signifies the infant's desire to explore the external world, provided the caregiver remains within close range. Practicing also signifies the infant's efforts to experiment with representations, thereby further controlling his ᵻnteractions with the world around him. It is particularly crucial that during this period the caregiver is conceived as a supportive partner to allay the infant's anxiety at the prospect of recognizing his physical separation.

As the infant grows accustomed to notions of an independent body image, he comes to explore his world with a newfound zeal. Explorations of the environment will only occur, however, if the caregiver has continued to adequately preview developmental achievement to the infant, thereby demonstrating that she will remain constantly available to the infant.

The infant's increased experimentation with the stimuli of the external world in the second half of the first year of life has been referred to as the consolidation of the *attachment system.* Bowlby (1982) and Bretherton (1987) describe this phase as one in which exploratory behavior, venturing forth from the safe orbit of the caregiver, and proximity-seeking behavior, returning to the orbit of the mother at a sign of danger, become integrated into a coherent system which motivates the infant's behavior. The key to understanding the attachment system, according to these researchers, is that infant's proclivities are now organized around a particular figure who serves as both a secure base, as well as a source of previewing future experiences.

Infants who lack a constant and consistent caregiving figure to serve as their secure base display extreme distress at seven months of age because they lack a stable representation to aid them in negotiating the anxiety aroused by the realization of being separate and by the prospect of future, and thus uncontrollable, development. As a result, the infant's capacity to predict the future is hindered. Yarrow (1967) observed this phenomenon in infants aged seven to twelve months who were transferred from secure foster homes to new adoptive homes. These infants displayed extreme and enduring distress at the transfer, evidenced by crying, clinging, apathy, eating and sleep disturbances. What is significant about these findings is that no such comparable distress is exhibited by infants who are adopted before six months of age, that is, prior to the consolidation of a relationship with an attachment figure.

Researchers like Bowlby (1980), Main et al. (1985), and Bretherton (1987) contend that the attachment figure exerts such a potent influence over the newborn because the infant has, by the second half of the first year, developed an entrenched and predictable *internal working model* of the relationship to the attachment figure. This internal working model represents a sophisticated coordination of the numerous representational schemes the infant has acquired during early interaction. By the second half of the first year, the infant has constructed a self-sustaining panorama of himself and the attachment figure. Moreover, the infant can use these representations to derive predictions about future development and future interactions, particularly during previewing episodes. As Bell (1970) asserts, the attachment figure has, at this point, acquired the status of a permanent person who is both emotionally supportive of and accessible to the infant.

The caregiver's role, then, has been dramatically transformed. Initially an interactional partner during the first months of life and subsequently a differentiated figure upon whom the infant can rely to help assuage anxiety, the caregiver finally becomes a *permanent object* who is of interest in her own right and who provides the infant with an indispensable source of information about imminent development through previewing. The caregiver is no longer merely a dependable partner whose presence will avert anxiety; the mother now acquires a new dimension. She is an interesting agent and companion for the infant, willing to engage in new forms of symbolic play and spontaneous representation, who serves to orient the infant's predictions about future development and about his own perceptions.

It is significant that the game of peek-a-boo surfaces at approximately this time. From this familiar childhood game one may extract numerous themes. First, the infant is deriving pleasure from a fairly sophisticated interaction with the caregiver that involves manipulation of the object's constancy in the environment. Second, the appearance of the peek-a-boo game suggests that the infant is moving in the direction of symbolic representation. Not only does the infant realize that external objects in the environment can be maintained on a constant internal panorama, but he is also experimenting with the notion that predictable objects and behaviors can be experimented with to derive at new meanings. When the caregiver hides from the infant during peek-a-boo, she is not really hiding but is only pretending in order to evoke the infant's desire to seek her out. By approximately nine months, the infant recognizes and predicts that the mother is only pretending. The disappearance of the caregiver's face from view during game playing, an occurrence that the infant begins to predict after repeated exposure to the game, merely *symbolizes* physical absence.

During the period when representational skills begin to consolidate the infant comes to realize that the caregiver serves as a vehicle for staving off anxiety and for exploring the external world through previewing episodes. This new attitude toward the caregiver is apparent not only in the infant's behavioral manifestations, but also in his emotional response during interaction and particularly during previewing. The quality of this emotional response is so distinctive that Stern (1985) created the label *affect attunement* to describe the emotional contours of interaction at this point.

Stern writes that the realization of subjective experience is rapidly followed by the understanding that attention, intention and affective states can all be *shared* with the caregiver. The infant begins to coordinate his subjective experience with that of the mother. Moreover, the infant's capacity to understand that the caregiver possesses her own intentions and emotions, qualities have been labeled *interintentionality* and *interaffectivity* comes to fruition during this period. A new form of alliance and intimacy is shared with the caregiver by means of affect attunement. No longer are imitation exercises sufficient for the infant; he now strives to approximate and share affective states with the caregiver, during which each member of the dyad will gradually modify and refine the temporal beat, intensity, contour and duration. Affect attunement is beyond true imitation, according to Stern, who notes that a new mood now suffuses the interaction resulting in a sequence of reciprocal behaviors distinctive for their almost orchestrated and rhythmic quality. This rhythm derives from the infant's facility in manipulating his internal representations of contingent behavioral patterns with the caregiver. Moreover, as the infant comes to understand that he can share experiences with the caregiver, so too does he eventually realize that predictions can be shared and that particular maternal behaviors can be elicited if the infant conveys the appropriate signal. Such experience allows the infant to share in a more refined sense of control over his interactions with the environment.

The affect attunement witnessed during approximately the ninth month of life is dependent on two phenomena. The infant's adaptational capacities must have evolved in an adaptive fashion so that initial interactive skills were mastered in the first months of life and the realization of separateness and its attendant implications was negotiated smoothly during the second half of the first year. One factor that will help ally the infant's anxiety during this period is the degree to which the caregiver has contrived to use previewing to convey to the infant that she will be a consistent, supportive interactive partner, despite his burgeoning development. The caregiver must then be a dynamic participant in the infant's progress toward more complex hierarchic adaptation and in particular, must guide the infant as he strives to enhance predictions about future interactions. If, for any reason, the caregiver has failed to evolve into a supportive partner for the infant, evidence of this defect will become accentuated during the ninth month of life when observers look for signs of affect attunement in the dyad. Bretherton and Bates (1979) report that during this time mothers sometimes underattune or overattune to the needs of the infant, falling short of genuine engagement or exaggerating responses to the infant's cues. If done consistently, these researchers report, the infant's ability to evaluate inner states and to respond adaptively may be undermined.

During the period where representational skills begin to consolidate, roughly spanning the third through the ninth month, one of the infant's main achievements lies in coming to terms with the realization of his status of independence from the caregiver. This initial realization provokes episodes of anxiety in the infant, as manifested by distress when confronted with a stranger or when the mother is absent. But assuming that the nurturing environment has been and will remain to be supportive, the infant will not only master his anxiety, but will also use this new realization to begin experimenting with his burgeoning ability to predict future interaction with the caregiver. In particular, previewing experiences will provide the infant with the opportunity to exercise this skill. The mother's separate status may initially be frightening for the infant, but gradually he comes to recognize that his newly discovered sense of differentiation means an entire universe is ready for his exploration and that he is capable of exerting control over his developmental capacities. Not only will he be able to explore this universe on his own, provided that he can return to the caregiver during periods of distress, but he can also engage in intimate interaction with the caregiver during periods of affect attunement which will infinitely expand the horizons of his predictive capacities.

The Effect of Representation on the Quality of Previewing

The period of consolidation represents another convenient classification to describe hierarchic adaptation in early life. As a footnote which will be further developed in a later chapter, interventive strategies designed to enhance infant-caregiver interaction will be more fruitful if they have occurred prior to consolidation, because this developmental period, by its very nature, appears to exert a powerful imprint on future behavior. The following discussion focuses on investigations of phenomena that occur during the consolidation period.

Social referencing, referred to earlier, acquires a new intensity during the period of consolidation. Campos, Hiatt, Ramsey, Henderson and Svejda (1978) discovered that by twelve months of age infants use the caregiver as a signaler who indicates or orients the infant to an appropriate behavioral response and as a figure of trust who will protect the infant from danger during periods of independent exploration. The infant has, at this juncture, transformed the caregiver into a landmark or beacon to assist in orientation as the infant begins to experiment with his own autonomy and manifests behaviors designed to elicit a predictable response from the caregiver.

In their study, Campos et al. investigated the level of confidence and trust with which the infant endowed the caregiver. These researchers created the optical illusion of a cliff existing at the end of the visual field. Infants were placed near the cliff and caregivers were instructed to display two separate forms of response. First, the caregivers were instructed to encourage the infants to move towards the cliff while smiles and other positive emotions were exhibited. They were then told to engage in nonverbal, emotional displays that they felt would inhibit the infant from moving to the cliff. When the caregivers displayed a positive response, virtually all of the infants were willing to negotiate the visual cliff. From this behavior we may infer that the infants used the caregiver response to predict that the visual cliff would be safe based on their referencing of the caregiver. Exhibitions of negativity resulted in infant reticence to move forward, suggesting the infant used the caregiver to orient his behavior. This study is significant because it demonstrates that although infants of one year are capable of engaging in sophisticated autonomous activity, at the same time their reliance on the caregiver to provide a coherent system of signals for predicting what new stimuli will be like is potent. The infant is also using the caregiver here to derive appropriate emotional responses to situations.

Mahler et al. (1975) also recognized these dual characteristics of infant autonomy coupled with dependence during the second year of life and labeled the period spanning from one year to twenty-one months *rapprochement,* during which the infant experiences a revival of separation anxiety reactions that first surfaced at seven months and later abated. The difference between these two versions of separation anxiety may be that the distress the infant experiences upon being confronted with a stranger at seven months represents the shock accompanying the realization of differentiation. The separation anxiety displayed during rapprochement stems from a different source, however. At this point the infant has accepted differentiation and has learned to use an awareness of his separateness in the service of making predictions about the world and achieving more complicated modes of interaction. But with this newfound autonomy comes a parallel realization of reliance on the caregiver as a barometer for testing and experimenting with new skills. If the caregiver is not present to orient and guide the infant in his predictions about the world, autonomy will be thwarted. Nevertheless, autonomy can proceed if the infant relies on the caregiver to help him preview upcoming experience, and an awareness of this reliance evokes strong anxiety in the infant during periods of maternal absence.

Nowhere is the awareness of reliance on the caregiving figure as an aid in predicting experience more evident than during the Strange Situation Paradigm devised by Ainsworth and Wittig (1969). The paradigm is designed to assess attachment patterns within the dyad and involves a sequence of episodes during which infant and caregiver interactions, as well as response to stranger and caregiver absence and reunion, are evaluated. During the paradigm infants of one year of age are permitted to explore various toys in the mother's presence. A stranger then enters, converses with the caregiver and invites the infant to engage in play. The caregiver then leaves for a brief period, returns and leaves again, this time after the stranger has departed so that the infant is entirely alone. Finally, the stranger returns and then the mother returns. Ainsworth and Wittig observed that reunion behavior following these sequences was particularly noteworthy in that distinctive patterns emerged.

Three identifiable patterns were documented. The first involved infants labeled as *securely attached*. These infants characteristically cried or evinced other forms of distress at separation from the caregiver. Upon the caregiver's return, the infants rapidly gravitated to her and expressed a desire to be comforted. A second category of infants, whom the researchers labeled as *insecurely attached-avoidant*, demonstrated no distress upon maternal separation and at maternal reunion characteristically snubbed or avoided the caregiver. A third category of infants displayed distress upon separation, but were angry or resistant when the caregiver returned. These babies were also labeled as *insecurely attached-resistant*.

Ainsworth and Wittig interpreted their data as indicating the developmental status of the attachment relationship by the end of the first year of life and report that patterns observed during the Strange Situation could be predicted by observing early patterns of feeding competence, face-to-face interaction and close bodily contact between the dyadic members. Infants who displayed a secure response during the Strange Situation characteristically had experienced gratifying and harmonious feeding sequences, fluid face-to-face interaction, heightened response to their emotional displays and an appropriate amount of intimate body contact. These infants, in other words, had learned to rely upon the caregiver as an aid in predicting experience. Infants who displayed an insecure response in the Strange Situation paradigm came from dyads in which the pacing of interaction was frequently less contingent, where affectionate body contact was minimal and where response to the infant during the first three months of life was muted. The infant's predictive abilities in this case were less developed.

The Strange Situation is valuable not only because it enables researchers to assess the attachment relationship and to derive inferences about previous levels of the dyadic interaction, but also because it reveals the intensity of the infant-caregiver relationship in cases where development has progressed in the direction of hierarchic adaptation and it suggests the degree to which the infant has come to rely on the caregiver in assisting him in predicting experience.

Paralleling the entrenchment of the attachment relationship during the consolidation period is the infant's evolving sense of *self-awareness*. Bertenthal and Fischer (1978) explored this facet of development in a series of investigations involving infants ranging from six months to two years. Infants were placed in front of a mirror and various manipulations were performed that involved the infant's capacity to differentiate between the mirror image of himself and the images of other objects. Based on their investigations, the researchers were able to observe how self-recognition evolves over time, emerging as a fairly coherent concept by approximately the end of the first year of life.

Among the most fascinating phenomena that occur during the period of consolidation is the integration of previously acquired skills into more sophisticated forms of interaction. Rutter and Durkin (1987) examined two types of skill—infant gaze and vocalization—consolidated during later infancy to accomplish such developmental landmarks as coherent speech and conversation. They studied dyads in which infants ranged in age from nine to twenty-four months. Two questions were posed for investigation at the beginning of the study. First, the researchers sought to determine when infants begin to play an active role in coordinating interactions with the caregiver. Investigation then focused on when infants begin to use gaze behavior to signal that they have completed their vocalization and to indicate attentiveness when the other person is speaking.

With respect to the first question, it was found that the majority of vocal exchanges between infant and caregiver occurred without interruption. At twenty four months of age, however, the level of infant interruptions diminished as they began to coordinate vocal response with the verbalizations, suggesting the emergence of predictive patterns of speech. In response to the second question, it was discovered that infant gaze behavior begins to resemble adult patterns somewhat earlier than does vocalization. It was determined that the most common time for gazing at the caregiver was during vocalization, a finding that remained constant throughout infancy. Such behavior on the part of adults is generally regarded as a signal of attention and the researchers reported that, at least in this respect, twelve-month-old infants behave like adults. As time progressed, the infants increased the number of looks they displayed when they finished vocalizing, which the researchers interpreted as similar to the "terminal look" adult speakers use to indicate that they are finished speaking and are ready to listen. This pattern became entrenched by the end of the second year, with the researchers reporting that by that time children were patterning their gazes in a replication of adult behavior. This discernible pattern suggests that in learning to speak, the infant must rely upon the caregiver to provide vocal cues which the infant eventually learns to predict and respond to. Thus, the pattern of reliance on the caregiver continues.

Conclusion

The diverse array of developmental skills manifested by the infant during the first year of life are outlined above. Findings of the above studies confirm that while development occurs gradually and incrementally, a distinct pattern characterizes the second year of infancy. By that point, the attachment system that has evolved during the first year of life becomes palable in the infant. The infant continues to rely upon the caregiver as a guide, enhancing his ability to predict upcoming experiences and to refine his predictions about what new stimuli will be like. Social referencing is one skill the infant uses to enhance and reinforce the appropriateness of his predictive responses. The caregiver's physical separation from the infant is fully acknowledged, but at the same time, the infant has transformed his global partner into an integral object who serves to predict discrete outcomes for his increasingly independent behavior. The caregiver attains heightened significance and the infant's perception of himself dramatically alters during this period. A full-fledged self-awareness now becomes apparent and the infant begins to experiment with internal representations with newfound zeal, deriving predictable variations and using the caregiver's response to confirm these predictions. Assuming consistent support of the infant's development to this point, the newly formed alliance between the caregiver and the self of the infant will evolve rapidly as the infant's personality fully unfolds. The infant is now capable of sustaining a stable and resilient representation of himself, of the other and of himself interacting with the other. Moreover, the ultimate achievement of this period remains the infant's capacity to predict upcoming development skills, to exert control over his burgeoning development, and to use the caregiver as a supportive guide to help him achieve these anticipated goals.

CHAPTER 4

Previewing: A Catalyst for Coordinating Developmental Functions

Introduction

Foremost among the questions confronting developmental theorists is the issue of how the infant perceives the stimuli impinging upon him from the external world and how this seemingly incomprehensible panoramic swirl of visual, auditory, and tactile imagery comes to be organized in a meaningful fashion. One way of probing this issue is to begin with information that is known about the neonate's developmental capabilities. It is known, for example, that even neonates just a few minutes old possess a degree of sensory awareness that acquaints them with the external environment. Various physiological tests have verified visual, auditory, and tactile awareness and sensitivity that is surprisingly acute, and such measures as the the Brazelton Neonatal Assessment have confirmed that indeed newborns are relating to the world with an impressive sensory apparatus. Nevertheless, it is still necessary to explain the process whereby the neonate's incipient perceptual skills mature to the point of enabling him to decipher the external environment in a sophisticated manner.

One of the most striking characteristics of the infant's developmental potential that has been reported in recent years concerns *multimodal perception,* a phenomenon which will be discussed in this chapter. Multimodal perception refers to the infant's capacity to coordinate input from a variety of perceptual domains in order to integrate comprehensive representations about objects and events. Thus, multimodal abilities allow the infant to discern that the particular color of a toy (a visual characteristic) and the sound emitted by the toy (an auditory characteristic) are somehow united such that both qualities combined constitute the identifiable features of the object. Similarly, it is through multimodal integration that the infant becomes familiar with the caregiver, who is perceived as having distinct features, a unique sound, and a characteristic smell. Such integration enables the infant to perceive and identify an object via one perceptual system even if the previous experience with the object was obtained through a different perceptual system. This capacity has been referred to as *multimodal transfer* and the actual recognition of the object—despite the perceptual system in which it is conveyed—is known as *multimodal matching*

Both multimodal transfer and multimodal matching necessitate that the experience perceived, regardless of the perceptual system in which it occurs, be equivalent to the experience in another perceptual mode, even if only on a symbolic level. There are two general theories concerning how this equivalence evolves, as will be discussed in this chapter. The first theory postulates that perceptions from different systems (i.e., visual, auditory, tactile) can only be related through experience, and that perceptual development is dependent upon other kinds of cognitive and affective maturation, such as the evolution of sophisticated memory sequences. According to this theory, perceptual equivalences must be achieved by the imposition of a mediation process that connects at least two sensory modalities and bridges the gap between them in some fashion. Visual and language perception have been suggested as two such mediators. For example, when using visual perception, the infant comes to understand that the visual features of an object are associated with the linguistic sounds emitted by the object because some form of mediating link has been forged between them. Nevertheless, this theory does not explain how infants who have not yet developed such capacities (e.g., the use of language) are capable of displaying multimodal awareness of the qualities of objects and significant others in their environment.

Thus, while the theory of equivalences in perceptual domains has some validity, we should also consider other hypotheses for explaining the phenomenon of multimodality as it relates to the development of perceptual integration. Another group of researchers has postulated that perceptual equivalences exist because different perceptual systems detect invariant qualities which serve as markers for identifying the same objects and events. Under this theory, there is no need for a *transfer* to occur between different perceptual modalities, since the individual already perceives the same object in both modalities simultaneously. This theory implies that the infant is equipped to cognitively extract abstract information from fairly specific types of stimulation. Such extraction abilities suggest the capacity of the infant to represent phenomena in several perceptual domains simultaneously and to experiment with variations of internal representations. As one example, researchers have found that infants demonstrate the capacity to transfer from tactile experience with an object to visual images of the object, despite the fact that the object may be new to them.

However, both of these theories (the notion that the infant gradually integrates perceptual information and the notion that the infant perceives sensory information simultaneously and gradually refines this information) appear to suffer from the same flaw: the infant's developmental capacities are viewed in isolation, as if maturation occurs outside the context of interaction with the caregiver. Although most infants will develop and eventually manifest these multimodal skills regardless of the nurturing atmosphere to which they are exposed, infants who share an optimal relationship with a supportive caregiver appear to develop this skill more rapidly and to exercise it more frequently. Moreover, previewing exercises initiated by the caregiver appear to play a particularly important role in fostering the infant's capacity to comprehend the environment in a multimodal fashion.

The issue, then, is how previewing interactions exhibited by the caregiver foster the emergence of the infant's perceptual capacities. As discussed in earlier chapters, previewing serves to acquaint the infant with imminent development by introducing behavioral manifestations that represent a consolidation of the incipient behaviors that the infant has already begun to express. While the process of previewing has previously been described, what will be highlighted in this chapter is the manner in which previewing fosters multimodal perceptual abilities. As important as the fact that previewing introduces the infant to imminent developmental trends is the fact that previewing takes place with a supportive caregiver who is attuned to the infant and who only previews skills that he is developmentally capable of sustaining and integrating.

As a result, a sensitive caregiver uses previewing to familiarize the infant not only with specific developmental trends, but also to provide him with insight into how to relate to a supportive "other." Moreover, previewing heightens the infant's awareness of the "other," because the infant comes to realize that he cannot coordinate certain skills on his own, rather, he must rely on the caregiver to guide him. As a result, previewing represents one way in which the infant comes to represent the notion of a supportive "other" who will guide his realization of *differentiation* and *autonomy,* both *between* himself and the external world, as well as *within* himself.

Some researchers have noted that the infant's initial recognition of this sense of differentiation and autonomy may be potentially traumatic. Such trauma is understandable from the infant's perspective. He is essentially confronted with the developmental events progressing in his own body, events which may often appear uncontrollable and unmanageable. If, however, the caregiver is present to guide the manifestation of these events and channel them in the direction of optimal skill through previewing behaviors, the infant's sense of helplessness about the inexorable pace of development will be assuaged. In this fashion, then, previewing performs two indispensible functions. First, previewing manifestations serve to alert the infant to the phenomenon of the "other" who possesses individual perceptions of the world and of the differentiated status of the infant; second, the shock or trauma that may attend an awareness of differentiation is eased, because the caregiver conveys to the infant through soothing gestures that she will help him regulate and control both the diverse perceptual phenomena and his burgeoning maturational capacities.

In essence, then, previewing behaviors foster and enhance more previewing behaviors. This is because once the infant is convinced of the benefits to be derived from previewing, he is motivated to perpetuate the relationship with the caregiver in order to experience further mastery and control over his emerging perceptual skills. The relationship with the caregiver thus becomes a prominent factor in the infant's life. Because of this, he will strive to enhance his ability to communicate and share with the caregiver; in turn, she will continue to guide his efforts towards self-regulation.

One way in which the infant enhances his communication with the caregiver is to develop better skills for conveying his awareness of and desire for stimulation. The infant strives, in other words, to convey his needs to the caregiver using the most elaborate capacities at his disposal. One of these capacities, the ability to represent, has been stimulated by repeated exposure to previewing on the part of the caregiver. When the caregiver previews imminent development adaptively to the infant, she coordinates a variety of perceptual messages in each previewing episode. Assume, for example, that the caregiver is previewing grasping behavior to the infant. She will touch and hold the infant's hand in a particular manner; she will often speak encouraging words to the infant as the previewing behavior is being performed and she will demonstrate the behavior in the infant's direct line of vision, so that he can observe what is taking place. Because the caregiver uses previewing episodes as an opportunity to integrate a diverse array of perceptions from different modalities into a single experience, the infant's representation of such episodes will also incorporate these different perceptions and actions into one unified experience.

Moreover, as the infant's representations accumulate, he will become aware of the fact that during interaction with the caregiver equivalent messages from different perceptual domains will be used to convey a similar or even identical message. For example, the caregiver's encouraging vocalizations communicate a message equivalent to the infant's visual image of his hand reaching for an object or the feeling aroused by the caregiver's touch as she guides the infant's gesture. And with each new previewing experience the infant will strive to discern the visual, auditory, gustatory and tactile input that is associated with the experience.

In this manner, previewing functions to enhance the infant's ability to represent experience in a multimodal fashion which integrates his diverse perceptual abilities. Moreover, as the infant's perceptual skills become more sophisticated, he will derive greater pleasure from previewing episodes, because he will experience the mastery derived from such episodes more comprehensively. As mastery is enhanced so, too, is the infant's motivation to engage in further experiences to heighten his perceptual awareness and devise even more complex ways of communicating his needs to the caregiver. The infant's multimodal perceptual abilities thus serve to both enhance the experience of previewing and to motivate the emergence of more complex functions that will facilitate the infant's experience of previewing.

Beyond notions of how multimodal capacities operate in young infants, an equally significant issue involves how these abilities evolve along the developmental spectrum. For example, some researchers believe that the infant's perceptual systems are initially *independent and unconnected* at birth, and that only after being exposed to numerous divergent experiences does coordination of these perceptual realms occur. Piaget (1952) is a prominent proponent of the view that the infant's different perceptual abilities have a discrete nature. Under this hypothesis, the infant devises separate representational schemas for each perceptual dimension (seeing, touching, smelling, tasting and hearing) and only after repeated exposure to environmental stimuli are these schemas eventually coordinated in a fashion that facilitates intermodal assimilation. Such coordination is thought to evolve in the following fashion: during the first weeks of life, the infant perceives equivalences of the object; within a few months, the infant begins to reliably understand that the tactile dimensions of an object are associated with the visual image of the object. Thus, those properties of the object which are modality specific are gradually merged to create the object's identity.

Other researchers, however, posit an *initial unity of perceptual capacities*. These researchers suggest that the neonate is equipped with an undifferentiated system of perception, so that he is oblivious to whether he is seeing, hearing, tasting, touching or smelling an object. Instead, the infant merely responds to the object in a kind of global and diffuse fashion, perceiving the object in several dimensions "simultaneously". As a result, the process of development essentially becomes one of *sensory differentiation and refinement*. Thus, certain phenomenal aspects of stimulation are initially perceived, regardless of modality, not because particular qualities of the object are extracted, but because the modalities themselves are not differentiated into separate domains.

It is virtually impossible to say with any degree of certainty whether development conforms to Piaget's view, that multimodal perception is largely a process of the coordination and regulation of different perceptual domains which begin independently and then converge or whether the views posited by Bower (1974), which rely on the gradual differentiation of function, are more accurate. In either case, researchers acknowledge that the neonate's perceptual capacities appear somewhat limited, and yet, by the time the infant is several months old, remarkable changes are apparent in the area of perceptual integration. As noted above, however, whichever theory is accurate, it is likely that previewing behaviors on the part of the caregiver serve to stimulate the degree to which the infant is able to integrate the multimodal perceptions attached to objects and to interaction. To clarify whether these changes are the product of the unfolding of the infant's *coordinating* capacities or whether these alterations reflect the infant's burgeoning abilities in the area of *differentiation* will be accomplished by future research. What is relevant, however, is that an internal *regulatory mechanism* seems to be operating that propels the infant in the direction of making more acute and distinct recognitions of the stimuli that surround him. The caregiver who responds to the infant's needs through the previewing of imminent development is encouraging the maturation of these regulatory skills in the direction of multimodal integration.

This chapter is devoted to exploring the intricacies of the infant's perceptual mechanism and to underscoring the seminal role it plays in the infant's development. Indeed, it may be argued that until the infant's capacities become more sophisticated in the area of multimodal perception, full communication with the external world, and ultimately, with the incipient self, will not be possible. This is because intermodal capacities are required for experiencing the full import of previewing exercises, of converting such experiences into representations and of using these representations to predict upcoming development.

Although it appears that the evolution of multimodal functioning is a normative aspect of development which occurs in virtually all infants, this chapter will ask and try to answer whether and to what extent the previewing skills of the caregiver contribute to the emergence of these abilities. Moreover, the way in which multimodal functioning impacts upon other developmental skills will also be explored. For example, how does the ability to perceive the various perceptual qualities of a stimulus supplement the infant's skill in acquiring awareness about his interactions with the animate and inanimate world for discerning predictable representational and interactive patterns? Each of these developmental acquisitions will be crucial as the caregiver guides the infant in the direction of autonomous functioning. Such functioning ultimately depends upon the capacity of the infant to make reliable predictions about the internal or external environments with which he continually interacts.

Moreover, developmental progress depends not only on the skill of anticipating or predicting upcoming events, but also on the related ability to develop strategies for dealing most effectively with these events. I have assumed the position that the infant can only predict future events and experiences if previous interactions have allowed him to experience similar or related phenomena, particularly during previewing exercises with the caregiver. As a consequence, the infant's developmental progress may rest on the representations he formulates during previewing episodes. Such representations permit the infant to regulate stimuli impinging on various perceptual domains, and then to formulate a coherent impression of the multimodal dimensions of the stimuli and of the interpersonal interaction with the caregiver. It is the contention of this chapter that previewing episodes tend to motivate the infant to coordinate experiences of even greater multimodal complexity until a sophisticated understanding of the external world and of internal developmental phenomena is attained.

The Development of Multimodal Integration

Although it appears that multimodal perception is an aspect of the infant's constitutional endowment, there is no doubt that the behavior of the caregiver contributes to the ease with which these this skill emerges in its full-fledged form (Bushell, 1981). In substantiation of this view, studies suggest that caregivers who are maladaptive or absent, as in the case of institutionalized infants, exert a deleterious effect on the evolution of the infant's multimodal capacities, often hindering the emergence of representational capacities and delaying the infant's ability to enjoy multimodal integration.

One study that investigated the effect of the caregiver's behaviors on the infant's subsequent development of multimodal capabilities was performed by Messer and Vietze (1988). These researchers studied forty-nine mother-infant pairs while the infants were ten weeks, twenty-six weeks and fifty-four weeks old respectively. Messer and Vietze reexamined earlier findings that indicated that the partner's gaze affects the likelihood of a mother or infant initiating or terminating direct eye contact. In reexamining this finding, the researchers discovered that dyadic gaze patterns do indicate intentionality and do not occur randomly or by chance. Nevertheless, it was not clear from the study whether gaze patterns emerged as result of the synchrony of the interpersonal interactions or rather, whether such patterns emerged because of individual organizational patterns. In either case, however, the ability of these young infants to visually coordinate and orient to the mother separate objects was definitely implied.

Messer and Vietze noted that the prime implication of their research was that earlier evaluations may have overestimated the influence of the partner in the initiation and termination of dyadic gazes and that caregiver-infant social gaze patterns may not be orchestrated in a fashion that promotes mutual gazing behavior. The researchers also commented that Stern's (1974) earlier findings of fairly distinct patterns of caregiver-infant gaze patterns may offer several insights. According to Stern, caregiver gaze patterns suggest that the infant is intentionally responding to the caregiver or, as Hayes and Elliott (1979) reported, the ostensibly integrated gaze behavior observed during dyadic interaction may reflect an independent arrangement of the frequency and duration of visual overlaps between caregiver and infant. Nevertheless, the correlations between the gazing patterns of the infants and mothers were far greater than would appear randomly or by chance, indicating that some form of perceptual skill and subsequent regulatory behavior inherent to the infant was at work during sequences of interaction. Thus, the infant may possess an innate capacity to gaze in the direction of the caregiver and the caregiver who engages in gaze behaviors may stimulate the infant's manifestation of this perceptual skill.

Other studies have demonstrated more precise patterns between caregiver cues and infant multimodal response as it occurs in the dyadic exchange. Kurzweil (1988), for example, was able to determine a specific difference between one-month-olds and three-month-olds in their capacity to "recognize" the caregiver based on cues that were emitted in a variety of divergent sensory domains, including the visual (face-to-face observations), the auditory (caregiver's speaking voice), and the tactile (touching) realms. This study demonstrated that even very young infants can associate and integrate different perceptual qualities of the same object.

According to Kurzweil, it has long been known that by three months of age an observable and characteristic form of recognition occurs in the infant that is detectable from facial expression, psychomotor gestures and affective displays. Recognition of the mother's voice and smell have each been found to exist to a certain degree in newborns (DeCasper and Fifer, 1980; Cernock and Porter, 1985). However, based on the findings of Haith, Bergman and Moore (1977) and Field, Cohen, Garcia and Greenberg (1984), facial recognition does not appear to emerge until three months of age. Facial recognition was detected in these studies by differences in visual fixation time when infants were shown reflections of a caregiver and stranger face, and by differential looking at the mother.

Researchers preceding Kurzweil have examined the complex operations of perceptual skill in the infant and have suggested that multimodal functions operate in an integrated fashion. After all, as noted in previous chapters, most of the hypotheses of the infant's early experience with the caregiver rely on visual exchange (face-to-face interaction); auditory exchange (vocalizations); tactile exchange (holding); and gustatory exchange (feeding behavior). Kurzweil's study contributes the notion that the coordination of these responses and hence, the emergence of multimodal perception, relies predominantly on typical mother-infant interactions involving several stimuli simultaneously. The question posed by this research was whether interactive sequences with a three-month-old infant would signal recognition of the caregiver. The experimental design included interactive sequences with the caregiver and encompassed a diverse array of stimuli (i.e., several interactive partners), multisensory stimuli involving face, voice, and physical handling simultaneously, and varying interaction conditions, including quiet and other more lively states. The infant's recognition was inferred from "multiple differential" responses (duration of gaze fixation, the length of time spent fixating visually and blinking) rather than from responses based on "simple discrimination," which only requires that the perception and discrimination of one stimulus be different.

Kurzweil's study involved a group of twenty-four infants of three different ages: two to three days, twenty-one to twenty-five days and twelve to fourteen weeks. The stimuli involved were the infant's mother and two female strangers, all of whom engaged in two types of brief, multisensory interactions with the infant, including a quiet, horizontal lull characterized by soothing vocalizations and touching. All interactions incorporated visual, auditory, tactile and kinesthetic qualities. Interactions were videotaped and then scored, with particular attention paid to the coordination of multimodal skills.

Kurzweil reported that by three months, infants demonstrated differential visual responses to mother and strangers, regardless of the multiple senses, stimuli, and conditions to which they were simultaneously exposed. These results occurred without a preliminary familiarization period and, according to the researcher, suggested that by the third month of life, a familiar caregiver can be recognized despite exposure to a variety of other sensory stimuli. Thus, it appears that infants are capable of perceiving a distinct visual stimulus, representing it on the stage of active consciousness, and recalling it from memory. Such infants may also be capable of recognizing the other perceptual qualities associated with their mothers or strangers.

This study implicates some of the hypotheses mentioned in the introduction of this chapter that dealt with the etiology of the infant's multimodal functioning capacities. As seen in the Kurzweil study, three months of age appears to signify a kind of demarcation period, at which point the infant's sensory perceptions are honed to a fairly sophisticated degree. The infant is no longer confused when bombarded with stimuli that impinge on different perceptual capacities simultaneously. Instead, by three months the infant can *coordinate* and *regulate* his attention span so that information that is stimulating a variety of sensory modes can be absorbed and integrated without confusion. The infant may be stroked, spoken to and held face-to-face, and it is likely that each of these perceptual domains will not only receive information, but will also coordinate the information to create an integrated, coherent representation that is capable of being retrieved at a later time. As noted earlier, it is not relevant to detect precisely whether this multimodal functioning capacity emerges as a result of a process of differentiation from a unified perceptual domain (Bower, 1974) or whether discrete sensory skills are gradually coordinated (Piaget and Inhelder, 1956). Rather, what is significant is that a dramatic change occurs by three months of age, enabling the infant to perceive phenomena multimodally and to respond in a fashion that indicates an awareness of the multimodal nature of experience.

This distinct change in the infant's functioning by the third month has several ramifications. First and foremost, it demonstrates that caregiver response during the first three months of life may be especially crucial to spark this form of multimodal development. The infant whose mother experiences postpartum mood disorders, then, may be especially deprived of experiencing the multidimensionality of sensory experience, as may the premature infant who is separated from the caregiver for long periods in the hospital (Trad, 1986, 1987). Second, these findings indicate that early intervention in the case of high-risk mothers may be warranted in order that the infant receives optimal stimulation during this peak period of the first three months of life to assure that intermodal functioning will emerge adaptively. Third, and perhaps most significant, these findings suggest that the infant has begun to organize perceptions and use them to generate representations, which in turn, can be relied upon to derive predictions about the world, and to exhibit behaviors designed to elicit a particular response from the caregiver.

Kurzweil's findings gain further credibility from the work of Lawson (1980), who investigated the spatial and temporal overlaps in audiovisual integration in infants, and the work of Bahrick and Pickens (1988) who attempted to discern whether five-month-old infants were capable of discriminating between the English and Spanish language.

The Lawson study provides compelling evidence that by six months of age the infant has developed a flexible ability to regulate phenomena that are experienced in the visual and auditory domains. Lawson reported that familiarization with an object that moved in synchrony with a periodic sound emanating from it resulted in the infants looking more at the familiar object than at a novel object, suggesting a visual-auditory association. According to Lawson, such findings indicate that six-month-old infants appropriately watch an object and sound from their previous experience that has been spatially congruent and has exhibited a synchronous pattern. The association of auditory and visual components as characteristics of a common object most likely requires an awareness of spatial congruity. Lawson commented that the results of the study point to the fact that by six months the infant can learn to understand an association between two formerly independent characteristics of a stimulus. This finding is significant because it suggests that the infant is not only responding in a multimodal fashion to the caregiver, but is capable of using this skill in relation to other objects in the environment as well.

In addition, Lawson's findings indicate that by this age infants are beginning to recognize *contingencies* in their environment. This phenomena and its significance for the infant's overall development cannot be underscored enough. Contingency awareness, reported by Watson (1966, 1972) and Watson and Ramey (1972), signifies the advent of the infant's capacity to connect two discrete events that have been patterned in a cause-effect sequence. An infant's cry and the subsequent appearance of the caregiver is one such cause-effect relationship. Thus, when the infant intentionally cries in order to evoke the presence of the mother, the infant is predicting that a contingent response will occur and is attempting to elicit that response.

Although on the surface the exhibition of contingency awareness may seem facile, it is important to realize that the process whereby the infant achieves this capacity is extraordinarily complex. First, as a skill that is precursory to contingency awareness, the infant must be able to perceive the characteristics of a single object or stimulus, and be able to perceptually integrate the object's diverse qualities. Next, the infant must be able to forge a temporal connection between stimuli. This requires capacities in the area of memory, expectation, differentiation, and, pertinent to this discussion, the ability to regulate intermodally the qualities of such stimuli. Hence, intermodal perception is a fundamental prerequisite for the infant's developing capacity for contingency awareness and for his using these contingencies to devise predictable sequences to explain and eventually control the world around him.

Indeed, the infant's manifestation of contingency awareness suggests not only that the infant is capable of discerning the multimodal qualities of stimuli external to himself, but also that the infant has some recognition of his own multimodal capacities as an initiator of action and a communicator of messages. For example, in the illustration referred to above, the infant uses his voice, in the form of a cry, to signal to the caregiver that he wishes to receive milk. The sensation of being fed may be characterized as integrating tactile, taste and smell perceptions. Thus, from this classic example, often used to demonstrate the infant's initial awareness and recognition of contingency phenomena, we can see how several dimensions of perception gradually become integrated.

Even more significant, this example reveals that the infant is coming to recognize that he can communicate to the world and evoke particular responses based on the different perceptual signals he emits. Eventually, a cry may be substituted for looking at the caregiver in a particular way or touching a particular object. What is of relevance here is that through the gradual repetition of such behaviors the infant becomes cognizant of his capacities in multimodal domains. Hunger may be communicated with a cry, a gesture or a look, or the infant may choose to integrate all three of these signals. In addition, the infant has come to recognize both that he himself possesses these diverse perceptual abilities and that multimodal functioning can be controlled and regulated in a manner designed to manipulate objects and persons in the environment.

The vital role played by contingency awareness in fostering the development of the infant's multimodal capacities also suggests why attuned caregivers may be so sensitive to exposing their infants to contingency experiences. As a result of such exposure, the infant practices his ability to understand and experiment with multimodal skills. In turn, the more the infant displays multimodal abilities, the more motivated the caregiver is to devise previewing behaviors designed to further elicit multimodal capacities. Previewing behaviors, which are designed to acquaint the infant with imminent development, also represent a form of contingency over which the infant has some degree of control. By manifesting particular cues to the caregiver, the infant conveys that he wishes to be exposed to particular behaviors at a given time. As a consequence, contingency awareness, a major developmental milestone achieved within the first three months of life, serves several significant functions in enhancing the infant's developmental skill. First since the stimulus-response sequence of the contingency episode often involves different types of perceptual signals (e.g., receiving a toy is contingent upon hearing a bell), the infant is challenged to begin representing interpersonal experiences in a multimodal fashion. Second, the infant is often a participant in the contingency experience, as when the infant emits a cry (stimulus) with the expectation of receiving milk (response). Thus, contingency awareness often requires the infant to actively partipate in the integration of different perceptual domains. Finally, previewing may be viewed as a form of contingency experience which further heightens the infant's sensitivity to the multimodal nature of experience.

The Bahrick and Pickens study referred to earlier investigated the capacities of five-month-old infants to respond to the bimodal dimensions of human speech. The researchers commented that young infants are adept at discriminating a wide variety of speech sounds, including consonants, vowels, single syllables and disyllables. For example, Kuhl and Meltzoff (1982, 1984) reported that four-month-old infants detected invariant relations uniting the spectral information contained in a vowel sound with the articulatory movements of the mouth when voice-lip synchrony was controlled. This finding led Kuhl and Meltzoff to hypothesize that speech is initially represented intermodally by infants, in a fashion that integrates visual and auditory perceptions. In turn, Kuhl and Meltzoff's conclusion has been confirmed by MacKain, Studdert-Kennedy, Spieker and Stern (1983) who found evidence of this ability in five- to six-month-olds, and Dodd (1979) and Walker (1982), who reported that infants of this age are able to match the sight of parent's face with the sound of the parent's voice during speech presentations.

Bahrick and Pickens reported that their research focused on a distinct aspect of the infant's perception of speech—the ability to discriminate and classify bimodal speech passages on the basis of language membership. Subjects included forty-eight five-month-old infants. Twenty-six of the infants came from homes where only English was spoken, and twenty-two infants came from bilingual homes where both English and Spanish were spoken. The procedure involved videotaped displays made of a woman reciting two different passages, one in English and one in Spanish. The displays portrayed a close-up image of the woman's face as she continuously recited the passage.

The researchers analyzed their findings and concluded that five-month-old infants could indeed discriminate and classify bimodal speech passages on the basis of language membership. This phenomenon was particularly evident when the infant was exposed to a new passage in a new language, although not when the infant was introduced to the new passage in the old, familiarized language. Bahrick and Pickens noted that this finding supported the conclusion that infants of five-months-old can discriminate and classify naturalistic, audible and visible speech on the basis of language membership.

In a follow-up study conducted by Bahrick (1988), three-month-old infants were provided with exposure to a single film and soundtrack under one of four familiarization conditions. Only those infants who were exposed to films paired with soundtracks that were synchronously related to the motions of the objects and appropriately related to the composition of the objects demonstrated intermodal learning capacities. The mean time looking at the sound-specified film for these infants during the intermodal learning test was significantly greater than that for the control group who had been exposed to noncontingent stimuli for the same period of time.

Among the conclusions drawn by Bahrick were that three-month-old infants were capable of learning the relation between visible and acoustic stimulation simply by watching a single, naturalistic audible and visible event. This intermodal learning occurs as a result of a single minute of exposure to each of two kinds of films and accompanying soundtracks. Since the test performance of the exposed subjects was significantly better than that of the control subjects, it was unlikely that performance was based on prior experience. Instead, the researcher concluded that it was the result of the two-minute familiarization period with these events. This study demonstrates the acuteness of the infant's skill in rapidly representing two perceptual dimensions, sight and sound.

Second, Bahrick noted that this intermodal learning was based on the infants' detection of a invariant modal relations. In other words, the infants abstracted two different kinds of modal relations that united the audible and visible stimulation from the filmed events during the two-minute familiarization period. According to Bahrick, this conclusion is supported by the finding that only those subjects exposed to the contingent stimuli displayed evidence of intermodal learning. In contrast, control infants did not. Moreover, the experimental condition differed from the control condition in only one way: it provided two levels of invariant audiovisual structure, because the soundtracks were both synchronous with the motions of the objects and appropriate to their composition. Infants exposed to the experimental condition must have detected the temporal macrostructure or synchrony uniting the sights and sounds of impact, and the temporal microstructure available at each synchronous impact specifying the composition of the moving object. In this instance, whether the object was composed of a single, larger unit or of an aggregate of smaller units did not appear to make a difference with respect to the infant's intermodal abilities. This interpretation was further confirmed by the finding of significant main effects of both synchrony and sound appropriateness on the infant's performance during the intermodal learning test. Once again, the infant's representational skills appear to lie at the root of capacities to integrate the various perceptual dimensions of stimuli.

As a third conclusion, Bahrick noted that the infants apparently learned to perceive a relationship between the concurring patterns of audible and visible stimulation when they detected invariant temporal structure uniting them, but did not learn to perceive a relationship between them when they detected any temporally discrepant audiovisual structure. Although infants exposed to the experimental conditions were given the opportunity to learn a relationship between a single film and soundtrack pair, only subjects who were exposed to synchronous and appropriately related film and soundtrack pairs displayed evidence of learning.

These studies indicate that even by three months of age, infants are coordinating intermodal capacities and converting them into internal representations. Significantly, Bahrick's investigations suggest that *infants may be particularly adept at making intermodal connections when stimuli are presented to them in a synchronous fashion.* This information is especially useful, because it is known that one characteristic that tends to distinguish adaptive caregivers from maladaptive caregivers is their capacity expose the infant to stimuli in an environment and atmosphere that is well-paced, rhythmic and synchronic. Moreover, such caregivers also employ synchrony when previewing to the infants, as well as when such previewing behaviors are being tapered off. These caregivers most likely manifest intuitive behaviors that stimulate the development of intermodal capacities. Since synchronic behavior is capable of being taught to caregivers who lack this skill, it may be possible to devise techniques for enhancing the infant's development of intermodal perceptual abilities through early intervention which teaches the caregiver to enhance her capacity for synchronic exchange with the infant.

The Contribution of Previewing to Multimodal Capacities

Even within the first few days of life, infants demonstrate the capacity to distinguish between discrepant stimuli. This capacity is referred to as *discrepancy awareness* and was first described by McCall and Kagan (1967, 1970), and McCall and McGee (1977). Discrepancy awareness refers to the infant's ability to recognize moderately variant stimulation in the environment and to respond to such stimulation by recognizing these moderate differences. Discrepancy can be demonstrated visually or through any of the five basic perceptual abilities. As can be seen in Bahrick's study, the ability to recognize discrepancies is an essential prerequisite for the infant's ability to integrate the divergent stimuli in his environment and to anticipate or predict upcoming events. This is because the infant must be able to retain memories of a stimulus, to represent it, to predict its reoccurrence and to engage in behaviors designed to reelicit this stimulus. The regulation of such abilities seems vital for the future emergence of developmental skills, including most significantly, the ability to represent.

In an imitation paradigm for happy, sad and surprised facial expression, Field, et al. (1982) found that neonates with a mean age of seventy two hours were able to discriminate and imitate facial expressions. From these data it is believed that such imitations may be due to an innate ability to compare the sensory information of visually perceived expressions with proprioceptive feedback. More recently, Reissland (1988) observed that neonates in their first hour were able to imitate two conditions (lips widened and lips pursed), confirming that the ability to imitate is present from birth onwards. Thus, as early as the neonatal stage, the infant "is already capable of storing abstract representations of perceptually absent objects and events" (Meltzoff (1981) p. 91). Such stored representations can be compared by the infant, as in the case of imitation (Meltzoff and Moore, 1977; Field, et al., 1982; Meltzoff, 1988), with his own unseen motor movements. Thus, the infant seems capable of transferring experiences perceived in one modality (Meltzoff and Borton, 1979; Kuhl and Meltzoff, 1982; Baldwin and Markham, 1989) into other modalities (e.g., from visual to motor). This ability to transfer information across modalities permits the evolution of an awareness that what is seen informs or is related to what will be heard or felt and vice versa. Stern (1985) describes this quality as amodal perception. Amodal perception is a function which allows the infant to take information received in one sensory modality and translate it into another sensory modality.

Previewing is a means for decoding information that helps the caregiver to perceive of the infant as an organism who conceives and translates external reality amodally, that is, by transcending any one particular mode. Through previewing, the caregiver's representations of the somatic-affective-cognitive and motivational perceptions of the infant can intersect, allowing the caregiver to realize how one domain of infant perception (e.g., affective) can transfer information from other domains (e.g., cognitive, somatic, etc.) and vice versa. Previewing exercises are designed to evoke this form of integration of the infant's amodal perceptual abilities. The caregiver's attribution of meaning to future experiences is one catalyst for previewing the current interaction and for supporting the infant's perceptual efforts to perceive external reality in an integrated fashion. In other words, previewing helps the caregiver convert temporary mental representations of the infant into stable constructs or schemas that emerge during interaction (Decarie, 1978). Transferring information from one mode to another permits caregivers to identify the variant and invariant behavioral features the infant is demonstrating. These episodes of previewing allow both the infant and the caregiver to experience continuity in their relationship.

Clinical practice with dyads suggests that encouraging previewing behaviors can prevent maladaptive patterns emanating from the caregiver's past experiences (i.e., conflicts) from impairing the infant's developing sense of self (Trad, 1989a,b). Previewing techniques signify the integration of various perceptual functions that permit the members of the dyad to convert information into an animated discourse within which both the present developmental status of the infant and his imminent development can be represented. Representation allows the caregiver to not only convert objective and subjective perceptions into systems of experience from which meaning can be derived, but also to organize and thus predict future interactions.

Given that multimodal integration is so vital to infant development, what are some of the definitive research conclusions in this area? Data from recent infant studies provide unambiguous evidence that language is not a necessary mediator for crossmodal transfer (Rose and Ruff, 1987). This finding is confirmed by studies showing that infants can recognize and represent both discrepancies and contingencies prior to the advent of language. In fact, rudimentary form of crossmodal ability is apparent even in infants of just a few weeks old, and investigations imply that amodal properties are readily detected by different systems of perception in very young infants. Finally, it appears that a kind of developmental spurt occurs between the third and sixth months of life, at which time visual and auditory, as well as auditory and tactile systems appear to be coordinated by the infant with greater facility, indicating that representational capacities are operating and that the infant is beginning to flexibly vary these representations to formulate predictions about his own behavior and the behavior of others.

Other researchers have demonstrated that not only can the infant coordinate properties of objects across two or more different perceptual domains by the first six months, but also that infants of this age are able to integrate such phenomena as temporal structure and motion without becoming confused or withdrawing their attention. Bahrick (1987), for example, focused on infant intermodal perception of two levels of temporal structure in naturally occurring events. The investigation involved four separate experiments. Films depicting a single object (a large marble) and a compound object (a group of several smaller marbles) colliding against a surface in an erratic pattern were shown to infants between three and seven and a half months of age. According to the researcher, these stimulus events integrated two levels of temporal structure, including the temporal synchrony uniting the sights and sounds of objects on impact and the temporal microstructure (defined as the internal temporal structure of each individual marble impact sound and motion).

In the first experiment, six-month-old infants were capable of detecting a relationship between the auditory and visual stimulation of events when both levels of invariant temporal structure guided their intermodal exploration. In a second experiment, five-month-old infants were able to discern the bimodal temporal microstructure specifying object composition. These infants gazed primarily at a film, whose soundtrack was played even though the motions of the objects depicted on the film were not synchronized with the soundtrack. The infants' sensitivity to temporal synchrony relations was assessed in a third experiment, which involved presenting two films depicting objects of the same composition, synchronized with an appropriate soundtrack. It was found that both four-and-a-half and six-month-old infants could detect temporally synchronic relationships under these conditions. Finally, a fourth experiment investigated how temporal synchrony and temporal microstructure interact in guiding intermodal exploration. To examine this phenomenon, the natural soundtrack of the objects was played out of synchrony with the motions of the moving objects. In six-month-old infants, no evidence of detecting a relationship between the film and its appropriate soundtrack was detected. This final experiment indicated that temporal dysynchrony is capable of disrupting the temporal microstructure specifying object composition.

Gibson (1969) has proposed that intermodal perception develops because some of the object's characteristics may be detected via more than one perceptual modality. As a typical example, most events that occur over time may be characterized by a temporal structure that is accessible to both visual and auditory perceptual channels. In addition, several types of invariant temporal relations may characterize a single event. Thus, the sights and sounds of a ball bouncing can share a temporal synchrony, a common temporal pattern or a rhythm. According to Gibson, infants appear equipped to detect certain kinds of invariant patterns of stimulation from birth and this nascent capability provides the foundation from which other perceptual skills develop.

More recently, data have suggested that young infants detect a variety of invariant temporal relations and are capable of extracting the visual and acoustical stimulation from single events. Spelke (1979, 1981), for example, found that infants of three to seven months are sensitive to temporal synchrony relations and discovered that infants of this age can perceive the simultaneity of sights and sounds of an object's impact against a surface. This finding suggests coordination of several perceptual realms. Walker (1982) found that infants younger than six months can detect the synchrony of voice and face movements during speech, while Spelke, Born and Chu (1983) concluded that such infants perceive the synchrony between sounds and changes in an object's trajectory of motion. The crossmodal transfer of rhythmic patterns has been established in seven-month-olds (Allen, Walker, Symonds and Marcell, 1977), as well as in four-month-olds (Mendelson and Ferland, 1982).

All of these studies confirm Gibson's original view of the neonate's intermodal capacities at birth, but raise questions as to how intermodal qualities develop and become more discriminating. Which perceptual properties of objects are infants innately prepared to detect and which are learned through perceptual experience? Moreover, how does differentiation of one type of perception lead to the detection of other types of perceptual qualities, and eventually to the simultaneous integration or discernment of all five intermodal capacities. Gibson's view is that perceptual development progresses along a pathway of increased differentiation to finer and more discrete aspects of sensory awareness. Objects and events possess hierarchically organized properties and the properties of objects are differentiated in order of increasing specificity. Adopting this view, Bahrick has suggested that audible and visible events may be characterized along hierarchic levels of temporal structure. The infant's detection of temporal structure may reveal an orderly progression from differentiation of more global to increasingly more specific levels of stimulation. Thus, obvious visual qualities captured by large size or vivid color are perceived more readily by the infant, while more subtle visual properties such as shading or pastel color are integrated later. Similarly, more exaggerated auditory characteristics such as loudness, clicks or elongated sounds may be perceived more readily by the infant than more subtle, softer sounds. Indeed, much of the early caregiver behavior described as being intuitive in Chapter 2 depends upon exaggerated cues which may be more accessible to the infant perceptually. For example, caregiver visual cuing tends to direct the infant to the caregiver's face and eyes in an accentuated fashion, caregiver vocalizations tend to exaggerate and over accentuate speech sounds and caregiver body contact tends to rely upon distinct and rhythmic behaviors such as stroking and rocking. Caregivers may repeat these behaviors because the infant responds positively, and it is through such repetition that intermodal integration is fostered.

To explore these views on intermodal integration in more depth, Bahrick hypothesized that most auditory and visual events can be characterized by at least two levels of temporal structure. For example, the sight and sound of a single object colliding with a surface represents two such levels, because the visual and auditory impacts are united by a synchronic relationship. The experiments devised by Bahrick sought to assess the infants' sensitivity to two levels of temporal structure in different audible and visible events. The events consisted of a single large marble and a group of smaller marbles colliding against a surface in an erratic pattern. In addition, the researcher investigated the infants' detection of a previously unexplored type of temporal microstructure, invariant temporal information specifying the composition of the object, in this case whether it was composed of a single solid substance or an amalgamation of smaller units. Moreover, the study extended the investigation of the infants' sensitivity to temporal structure to several age groups so that the emergence and developmental pathway of intermodal sensitivity might be revealed more distinctly. Finally, the researcher investigated how the two levels of temporal structure interact to influence exploration and the acquisition of intermodal relations.

Among the key findings of Bahrick's investigations were that it is likely that by six months, infants are capable of detecting a bimodal temporal invariant and are sensitive to the internal temporal structure characterizing the audible and visible impact of an object against a surface. This temporal microstructure, whether detected visually or acoustically, specifies the composition of the moving object—in this case, whether the object was composed of a single, solid substance or of a group of smaller units. The pattern of change over time characterizing the sound and visual trajectory of the object around its point of impact must clearly differentiate the single from the compound object. By this age, then, infants are not only capable of integrating the visual and auditory properties of a stationary object, but they can also maintain this integration over time. Second, infants are sensitive to the temporal macrostructure or synchrony between the visible and audible impacts of such events. Although of four and a half-month-olds displayed this capability under some conditions, observations of six-month-olds have provided strong evidence of this capability. These findings tend to further substantiate the data from earlier research indicating that young infants detect temporal synchrony uniting visible and audible stimulation under a variety of conditions and across a diverse set of stimulus events.

Bahrick's research also supports conclusions of other recent studies that young infants appear capable of learning about audiovisual relations on the basis of a single familiarization period. According to Bahrick, infants can display this capacity because they abstract invariant temporal structure. Bahrick explains that infants' sensitivity to temporal invariants enables them to determine which of two simultaneously presented visual images correlates with the soundtrack. Based on repeated exposure to invariant properties, infants develop intermodal knowledge about the visual properties of acoustically detected events. Subsequently, they search in the direction of sound-specified objects upon hearing a brief, nonsynchronous sound. In contrast, control subjects who are not exposed to a prior familiarization period do not display comparable searching manifestations.

Bahrick concluded by noting that it is evident from these studies that young infants are capable of detecting a wide range of invariant intermodal qualities, from global to specific, and of extracting these qualities from the experience of natural events. Nevertheless, while these studies provide heightened insight into the capacities of such infants, it is still unclear precisely how these capacities emerge and evolve, leading to the perception of meaningful objects and events. Bahrick's framework for analyzing the multiple levels of natural events offers a valuable guide for future explorations of perceptual development. Studies such as these permit clarification of the theories of Gibson, who argues for the differentiation of the perceptual properties of objects in order of increasing specificity.

One reason why an understanding of the development of intermodal capacities is so vital is that these skills are, to some degree, prerequisites for the infant's ability to exhibit more complex developmental abilities designed to exert control and mastery over the environment. Among these latter skills are combinatorial skills which reflect the coalescence of a cluster of developmental abilities that emerge by the end of the second year of life. Brownell (1988) examined these combinatorial skills over several behavioral domains as a function of age and task demands. Toddler combinations were observed during elicited imitation in four domains (object play, pretense, social play and motor play) and the spontaneous production in two others (language and peer-directed social overtures). Relative to younger children, older children produced more combinations of at least two or three discrete behaviors in every domain.

The role of previewing in stimulating all of these perceptual skills should, once again, be emphasized. Previewing behaviors engaged in by the caregiver tend to heighten the infant's ability to discern the varied perceptual dimensions of experience and to integrate discrete perceptions in diverse ways. It should be remembered that previewing exercises attempt to isolate specific developmental precursors that the infant is on the verge of manifesting in the form of a full-fledged skill. In devising these behaviors, the caregiver seeks to acquaint the infant with a realistic perceptual awareness of how the developmental skill will be experienced and affect the infant's interpersonal relationship with the caregiver. To do this, the caregiver creates behaviors that appropriately simulate the emergence of each imminent milestone, and particularly accentuates the perceptual dimensions of the milestone.

The caregiver's contributions to the integration of perceptual dimensions during previewing episodes becomes apparent through careful observation of such episodes. For example, the caregiver will not merely preview speech for the infant. Instead, speech, which relies on auditory perception, will be integrated with stroking of the infant, as well as with exaggerated facial expressions designed to simultaneously capture the infant's visual attention.

Moreover, as noted in Chapter 2, previewing manifestations emerge from such intuitive caregiver responses as visual cuing, vocal cuing, touching behavior and feeding competence. Each of these manifestations focuses upon perceptual capacities, and the adaptive caregiver will strive to coordinate all of these perceptual qualities when engaging in intuitive manifestations. As a result, the capacity of previewing to enhance the infants multimodal perceptual capacities becomes apparent.

Conclusion

This chapter has examined the phenomenon of multimodal perceptual capacity, the ability to integrate sensory awareness which derives from different domains into a unified representation of an object, person or interaction. While various theories have been proposed suggesting the origins of this development skill in the infant, it seems clear that contingency and discrepancy awareness both play key roles in facilitating the infant's multimodal functioning. As a result of discrepancy awareness the infant learns to distinguish between invariant characteristics conveyed in the same or different perceptual domains. For example, discrepancy awareness heightens the infant's sensitivity to differences between related sights, sounds and tastes. Contingency awareness, on the other hand, promotes the capacity to transfer messages crossmodally. For example, the infant may come to realize that a particular caregiver facial expression (visual) signals the onset of tickling manifestations (touch). Thus, contingency enables the infant to associate events and objects whose perceptual qualities are, or may be, different.

Studies detailing the infant's gradual acquisition of multimodal skill have been reviewed in this chapter. These studies reveal that even after only a few months of life, the infant's capacity to engage in multimodal abilities is present. Nevertheless, the prime motivator of multimodal perceptual skill appears to be the previewing exercises the caregiver engages in with the infant. As a result of such previewing, the infant comes to integrate and represent large segments of behavior that incorporate various perceptual dimensions. When previewing exercises are repeated, the integration of perceptual phenomena is reinforced for the infant. Eventually, the infant comes to represent experience as encompassing diverse perceptual elements which can be regulated to create a unified and coherent panorama of experience.

CHAPTER 5

Play: A Paradigm for Tracing Previewing Behaviors

Introduction

Play is among the most distinctive activities manifested by infants and young children. Indeed, it is perhaps the sole behavior that is clearly relegated to childhood and that is viewed as being an essential prerequisite to the child's development. Given the characteristic features that are associated with this activity, we may ask what constitutes play and how can it be defined during the early years of life. Moreover, how are the behaviors associated with play different from the myriad of other behaviors manifested by the infant? As will be seen below, there are three predominant qualities of play that have been isolated by researchers who have investigated this phenomenon in infants and young children. These are: (1) a cognitive element, (2) an emotional element, and (3) a social element, all interwoven in a sequence of activity that is filled with joy and delight.

The cognitive element emerges when play requires the infant to reenact representational sequences he has learned from prior experiences and to experiment with these sequences in new and different ways. During other kinds of activities the infant merely uses representational sequences to reinforce what he has already learned. In contrast, play requires the infant to use representational sequences in a very unique fashion. For example, representations that have been learned previously are reinforced through reenactment during play activities; but representations that are already familiar to the infant are varied or experimented with during play, in order to derive new patterns and new activities. Moreover, the cognitive component of play is analogous in several respects to previewing behavior engaged in by the caregiver. As has been noted in earlier chapters, previewing behaviors expose the infant to sequences of imminent developmental achievement. To acquaint the infant with such upcoming developmental trends the caregiver devises behaviors that enable the infant to simulate new manifestations and provide the infant with support in areas where maturational skill is deficient. As a result of these exercises, the infant begins to formulate representations of what future development will be like and of how the nature of the relationship with the caregiver will change as a result of this development. Through play, the infant experiments with these representations either by reenacting them or by varying them into new patterns. In this sense, play may almost be viewed as a means of infant previewing, whereby the infant shapes and implements what he has learned from the caregiver to devise his own representations of imminent development.

The second major element of play, the affective component, is also reminiscent of the emotional atmosphere that prevails during a previewing episode. Both play and previewing are associated with positive affective states and, in both instances, this positive emotionality appears to derive from the same source, the sense of mastery and control the infant acquires as a result of engaging in these activities. During previewing episodes, the infant achieves mastery as a result of experimenting with a new developmental milestone; during play, the infant achieves mastery over a situation which he has devised for himself as a result of experimenting with familiar representational patterns. This sense of mastery produces positive emotion. Researchers have speculated that these pleasurable feelings stem from the fact that play episodes reinforce the experience of contingency and expectancy, and that such reinforcement results in pleasure. This author believes that the positive emotions associated with previewing spring from a similar origin. Particularly when previewing behaviors are repeated by the caregiver, the infant's sense of anticipation is rewarded and he experiences a pleasurable affect.

Finally, the third element of play concerns the fact that this activity, at least initially, occurs during social interaction with a supportive other, generally the caregiver. As will be seen from the following discussion, during the first year of life play occurs primarily in the context of dyadic interaction. The first indication of full-fledged play behavior surfaces at approximately the third month of life, when the infant has acquired a sense of discrepancy, contingency and expectancy awareness. Play episodes at this time, like previewing episodes, are generally initiated and curtailed by the caregiver. Indeed, in some instances we may even label early examples of previewing as being a form of simulated play. As the infant progresses developmentally, however, play becomes more of an independent activity. During the second year of life, it is not unusual for the infant to be found playing by himself. Eventually, with the onset of toddlerhood, the infant once again engages in play as a social activity, this time with peers of his own age.

This chapter explores these three features of play-the cognitive, social and affective components-and seeks to delineate the ways in which play most resembles previewing during the first two years of life. This comparison makes it evident that play represents a unique form of behavior whereby the infant familiarizes himself with the skills learned during previewing and even reenacts previewing experiences within the arena of play to attain feelings of mastery and control over developmental phenomena. In this sense, previewing functions as a kind of punctuation to the experience of maturational change which heightens and enhances the accomplishment of development by contributing to other maturational phenomena such as play.

Defining Play

Any meaningful discussion of play must begin by defining this concept and explaining how this activity originates during the early months of the infant's life. Papousek, Papousek and Harris (1987) have emphasized that play behavior is composed of three interrelated components: an *affective* or *positive emotionality* element, a *cognitive* or *didactic* element, and a combination of these two elements which emerges within the context of the *social interaction*.

Vygotsky (1962), who concentrated more on the cognitive aspects of play, observed that full-fledged play involves the formulation and detection of rules, the creation of symbolic associations and the manifestation of exploratory behaviors. For Piaget (1951), too, the cognitive dimensions of play assume the utmost significance. Piaget views play as the fundamental activity whereby the child learns to accommodate and assimilate lessons gleaned from experiences with the external world. Bruner (1974, 1983) has theorized that play activities enable the infant to experience the consequences of error without enduring an excess of negative emotion. Thus, the cognitive dimension of play appears to facilitate a number of intellectual skills. It permits infants to establish the connection between means and ends, thereby facilitating the reinforcement of contingency associations and enhancing the infant's ability to anticipate and predict future events. Play also fosters experimentation, an activity that involves the manipulation of representational patterns, which, in turn, enhances the infant's ability to anticipate and predict upcoming events.

Interestingly enough, many of these same cognitive features are embedded in previewing experiences. For example, through previewing, the child learns that the developmental forces of his body can be controlled and conformed to particular rules of behavior. Moreover, previewing provides the infant with an opportunity to explore not only his external environment, but the environment of his own body as well. Finally, since previewing exercises are generally repeated by the caregiver over time, they facilitate the infant's understanding of connections between the gestures and gropings of his body and the measured behaviors to which the caregiver is introducing the infant. Thus, in many respects previewing resembles the cognitive dimensions encountered in play activity.

While the researchers mentioned above have emphasized the cognitive

features associated with play, others, such as Erikson (1963) and Winnicott (1971), have highlighted the distinctive display of pleasurable affect,
including smiles and laughter, which imbues playful interaction with an
emotional aura. But whether researchers have stressed the cognitive or
the affective components of play, virtually all who have written about the
phenomenon have underscored that, initially, play behavior is a fundamental by-product of social interaction with the caregiver. Although beyond the first year of life children tend increasingly to exhibit the capacity
to play by themselves, researchers have noted that such self-initiated play
represents the *outgrowth* of earlier routines and patterns that were first
established in the child's early relationship with the caregiver.

We may, therefore, consider play as being primarily an activity that
encompasses a cognitive and affective component. In addition, at least
during the first year of life, play is a social endeavor in the sense that it
is participated in jointly by caregiver and infant. The following discussion
of play and its significance as a tool for optimizing infant and early childhood development will concentrate on the social dimension evident in
this form of behavior for two main reasons. First, as Papousek, Papousek
and Harris and other researchers have indicated, during the initial months
of life playful behavior is triggered by the gestures and nuances of the
caregiver. That is, the mother's intuitive behaviors in the form of visual
cues, vocalizations, stroking and holding behaviors, as well as the degree
to which she provides adequate stimulation for the infant serve as catalyz-
ers which eventually spark a playful response in the infant. As has been
discussed in earlier chapters, these behaviors form the essential components of previewing. Such interactions promote adaptive development by
expanding the infant's representational horizons, enabling him to formulate predictions about behavioral strategies. Thus, previewing behaviors
reach their pinnacle during play activities. As a consequence, if we are
to probe more deeply into the nature of play and its significance for neonatal and infant behavior, we must first examine the origins of these maternal manifestations. Equally as significant, if play emerges as a particular by-product of social interaction, perhaps by modifying the initial
interaction we may modify the kind of playfulness that emerges, thereby
influencing the infant's developmental course.

However, although previewing and play activity share much in common, the two behaviors should not be confused. One prime difference
between these behaviors is that the purpose of previewing is to acquaint
the infant with a specific impending developmental skill. Previewing thus
familiarizes the infant with an upcoming experience he would not ordinarily attain on his own until later in his developmental course. In contrast, the prime purpose of play as it emerges during the first year of life
is to help the infant experiment with skills and experiences already attained and to do so in a pleasurable atmosphere.

Having articulated what I believe is the most challenging aspect of play behavior, namely, its social interactive quality, it is necessary to explain how the concept of play will be used in this chapter. I contend that play behavior occurs when the caregiver is able to represent the infant in a multidimensional fashion. Representation here refers to a visual image and also includes having a simultaneous awareness of the infant's somatic, affective, cognitive and motivational perceptions. A caregiver who is representing her infant responds on a primal level to the myriad signals the infant may emit, signals that are often imperceptible during standard observation. As one illustration of how the integration of these perceptions occurs, Papousek and Papousek cite a common practice displayed by the mothers of newborns, who often play with their infant's hands during transition periods between waking and sleeping states. Monitoring of the infant's hands permits the caregiver to assess muscle tone as a state parameter and then to make a correct decision about further nurturing behavior. Depending upon the temperature and responsiveness of the infant's hands, the caregiver may proceed to soothe the infant in preparation for sleep or may instead gently stroke the fingers in an effort to initiate a playful exchange. This form of maternal responsiveness appears to be highly intuitive and, as demonstrated by caregivers who are attuned to their infants, is a convenient method for ascertaining the infant's physiological and psychological needs, while smoothing the transition to another state of consciousness without causing unwarranted distress. Intuition arises from the caregiver's ability to experience the infant's needs vicariously, as well as to predict the effect her ministrations will have upon the infant. A similar kind of monitoring is present during previewing exercises, when the caregiver intuitively assesses the infant's developmental status in order to determine the kinds of interactions to which he will be receptive.

Play behavior occurs when the caregiver's overall mood is one of profound receptivity, enabling her to experience the myriad aspects of the infant's experience. This mood encompasses not only a distinct and highly sensitive impression of the temperature and flexibility of the infant's fingers, but also perception of the infant's emotional, cognitive and motivational states at any given time. As this ability for empathic receptivity is shared with the infant, the infant will eventually begin responding to the caregiver. Gradually, the pair develops a rapport which is typified by sequences of predictable behaviors exchanged within the dyad. Although initially these sequences are new for the infant, he becomes accustomed to a specific pattern of response as time goes on and new developmental skills emerge. This pattern of maternal responsiveness to the infant's cues comes to be understood as a *contingency* relationship from the infant's perspective. Subsequently, after having mastered such contingencies, the dyadic members begin to vary the contingent responses solely for the purpose of experimentation. One can see from this description how play can foster the emergence of previewing exercises. Indeed, play may signify the most prolific arena within which previewing interactions occur and may be the preeminent behavior that encourages the caregiver to preview events to the infant. Although the ultimate goal of previewing remains to acquaint the infant with imminent developmental trends and the ultimate goal of play remains the experience of pleasure through the replication and variation of already familiar experiences, in many respects the outward manifestations of both of these interactions may appear identical to the external observer.

Developmental Changes in Play and Play-Related Behaviors

This section outlines the progression of infant play. Discussion is devoted to typical play manifestations evident during the first two years of life and to how such behaviors resemble and contribute to previewing exercises. Also explored is perhaps one of the most challenging issues posed by infant play: how such behaviors, which in the normally developing infant appear with spontaneity and joy, can be used as models for instilling previewing in mother-infant pairs in which the optimal channels for development have been impaired.

Although the affective dimension of play is generally the most familiar, play should also be considered as a developmental phenomenon. As such, play behaviors evident during the first three months of life are governed and mediated by the infant's somatic, affective, cognitive and motivational repertoire during this developmental phase. Thus, play for infants of this age incorporates such behaviors as repetitive and rhythmic vocal exchanges, the matching of emotional expressions, finger and body touching and occasional tickling. More often than not, the caregiver initiates these sequences, relying on the infant's developmental status to devise various exercises to entertain the infant. From six months of age onward, however, distinctive changes occur in the types of behaviors the infant displays during play. Now the infant's heightened mobility and enhanced vocal manifestations propel him towards play behaviors focusing on environmental exploration and ritual games which rely upon repetitions and imitations of verbal sequences. It is clear why these play behaviors are appealing to the infant. Environmental exploration is appropriate as the infant's burgeoning motor skills emerge and the repetitions of verbal sequences help the infant exercise inchoate language skills. Papousek, Papousek and Harris also report that, although in the second half of the first year play remains a social activity, it is the infant, rather than the caregiver, who initiates the majority of play behaviors. At this juncture, play reaches its pinnacle.

Other researchers have emphasized not only that, as the baby matures, developmental skills are increasingly envinced in the infant's play, but also that the forms of play become more complex. Zelazo and Kearsley (1980) point out, for instance, that during the first few months of life the infant engages in *stereotypical play*, which is characterized by such diffuse and ostensibly disconnected behaviors as mouthing, fingering, waving and banging toys. To the casual observer, such manifestations may not seem playful at all; it is only when we notice that these behaviors-often motivated by a caregiver stimulus-occur in an atmosphere of positive emotionality and that they signify repetitions or predictable variations of earlier learned responses by the infant that the label of play behavior seems to apply. This form of stereotypical play emerges by approximately eight months of age. Play behaviors now reveal more sophisticated associations on the part of the infant, suggesting that the infant is using new skills from dyadic interaction and integrating them into play sequences. After stereotypical play has been mastered *relational play* emerges. Relational play has been defined as the simultaneous association of two or more objects in a functional manner during a sequence of pleasurable interaction. For example, the infant begins to mingle both a doll and a spoon during play. Likewise, disparate toys and objects are used in a manner appropriate to their intended function. Finally, by the second year of life, *make-believe* games become evident, indicating an ability to manipulate objects in both their literal or functional sense and their symbolic sense. During these make-believe sequences, the infant devises imaginary scenarios and manipulates the activities of pretend characters. *Role play* also surfaces during this period.

These progressions, in the specific, discrete behaviors manifested during play and in the substantive dimensions of the play itself, are both clearly the outcome of developmental progression. Interestingly enough, these are the kinds of behaviors that the infant may manifest during previewing as well. By studying play manifestations exhibited within a particular dyad, we can gauge whether the infant's somatic, affective, cognitive and motivational capacities (as well as whether the nature of the relationship with the caregiver) are moving in the direction of previewing in that the capacity to engage in more sophisticated predictions is being instilled and reinforced.

Factors Contributing to Developmental Transitions

The Contribution of Mood States

In what other respects does previewing resemble play activity? Haviland and Lelwica (1987) investigated the capacity to respond to emotional displays in ten-week-old infants whose caregivers were instructed to display happy, sad, and angry faces. The researchers interpreted the data as supporting three main conclusions. First, infants of ten weeks of age are capable of responding differently to three distinctive maternal affective presentations (joy, anger and sadness) when the presentation includes simultaneous facial and vocal elements. Second, infants of this age exhibit a tendency to match happy and angry, although not sorrowful, expressions. This matching skill is a precursory milestone for interacting during previewing exercises. Third, Haviland and Lelwica noted that infant imitations in response to maternal emotive expression became predictable, suggesting the capacity for self-regulation and cognitive awareness of responses.

According to these researchers, the findings indicate that ten-week-old infants respond differently to discrete emotional expressions, can match maternal expression, and can respond in meaningful ways to specific emotional displays. Two additional comments can also be made about these findings. Infants generally displayed a response upon the first presentation of the emotion, they exhibited a minimal reaction during the second display of the same emotion and manifested a full response when the emotion was presented a third or fourth time. This pattern suggests that infants are rapidly habituated to affective displays. The first time the expression is displayed the affect is novel and invites a response, while at the second presentation, the emotion has become familiar and provokes little interest. Why then does the infant respond with renewed vigor at the third presentation of the emotion? One explanation may be that once a response has been learned or mastered by the infant, he displays a propensity to begin experimenting with the response in order to create a variation of what has become an ingrained pattern. This form of experimentation is the hallmark of both play and previewing, and the desire to experiment and thus master inchoate forms of learning on the part of the infant emerges in both of these activities. Thus, it becomes apparent that the development of play influences the social exchanges between the members of the dyad during previewing exercises.

Another pertinent finding in Haviland and Lelwica's study involves the kinds of responses the infants displayed when presented with happy and angry faces, as compared with sad expressions. Because these infants tended to mirror joy, while avoiding imitation when confronted by the sad expression, it may be argued that infants are constitutionally primed or predisposed to experience positive emotion. It should be remembered that such positive emotions represent the affective foundation fueling play and thus, even very young infants may be emotionally equipped to participate selectively in playful interactions. If this interpretation is correct, then infants exposed to positive emotions may be more prone to predict and replicate interactive sequences during previewing exercises. This finding also suggests that caregivers who expose their infants to sufficient positive emotional expression during play are preparing the infant for the experience of being previewed. Although positive emotionality is characteristic of both play activity and previewing, it should be remembered that pleasure during play emerges as a result of the infant's recognition of already familiar contingencies, while pleasure during previewing is due to the infant's exposure to new experiences.

A recent study by Campos, Campos and Barrett (1989) indicates that emotional expression may play an even greater role in facilitating such activities as play than has been previously supposed. According to these researchers, earlier developmental theorists considered emotions to be feeling states indexed by behavioral expression. In contrast, more recent researchers have posited that emotions are processes of establishing, maintaining or disrupting the relationship between the organism and the environment. Emotional development is, therefore, an aspect of the relational processes that emerges as a result of interaction with the caregiver.

According to Campos et al., emotions are beginning to be viewed as a series of three processes which make an event significant to an individual. These processes are based on (1) the relevance of the event to the goals of the individual, (2) the degree of communication the event creates significant others, conveyed through facial, vocal and gestural actions, and (3) the hedonic nature of certain types of stimulation. Thus, cognitive factors such as object permanence and self-recognition are not, in themselves, affectogenic. Instead, in order for cognition to produce emotion, the cognition must be about significant events.

From this new concept of emotional regulation, we can begin to understand how crucial play and previewing are to the enhancement of the infant's development. Both of these activities emerge from the context of interaction and in both instances, positive affective states are characteristic and indeed emblematic of these activities. It may be argued that such activities fuel the infant's burgeoning emotional repertoire, and in particular, enhance the capacity to experience pleasurable emotions. It may be argued that if such activities do not occur, the infant will be deprived of learning how to experience positive affect within a relational context. This theory bears credibility, particularly in light of Spitz's (1945) observation that institutionalized infants who were deprived of consistent care tended to lack the expression of positive emotional states.

By focusing particularly on the kinds of emotional responses that emerge during dyadic interaction, researchers have isolated other elements that are evident during early mother-infant exchanges. Keller and Scholmerich (1987), for example, examined how caregivers respond to infant vocalizations during the first months of life. They discerned four types of infant vocalization based on affective expression in a group of infants ranging in age from two to fourteen weeks. These categories included physiological vocalizations which incorporated respiratory responses such as deep inhalation to express surprise, throat-closing sounds, clicking and drinking sounds. In the category of negative vocalizations, they categorized all sounds that began with a cessation of respiration followed by a quick series of rhythmical sounds. Whining, fussing, crying, sighing and sounds of discomfort were grouped in this classification. In contrast, positive vocalizations were those sounds uttered with low to moderate intensity emitted during the process of gentle exhalation. Such sounds are commonly interpreted as expressing positive emotions and include, babbling, cooing, consonant-vowel groups, laughing, strings of "r" sounds, and repetitive sounds. Lastly, the researchers delineated effort vocalizations which encompassed motor sounds and consonant-building sounds.

Among the key findings of the study were that parental verbal reactions to the four types of infant vocalizations increased over time, while tactile responses diminished. According to Keller and Scholmerich, the results indicated that infants perform different kinds of vocalizations to communicate affective states from the second week of life onward. This trend suggests an effort on the part of the infant to predict caregiver response and to manifest a disposition designed to elicit previewing interactions from the caregiver. Such vocalizations serve a communicative purpose as well, as demonstrated by the fact that their occurrence varies with the mood of the dyad. Furthermore, direct eye contact between dyadic members seems to be a crucial factor in determining the frequency and nature of the vocalization emitted by the infant. For example, during periods of sustained eye contact, infant vocalization not only increased, but was also common; in contrast, when eye contact initiated by the caregiver diminished, vocalization also diminished substantially. Here we see how the coordination of intuitive behaviors, visual and vocal cuing, is used to engage the infant in interactive sequences which gradually introduce the infant to imminent developmental trends through previewing. Moreover, these intuitive skills engaged in by the caregiver serve to enhance both the nature and degree of play and previewing activity.

The researchers summarized the results of the study by concluding that caregivers understood the messages infants conveyed through different vocalizations and reacted appropriately. They also noted that those infants who expressed more positive vocalizations received a greater degree of verbal feedback and more verbal stimulation, and further, may have experienced the verbal feedback as being a contingent response to their vocalization. Positive emotion was thereby reinforced, motivating the infant to seek more dyadic experience. This finding indicates that caregivers who reinforce the infant's predictive abilities through the integration of various forms of stimulation such as eye contact and vocalization may foster previewing interactions with their infants. Keller and Scholmerich hypothesized that in optimally functioning dyads there may be no quiescent stage; instead, from the first weeks of life onward social relationship develops through a series of developmental tasks. This study offers convincing evidence that almost from birth, infants and their caregivers establish systems of communication to convey not only physiological needs and psychological states, but also to engage in predictable interactions about what future behavior will be like. It is from these incipient predictive abilities that the behaviors we associate with play emerge. Moreover, it is within this arena of communication that both play and previewing emerges.

Cohn and Tronick (1987) have further investigated specific mechanisms of the intimate exchange occurring between infant and caregiver in the early months of life. One goal of their study was to further clarify the nature of the exchange of emotional states between infant and caregiver. For example, Cohn and Tronick describe a sequence that has been observed in two- to three-month-old infants in which the caregiver initiates the exchange by passively watching the infant while the infant's attention is directed away from her. Eventually, the mother elicits the infant's attention by displaying positive affect in the form of a cheerful, animated facial expression which may be accompanied by bursts of animated vocalizations. The infant responds to this display first with a neutral affective expression which is gradually transformed into a positive affective expression as engagement is successfully achieved. The mother and infant then enter what has been referred to as a *positive dyadic state* which endures until the infant resumes a neutral expression and turns attention away from the mother who remains positive. During this sequence, the infant has learned a contingency experience which will later be used by the caregiver to initiate play with the infant and subsequently to devise new previewing behaviors that rely on these emotional responses.

To further explore this phenomenon, the researchers followed dyadic pairs during periods when the infant was three, six and nine months of age. Videotaped sequences between the caregivers and infants were analyzed. The researchers found that caregivers and infants engage in a reciprocally mediated form of regulation that is sensitive to the nuances of the other partner. At three and six months, maternal positive emotional expression generally functioned as a prelude to the positive emotional expression of the infant. In addition, caregiver receptivity to infant affect during this period was demonstrated by the caregiver's replication of the infant's positive emotional expression until the infant disengaged. It was also found that at six and nine months, the caregiver was the primary initiator of positive emotional expression and would often attempt to attract the infant's attention with displays of pleasant emotional states if the infant was disengaged. By nine months, however, this pattern reversed itself and the infant became the more frequent initiator of positive affective episodes. By this age, then, the infant has become more adept at predicting interactional exchanges and, hence, initiating behaviors designed to elicit expected responses from the caregiver. It is during this period that the infant comes to actively communicate his needs to the caregiver. The caregiver will sense either that the infant is ready to have a new play episode or that the infant wishes to end the previous episode. A similar kind of mood prevails during previewing exercises, where the caregiver organizes the interaction without overwhelming the infant. This study offers vital information regarding the developmental pathway of both play and previewing behavior. It is important to note that during the first year of life the caregiver is the primary initiator of these forms of response. Over time, however, the infant displays an eagerness to begin experimenting with learned skills (manifested by play) and to experience new, imminent developmental skills (manifested by behaviors designed to elicit a previewing response from the caregiver). In other words, a transformation occurs by the second year of life as the infant becomes the prime initiator of interaction.

Although the above studies confirm that even from a very early age infants respond to facial expressions denoting different emotional states, we must ask whether such expressions are cognitively differentiated by infants in the same way that adults construe these emotional messages. Nelson (1987), among others, has argued for caution in this area, noting that the infant's ability to recognize emotional expression undergoes a lengthy period of incubation and does not generally achieve fruition until well into the second year of life. But even if, as Nelson indicates, the process of emotional maturation is gradual and depends on such peripheral factors as cognitive development and caregiver nurturing skills, we may still chart the route whereby the infant attains the capacity to comprehend and respond appropriately to an affective cue.

Clearly, some infant capacity for recognizing and discriminating facial expressions appears relatively early in life. This skill is crucial to the eventual ability to formulate predictions about the environment. For example, Field, Woodson, Greenberg and Cohen (1982) have documented the ability of one- to two-day-old full-term infants to discriminate and imitate such basic facial expressions as happy, sad and surprised. Nelson and Horowitz (1983) found that two-month-olds could discriminate between a happy face and a neutral face, while Young-Browne, Rosenfeld and Horowitz (1977) reported an ability to distinguish happy, sad and surprised expressions on the part of three-month-olds, and Barrera and Maurer (1981) found that such three-month-olds were also able to recognize differences between smiling and frowning faces. Nevertheless, such researchers as Caron, Caron and Myers (1982) and Nelson (1985) advocate caution with respect to these findings. The visual capacities of an infant less than three months of age are known to be limited, and it is uncertain whether such newborns are responding to an entire facial presentation when they react to a particular expression. As Haith, Bergman and Moore (1977) have stressed, newborns of less than four months of age rarely scan full faces and when they do, such scanning activity is generally confined to the hairline and chin areas. It is not until four months of age, according to Caron, Caron, Caldwell and Weiss (1973), that an ability to examine all the features of the face becomes apparent. This type of scanning ability suggests that representational capacities are functioning. In other words, the infant is beginning to develop an internalized schema or image of the caregiver's face and of the changing impressions of her face. This form of discriminatory ability will be vital as the infant begins to engage in play behavior. This is because during play, the infant derives pleasure from slightly varied or discrepant patterns.

Between four and seven months, however, a qualitative progression in the infant's visual and perceptual capacities appears to occur. Several studies have confirmed that infants of this age readily classify emotional expression, indicating full-fledged discriminatory abilities, even when the models displaying these expressions vary on several dimensions. Thus, Caron et al. (1982) report that seven-month-olds can generalize their discrimination of surprise expressions despite changes in same-sex models, while happy faces can be distinguished over changes in models of both sexes, according to Nelson and Dolgin (1985). In a related investigation, Nelson and Ludemann (1987) found that happy and fearful faces that vary in intensity with each expression will, nevertheless, be identified as happy faces by four- to seven-month-olds and as fearful faces by four-month-olds. Displays of a frowning face were responded to with exhibitions of distress by eight-month-olds, but not in younger infants, according to Ahrens (1954). Finally, Sorce, Emde, Campos and Klinnert (1985), in their experimentation with the visual cliff paradigm in twelve-month-olds, discovered that by this age, infants easily distinguish between the positive and negative emotional expressions of their caregivers. But since responses to the angry and happy faces differed little and response to a sad face was ambiguous, they concluded that the infants may have been reacting to broadly defined, rather than narrowly drawn, categories of affective display. Clearly, however, positive emotion was found to motivate further infant interaction, while negative emotion resulted in withdrawal.

What are the implications of these data for play behavior in infants during the first year of life? In Chapter 2, it was noted that several significant kinds of intuitive caregiver behavior (meaning attribution, the provision of adequate stimulation and the support of the infant's integrative processes) emerge during the first months of dyadic interaction to fuel the caregiver's displays of play and previewing behavior. It may be argued that meaning attribution (the maternal tendency to provide an interpretation for infant response) acts in the service of emotional maturation by enabling the caregiver to compensate for the infant's limitations and to provide developmental impressions to the infant. For example, if the caregiver smiles at the infant and the infant responds by emitting cooing or gurgling sounds, the caregiver may interpret such a display as meaning that the infant appreciates the positive affect and seeks to experience more of it. Moreover, the caregiver's response helps the infant formulate predictions about future change. In fact, an infant of less than four months of age may only be reacting to a visual discrepancy in the caregiver's lip movements. Nevertheless, because the caregiver *believes* the infant is responding to her positive affect, she will be motivated to replicate the behavior intermittently in order to attain a positive infant response. Gradually, as the infant matures, his reaction to his mother's smile will approximate the meaning she originally attributed. Once this congruity of meaning between caregiver and infant occurs, a shared feeling suffuses the interaction.

But to arrive at this point of mutually understood emotional states, the caregiver must engage in repeated exhibitions of emotion during interaction with the infant. These long-term and repetitive presentations of emotional expression are necessary in order for the infant to begin developing representational schema pertaining to the interaction with the caregiver, who will be his partner during play. Since the dyadic exchange tends to create an atmosphere of positive emotionality, the caregiver's ministrations stimulate the infant to represent and predict a full facial expression. When the entire interaction takes place within the dyadic social context, this predictable pattern of emotional display, along with its corresponding infant response, may be categorized as *play* because all the prerequisites of playful behavior articulated by Papousek, Papousek and Harris (including the cognitive element, positive affect and social interaction) are present. The emphasis on behaviors that the infant has already experienced also enables us to characterize this activity as play.

Field (1978) has described how the caregiver's ability to provide adequate and predictable sequences of stimulation for the infant, as well as support of the infant's *integrative* capacities, can be converted into a form of play which encourages the development of the infant's emotional repertoire. By the time infants are approximately three months of age, the caregiver's repertoire of responses includes a number of common games that emerge during face-to-face exchange. Among such playful exchanges are "peek-a-boo," "I'm gonna get you," "so big," "itsy-bitsy spider" and "pat-a-cake" (Sroufe and Wunsch, 1972). Each of these games represents a predictable sequence that helps the infant to anticipate the responses that may be expected from the caregiver. Once again, here play serves to stimulate the kinds of capacities that will be used during previewing, particularly the capacity to predict upcoming interaction. Moreover, Field stresses that the development of such a series of playful sequences evolves gradually, as the caregiver acquires an understanding of the infant's emotional range. If a caregiver is not attuned to the needs of her infant, such play sequences are often disrupted, as for instance, when a mother initiates "peek-a-boo" with a six-week-old, rather than with a twelve-week-old. A similar situation has been observed in caregivers of failure-to-thrive, atypical and developmentally delayed infants; caregivers do not play age-appropriate games or display developmentally appropriate behaviors with their infants (Greenberg, 1971).

This discussion has highlighted some of the major similarities between play activity and previewing. As has been seen, in both activities the predominant emotional state suffusing the interaction is one of pleasure. Moreover, as discussed, both play and previewing tend to encourage the infant's predictions about the future course of interaction with the caregiver and about the course of his overall development. Play, however, tends to focus more on enabling the infant to exercise learned skills within his developmental capacity, while previewing focuses on imminent skills the infant has not yet achieved.

The Contribution of Socialization

A distinctive aspect of play behavior mentioned by Papousek, Papousek, and Harris is the role of social interaction and the participation of an *active and responsive partner.*

Fenson, Kagan, Kearsley and Zelazo (1976) have pointed out, during the later portion of infancy children tend to play more and more by themselves. Certainly well into the second year, play remains a phenomenon of dyadic interaction. It may seem obvious that the infant relies on the caregiver, even from the first days of life, to acquaint him with the alien universe in which he finds himself, or phrased differently, to convert the world into a *predictable domain,* but several researchers have sought to probe more deeply into the motives propelling early interaction and the crucial role played by the caregiver. Trevarthen (1985) notes that the infant's self-regulatory capacities, such as proclivities to alter mood-states, reveal themselves initially through changes in emotional displays. The interpersonal relation with the caregiver serves to teach the infant how to better communicate self-regulatory needs via affective displays.

The caregiver's affective disposition during infant stimulation is so potent that numerous researchers have delineated the connection between early interaction patterns and such behaviors as cognitive behaviors (Brazelton and Yogman, 1986), imitative behaviors (Field, Goldstein, Vega-Lahr, and Porter, 1986), language acquisition (Kuhl and Meltzoff, 1982; Tamis-LeMonda and Bornstein, 1989), contingency learning (Lewis, Wolan-Sullivan and Brooks-Gunn, 1985) and object relations (Legerstee, Pomerleau, Malcuit and Feider, 1987). In sum, it appears that the infant's early and consistent interaction with the caregiver will determine, in large part, the degree to which the child is able to represent and predict both behaviors and the caregiver's corresponding response to the infant. Indeed, the supportive dyadic environment appears a prerequisite for stimulating virtually all developmental skills, including the infant's ability to engage in predictions about the future.

As Stern (1974) suggests, during interaction the infant strives to gratify his own needs, while the caregiver regulates and occasionally guides displays in order to provide the infant with an optimal level of arousal. This modified push-and-pull between the dyadic members, similar to a harmonious tug-of-war and reminiscent of the push-pull motivations toward play described by Papousek, Papousek and Harris, results in a kind of compromise between infant and caregiver. Each member will seek to ful-fill the other's needs by developing a mutual system of communication in which predictive interaction is facilitated and in which the parent and in-fant continually guide one another's affective states. Trevarthen (1985) explains this reciprocity by noting that the infant innately focuses on the caregiver as his communicative partner and modulates his predictive dis-plays with those of the parent. While Stern (1985) labels the quality suf-fusing this interaction *affect attunement,* Trevarthen dubs it innate *inter-subjectivity,* which, he says, refers to the shared and trusting aspect of an exchange based on mutual identification and recognition. Regardless of the label used to describe this activity, however, what is significant is that the caregiver sufficiently stimulates the infant with appropriate posi-tive affect.

Within the confines of dyadic interaction, is it possible to identify cer-tain specific behaviors and label them as play. Assuming this is the case, what playful behaviors are caregiver-initiated and which behaviors are infant-initiated? Stern (1974) has cataloged a series of manifestations that originate with the caregiver and which fall into the category of play be-cause they assist the infant in formulating predictions about upcoming behavior and because they elicit pleasurable responses. He comments, for example, that parents tend to exaggerate their facial features, vocal-izations and body movements, speeding up and slowing down their be-haviors in order to stimulate and arouse the infant. One reason caregivers may intuitively slow down the speed of interaction may be because of the perception that the infant incorporates and comprehends information in a relatively slow-paced fashion. The parental tendency to adopt one facial expression for a prolonged period or to exaggerate an expression may provide the infant with a sufficient amount of time to represent the mes-sage that the numerous expressions displayed by the caregiver are all linked to one facial structure. From the perspective of the parent, one goal of play is to maintain an optimal level of arousal and attention in the infant in order to elicit smiles, coos and other pleasurable signs which, in turn, lead to feelings of effectiveness and achievement in the parent. Thus, the caregiver regulates her own behavior during play to keep pace with the infant's developmental status.

But the dynamics of parentally initiated play are likely somewhat more complex than this model suggests. Stern comments that during these first months of life, the infant can become as highly attentive and aroused as possible when experiencing a positive affect. To achieve this peak of arousal, the parent either intensifies stimulation or behaves in a manner slightly discrepant from what the infant has come to expect, thereby prod-ding the infant on to new representations, with which the infant becomes able to predict new caregiver responses. Parents may inadvertently per-form behaviors that are either too complex or too discrepant from already established interactional patterns. If caregivers engage in such behaviors, they may press the infant beyond the optimal level of stimulation and evoke a negative affect.

It is important that parental playful interactions somewhat alter the previous patterns to which the infant has grown accustomed. Such modifications stimulate the infant's ability to formulate predictions and introduce the infant to the kind of experimentation that is a hallmark of play behavior. Moreover, such play activity prepares the infant for the kind of experimentation that will occur during previewing. In other words, the infant has an incessant need to be stimulated and previewed. The caregiver who fails to fulfill this basic need may deprive the infant of experiences in which he is given an opportunity to rehearse and begin mastering, and thus coordinating, his representations. The adaptive dyad, therefore, is an interactional arena in which the infant begins to manipulate mental representations in order to devise and gradually test predictions based on these representations. It is clear that during the play behavior of the first six months of life the caregiver is involved in the complex task of modulating behaviors in order to adequately stimulate the infant's representational skills, while aware that overstimulation may hinder such stimulation. To arrive at this delicate balance, the caregiver must be attuned to the infant and be willing to experiment with flexible forms of interaction.

What, then, is the role of the infant during play sequences in the first months of life? Just as the parent regulates the interaction through stimulation and arousal of the infant, so too does the infant exert control over the interaction through absorption or rejection of the stimuli presented. In this fashion, the infant's early efforts to regulate his perceptual input represents his first means of manifesting a desire for predicting either overstimulation or understimulation during interpersonal engagement. By continually regulating his responses, the infant seeks stimuli within his optimal range while withdrawing from stimuli which fail to meet such qualifications.

Infant responsiveness affects caregiver behavior as well, because by regulating his level of arousal and thus attention span, the infant provides the caregiver with a means through which to modify behavior in order to engage the infant harmoniously. In other words, by monitoring the infant's response, the caregiver begins regulating and modifying her behavior appropriately. Trevarthen (1985) observes that eye contact behaviors begin to be incorporated into the infant's visual repertoire by five weeks. By six weeks, it is hypothesized that the infant has begun to form a mental representation of the caregiver's face and by two months infants can interact with a parent through the use of facial expressions and vocalizations. Trevarthen reports that between six and twelve weeks, the infant will display silent lip-and-tongue and hand movements. These behaviors are believed to be a form of prelinguistic communication through which the infant strives to convey verbal messages to the caregiver. According to Trevarthen, such prelinguistic speech behaviors, relying on both oral and motor skills, are most likely precursors of the babbling behavior exhibited in later months. As each pattern of development flourishes, the infant's predictive abilities have a cumulative effect during social interactions. Stern notes that by the fourth month of life, the infant has developed sufficient skills to represent the multiple expressions and gestures of the caregiver, and can predict the myriad ways in which the caregiver can alter vocal patterns while interacting with the infant. This enhanced responsiveness on the part of the infant encourages the caregiver to introduce the infant to more sophisticated developmental skills during previewing exercises.

Now that this pattern of progressively more complex interactions has been established, we turn to the specific behaviors involved in play during the first year of life. Such manifestations essentially fall into three categories: first, facial expression and gaze behaviors; second, the manipulation of the body (movements and gestures); and third, language manifestations (vocalizations). By coordinating these interactive behaviors, the infant is able to rehearse and master socioemotional and cognitive skills which will be of later use to him during episodes of pretend and make-believe. Thus, mastery of communication skills in the three domains mentioned above, as well as the caregiver's readiness to support the infant's predictive manifestations, is crucial in order for genuine play behavior to occur.

How are these apparently discrete behavioral manifestations woven into the fabric of play? Stern and Gibbon (1980) report that the infant uses gaze behaviors when he wishes to initiate or terminate a playful interaction. The infant gazes in the caregiver's direction, striving for direct eye contact, as the play behavior commences and averts his gaze when the behavior no longer stimulates him. A rudimentary form of communication thus begins to develop between infant and caregiver. Gaze behaviors are thus one vehicle with which the infant can control the amount of incoming stimuli received and convey to the caregiver the need to modify the level of stimulation. This form of infant regulation during play is similar to the caregiver's observation of and response to the infant's status during previewing. Fogel (1980) contends that the infant's early motor behaviors of pointing, grabbing and reaching indicate his attraction to specific persons, behaviors or objects observed within the immediate vicinity. At some point between three and six months of age, the infant acquires the capacity to control his neck muscles and this is subsequently incorporated into his repertoire of communicative behaviors. The infant may either orient his entire face toward the caregiver or avert his face from parental view. Facial aversion signifies the infant's desire that the interaction cease. He has either achieved an optimal amount of stimulation or he is underaroused and needs the caregiver to readjust the level of interaction.

Body gestures and movements are the second key components in the repertoire of infant play manifestations during the first year of life. Stern and Gibbon (1980) report that between five and twelve months of age, the infant achieves upper body control. Just as the infant earlier relied on head motions to signal an eagerness or a reticence to play with the caregiver, now the entire upper body may be used to convey such a message. These motor skills are initially used to attract the attention of the caregiver, but as more complex and expressive means of predictive skill come to the fore, such behaviors may decrease or become aspects of future play behaviors like pulling, climbing and rolling. The incipient communications network between caregiver and infant during the first months of life has now been consolidated. As these skills of mobility proliferate, the infant also becomes more assertive with respect to initiating play interaction. This assertion may result from the infant's increased ability to devise predictions and to elicit a desired response from the caregiver through previewing exercises. Fogel reports that while the six-week-old infant passively awaits the encouraging gestures of his caregiver before commencing a play episode, the six-month-old infant who has attained body control begins to actively use his representations to initiate play episodes with the parent. The ability of the infant to initiate interaction may predict subsequent previewing episodes designed to explore impending achievements. Indeed, infants who fail to initiate play after the sixth month of life may be at risk for later developmental deficits.

In a study conducted by Hornik, Risenhoover, and Gunnar (1987), infant responsiveness to caregiver's signals at one year of age was examined. These researchers investigated how twelve-month-old infants would respond to three stimulus toys based on maternal response to the toys. Each toy had previously been demonstrated to evoke a particular response. The first toy, a musical ferris wheel, triggered a positive emotional response; the second toy, a stationary toy robot that recited facts about outer space in a machinelike voice, evoked neither strong approach or avoidance behaviors, and hence, was labeled as ambiguous; the third toy, a mechanical cymbal-clapping monkey had elicited avoidance responses in earlier work (Gunnar and Stone, 1984) and was labeled aversive. Mothers involved in the study were taught three types of responses. The first response involved a display of positive affect manifested through face, voice and gestures; the second response was characterized as a negative one in which the mothers were instructed to display disgust by imagining that insects were crawling up the toys; in the third response, the caregivers were asked to remain silent and neutral. The sample consisted of twenty-seven male and twenty-seven female infants, ranging in age from twelve to thirteen months. Infants were randomly assigned to three groups of simulated maternal affect. Mothers in the groups simulated positive affect, negative affect and neutral expressions. After the toys had been presented once, infants in the first two groups were shown the toys again in the same order in which they were initially presented. During this second series of toy presentations, however, the mothers were silent and neutral.

According to Hornik et al., issues involving social referencing were the focal point of this study. Infants whose mothers exhibited negative, disgust reactions played less with the stimulus toys than did infants whose mothers exhibited positive or silent/neutral reactions. This response suggests that infants use caregiver behavior as a model for a representation which was later used to determine their own response. Second, the results provided some support for the notion that infants respond more immediately to negative, rather than positive, maternal communications. Third, the results indicated that twelve-month-olds maintain their initial appraisals of novel toys the second time the toys are presented. Each of these findings suggests that during play interaction the affect by the parent projected will have a strong predictive effect on the kind of infant behavior that is or will be manifested. It is clear that by this age the communicative network between infant and caregiver is firmly in place. The infant's reliance on the caregiver will now be especially helpful as the caregiver begins to introduce the infant to more complex behaviors through previewing.

Legerstee, Pomerleau, Malcuit and Feider (1987) investigated the age at which infants would respond differently to a doll as opposed to a person. They found that by two months of age, infants express positive affect towards a person, but not towards the doll. By twelve weeks, as the infant's motor skills have developed, he directs more motor behaviors toward the doll, although social behaviors remain primarily directed towards the caregiver. At seventeen weeks, as the infant's motor skills developed further, more attention is directed toward the doll, although social skills remain oriented towards the caregiver. Legerstee et al. hypothesize that the interaction occurring between the dyadic members provides the infant with contingency experiences which regulate response. These sequences enable the infant to devise predictable representations of caregiver response. Dolls, in contrast, do not regulate the infant's state, but provide the infant with a means through which to rehearse the social behaviors acquired during the initial caregiver-infant interaction. By nineteen weeks, the infant displays more interest in the doll than in the caregiver.

This shift may be attributed to the fact that the infant has now developed full-fledged representations of predictable sequences of interaction with the caregiver. These representations may now be experimented with by the infant through use of his motor skills, with which he seeks novel stimuli for experimentation and exercising of cognitive skills, as opposed to merely responding to the cues of the caregiver. The overlap between play and previewing in this form of infant behavior is now apparent. The infant is provided with an outlet for manipulating social interactions and uses these interactions to make predictions. The arena of infant-caregiver interaction now expands to include the environment beyond the physical dimensions of the dyadic members. Stern (1974) observes that by six months of age, the infant has lost interest in the parent's facial expressions, vocalizations and behaviors and is now primarily motivated by a desire to manipulate objects. The caregiver assumes the role of a partner for the infant, providing a reference point for all the infant's play behaviors. This transition occurs because the infant seeks to test the predictions acquired during dyadic interaction with the play arena by initiating his own behaviors.

Such data suggest that play behavior, initially engaged in spontaneously by the caregiver, represents a vehicle through which the infant is encouraged to exercise predictive capacities to the fullest extent. Play not only reinforces the skills the infant has acquired, but also assists the infant in acquiring the ability to recognize and distinguish between differing emotional states and subsequently to display a particular response to elicit a desired reaction. It is from such interactions that the infant acquires a sense of mastery over his environment and begins to reconcile his predictions. Complementing these play sequences is the simultaneous caregiver previewing which serves not only to reinforce some of the experiences the infant has learned through play, but also to introduce the infant to upcoming skills that may be incorporated into experimental play episodes to see how these future skills will impact their relationship. If the caregiver has provided the infant with optimal stimulation, the transition between play and previewing will occur smoothly.

The Contribution of Cognitive Processing

The above discussion focuses on how play behavior can contribute to and reinforce infant socioemotional functioning during the first year of life. We turn now to an examination of how play behaviors are related to the infant's cognitive maturational processes. Numerous researchers, including Stern (1985), Tronick, Cohn, and Shea (1986), Field, Woodson, Greenberg and Cohen (1982), Meltzoff and Moore (1983a,b), and Tamis-LeMonda and Bornstein (1989) have commented on a phenomenon observed from the first days of life onward involving the infant's proclivity to create active, mental representations of the interactions with the environment. This tendency, which begins to surface gradually during the first few weeks of life and becomes more prominent as the infant develops, has been referred to as the mechanism of *intrinsic motivation*. Intrinsic motivation describes the infant's compelling desire to gain knowledge about the external world and to engage in problem-solving which results in mastery over the environment. Indeed, this tendency may be viewed as the analog of the caregiver's desire to represent future achievements and to stimulate the infant through previewing exercises. The developmental progression that occurs during infancy involves the acquisition of knowledge and the formulation of a series of representations, facilitating the infant's transition from situations with which he is familiar to situations with which he is unfamiliar. This shift entails the coordination of various cognitive operations. The motivation for mobilizing or demobilizing such operations is catalyzed by the degree of positive affect infants experience upon exposure to either too much or too little novelty. A kind of push-pull effect between pleasure and displeasure, stimulates infants to progress cognitively. To enhance his pleasure, the infant also begins to manipulate representations to devise predictable sequences. Play serves to reinforce the pleasurable affect associated with the experience of a predictable outcome and propels the infant to seek more novel experiences. Play and previewing behavior, therefore, serve as synergistic forms of activity in the sense that each stimulates more of the other kind of behavior.

Contingent stimulation is significant during play behavior because, as was noted in an earlier chapter, contingent stimulation elicits positive affect and this positive emotional atmosphere is an indispensable ingredient of play, as observed by Papousek, Papousek and Harris. A caregiver who repeatedly alters play behaviors prior to the infant's ability to represent them hinders the infant's abilities to perceive contingent relationships. Failure to acquire an understanding of contingency relationships during infancy may, in turn, lead to subsequent experiences of helplessness. This is because the infant has been deprived of the experience of learning to predict the caregiver's responses and may, as a result, come to view the caregiver as an uncontrollable force whose manifestations are beyond prediction, and hence, control. During the first months of life, the infant needs to receive specific responses to his behaviors. The caregiver's responses during this period will either support the infant's predictions or provide him with a series of disjointed, noncontingent experiences. In order for genuine play sequences to occur, infants need to be able to test their predictions about the world within the confines of the play activity and to anticipate future courses of action manifested in this form of play, which is a kind of previewing. These capacities enable the infant to feel that he can effectively predict and control the environment to meet his needs. To arrive at this point, the caregiver-infant interaction must provide the infant with a significant number of contingency experiences from which mastery and control will later be derived.

Researchers have emphasized the role of imitative behaviors during play in the first year of life. Trevarthen (1985) writes that infants often imitate their caregiver's facial expression by exaggerating the mouth or protruding the tongue, thereby manifesting a capacity to correlate the facial structure and motivations of another with their own motivations and facial structure. Field et al. (1986) state that imitative behaviors may be observed within the first weeks following birth, and that these behaviors increase to an optimal level at two months and then decrease as infancy progresses. They note that it is not clear why imitative behaviors decrease in this fashion, although it may be that the infant has habituated to the behavior and is motivated to find more stimulating challenges. One reason why imitative behaviors may eventually diminish is because the infant begins to initiate behaviors on his own. It is, in other words, no longer imitation per se that stimulates the infant. Rather, he varies representational patterns to elicit a previewing response from the caregiver.

The imitation behaviors engaged in by young infants suggest that they are formulating internal representations about visual perceptions. Once the ability to imitate the expressions of the caregiver is attained, along with the concomitant capacity to control facial muscles, the infant may prefer to communicate his own feelings rather than to imitate those of another. Thereafter, although the infant remains dependent on the parent for interaction, he relies upon his own ability to self-regulate. Imitative behaviors may, however, also diminish for another reason. As the months pass, the process through which the infant previously imitated behaviors may have been inculcated, assuming the form of a mental representation or schema. This schema can be readily recollected by the infant throughout childhood as numerous novel play tasks begin to appear. Thus, when the infant begins playing with paints, blocks or even peers, he may initially imitate the social and cognitive behaviors of his playmates. Once mastered, however, these skills may decrease as the child now possesses the capacity to represent and incorporate imitated skills into his own repertoire of behaviors. Gradually, as the infant develops and the imitative behaviors subside, the imitative process becomes divorced from the play skill learned. Imitation thus becomes a vehicle whereby new representations are acquired; once the skill is acquired, however, the amount of imitation recedes and the behaviors are incorporated into the infant's or child's personal play repertoire.

Vocalizations represent the third behavioral feature of early play interaction. As noted in Chapter 2, caregivers intuitively alter speech patterns in the presence of their newborns by exaggerating tone and pitch patterns, elongating vowels and, in general, modulating vocalization to a form that can be experienced meaningfully by the infant. Stern (1979) has reported that the three- to four-month-old is capable of discriminating vowel sounds from other sounds. Evidence suggests that by six months, the infant can differentiate between pitch, sound levels and speech patterns and that by approximately seven months, the infant can begin to predict the parent's vocalizations when they are accompanied by a gesture. Finally, by one year, vocalizations are comprehended without their gestural counterparts. Stevenson, Ver Hoeve, Roach and Leavitt (1986) found that caregivers may employ vocalizations both to orient the infant's attention and to communicate. At least during the first six months of life, it is probably not that significant whether the infant understands linguistically the precise meaning of the vocal sounds. Rather, as Trevarthen (1985) points out, what is important is that the infant begins using his own vocalizations-in the form of cooing, laughing or crying-to predict a desired response from the caregiver and to convey to the caregiver the need to regulate the degree of stimulation. These responses are known to result in pleasurable affect, a key characteristic of both play and previewing behavior.

Contingency responses manifested by the caregiver can also affect the development of language, according to Stevenson et al., and based on the research of Lewis et al., may impact on the subsequent unfolding of socioemotional and cognitive skills. Stern and Gibbon (1978) argue that the infant depends not only on the contingent behaviors of the caregiver, but also on the specific timing of these behaviors. They posit that during dyadic interaction, the infant learns to predict responses within the given time span based on previous responses. The infant tests his expectancies against the stimuli received and then regulates or modifies expectancies to the stimulus response to generate a previewing behavior. Contingent responses are thus necessary to provide the infant with a foundation upon which to anticipate and form hypotheses concerning future experience. Moreover, it is the caregiver who must stimulate the infant's contingency awareness by exposing him to sufficient stimulus-response sequences.

Substantiating the observation that mastery of new situations and cognitive challenges results in enhanced predictive abilities and that play, in turn, provokes the infant to seek out new challenges, is the work of Messer, McCarthy, McQuiston, MacTurk, Yarrow and Vietze (1986). This team observed infants aged six to twelve months during twenty-four-minute play sessions. McCarthy's Scales of Children's Abilities (McCarthy, 1972) were used to evaluate their performance at thirty months. It was found that infant mastery behavior demonstrated during play strongly predicted scores of the McCarthy scales. The researchers emphasized that infants who spent more time investigating toys at six months and who devoted greater persistence to solving tasks at twelve months revealed higher McCarthy scores. These findings suggest a relationship between mastery behavior and subsequent displays of cognitive functioning in the direction of prediction. The inclination to engage in previewing exercises and to master new problems, which can emerge most clearly in a play setting, may then represent an important contribution to the process of development.

Further evidence that both members of the dyad influence the outcome of developmental achievement comes from studies with premature infants. One research team who investigated this issue, Landry, Chapieski, and Schmidt (1986), examined the relationship between maternal attention-directing strategies during play and corresponding infant responsiveness to such behaviors in forty preterm and twenty full-term infants of one year of age. The findings of the study indicated that, in fact, mothers of preterms employed attention-directing strategies that were significantly different from the strategies manifested by mothers of full-terms. It is important for therapists dealing with caregivers of preterm infants to recognize that such differences exist and to help foster acceptance of what may be temporary developmental delays in infant responsiveness. Such infants may be slower in developing the capacity to formulate representations and predictive sequences, and, as illustrated in Chapter 3, the caregivers of such infants may be hesitant about providing appropriate developmental stimulation. Landry et al. found that, when health care personnel explained the infant's condition, such caregivers were better able to manifest an appropriate response. Despite the developmental lags that may be encountered with premature infants, the caregiver's stimulation remains vital in order that appropriate play and previewing behaviors emerge at a pace attuned to the infant's development.

Symbolic Play

The above discussion has highlighted the numerous mechanisms involved in play sequences between the infant and caregiver during the first months of life. Yet, it is not sufficient to simply declare that exaggerated vocalizations, facial expressions and soothing gestures, all packaged within a segment of interaction between caregiver and infant, comprise the main elements of play. Nor is it enough to say that play behavior is distinctive because it creates a positive affective mood within the dyad or because during a playful exchange infants are engaging in a more advanced cognitive operations. We may say that play is different because, although cognitive skills are being exercised, no precise goal is attained; that is, infants and their caregivers engage in play solely for the sheer pleasure and exuberance that is generated by sharing an experience. Part of this pleasure derives from the fact that during previewing exercises the infant is generating representations to formulate predictions about future interactions. Both the emergence of representations and the validation of such predictions allows the infants to assert control within the interpersonal arena; in other words, the infant *assesses* the present, represents how he is going to *assert* himself in the future and finally, *validates* such predictions. Indeed, play may be viewed as an arena within which previewing emerges.

One feature of play that first surfaces and consolidates in the second year of life is its *pretend* or *symbolic* quality. According to Lowe (1975) symbolic play presupposes not only that the child's actions have acquired meaning in relation to the objects around him, but also that his ability to represent an absent object or experience by means of his own action, usually with the aid of objects that resemble the represented content of the object or experience that is absent. Moreover, one significant developmental phenomenon associated with this type of play is the emergence of language, which also relies upon the acquisition of symbolic representation. This is because with language particular words or symbols which are arbitrarily chosen come to represent persons or things. As language evolves, the infant acquires the capacity to engage in digital forms of communication.

What is meant by symbolic in this context? Essentially, symbolic play emerges from developmental progression. Hughes (1987) argues that first the child engages in manipulative play activities, during which objects are explored and representations of the object are learned. Manipulative play eventually yields to representational play, during which the child repeats behaviors that he has seen enacted by others, such as cleaning the house or drawing a car. Symbolic play surfaces as the child begins to integrate the reenactments he has experimented with during representational play around one creative theme, as for example, the acting out of doctor and nurse roles or the pretence of an expedition to a foreign land.

Both symbolic play and language represent ways in which the child exerts control and mastery over his experience. De Gramont (1987) writes that if the child obtains sense of participation and control through the organizational experience of language, then anxiety will be staved off, since feelings of helplessness are only present when meaning has broken down. The researcher explains that the symbolism inherent in language emerges when a *functional relationship* exists between the symbol and its felt experience. That is, the experimental persona that has undergone the event is capable of reflecting upon the event and has become an objectified "me." This transformation of perspectives from the subjective (the experimental "I") to the objective (the objectified "me") lies at the core of symbolic thought.

As has been noted, during the first months of life play is initiated by the caregiver who uses a variety of intuitive behaviors (including visual cuing, vocal cuing and touch) to stimulate a reciprocal reaction in the infant. This reaction creates pleasurable affect in both the caregiver and the infant. The caregiver's pleasure derives from the fact that she obtains a reaction from the baby. The infant's pleasure involves the repetition of these sequences, as he represents the interaction cognitively and predicts how the caregiver will behave. When these predictions or expectations are fulfilled the infant experiences gratification and a sense of mastery over previously unpredictable and uncontrollable events. Eventually, the caregiver will repeat these sequences to reinforce the positive feelings she shares with the infant and these kinds of repetitive sequences may be characterized as "play."

It takes approximately six months for this type of play to emerge. Thereafter the caregiver's focus will shift to more functional and relational play, whose goal it is to acquaint the infant with the variety of objects and people he encounters in the world. During this phase, the cognitive aspect of play moves to the fore, as the caregiver strives to teach the infant various gestures and introduces him to an array of objects and their functional uses. Cognitive capacities and physical manifestations here become associated with one another and this form of association paves the way for subsequent symbolic abilities. The caregiver now uses the developmental skills the infant has already displayed to engage in this form of play and, therefore, such play can be distinguished from previewing, whereby the caregiver strives to acquaint the infant with his own imminent, although not yet realized, developmental capacities.

Functional and relational play tend to dominate from the later half of the first year through well into the second year. However, by late in the second year, a distinct change may be noted in the infant's play activities. Now he initiates more of such behaviors than the caregiver and, significantly, creativity emerges, as the infant begins to vary and experiment with patterns on his own. At this point, the infant is displaying the distinct qualities of symbolic representation. The infant feels secure and familiar with these schemes. But new developmental skills of discrepancy, contingency and expectancy have taught the infant that these skills can be experimental and that the objects in the world may be manipulated. Moreover, by this juncture the infant has come to recognize that his "self" is distinct from the "self" of the caregiver, a recognition of the delineation of boundaries. If the caregiver is supportive, the infant's recognition of this "self-other" differentiation will not be traumatic but will instead motivate the infant to develop even more sophisticated means of interacting with "other" of the caregiver. One way of motivating such interaction involves adopting the perspective of the other. Hence, the infant begins experimenting with the notion that he can initiate behaviors in the same way that the caregiver previously initiated behaviors. Eventually, the infant recognizes that he is not only capable of imitating the "other," but also that he can view himself as an "other" and can plan or create new activities for himself. The caregiver who provides the infant with sufficient stimulation fuels this capacity. With this realization on the part of the infant, symbolic representation is born.

Symbolic thought means that the infant understands that one object which has a particular function or meaning can also have another very different function or meaning simultaneously and without confusing its identity. A spoon, for example, may be an eating utensil but at the same time, may also serve as a different object that the infant has devised. As will be seen in the following chapters this ability to engage in symbolic thought correlates significantly with the child's capacity to understand the fundamental principles of language. Language, after all, is composed of arbitrary symbols (in the form of words) that stand for objects and ideas. Until the infant comes to recognize that one object can have more than one meaning simultaneously, the intricacies of both symbolic thought and language will escape him. As has been seen in this discussion, play is one way in which the child is able to exercise and experiment with his novel ability to engage in symbolic thought.

Role-Playing

During the first months of life, the play sequences occurring within the dyad are characterized by *reciprocity,* which reinforces the infant's predictive abilities. Reciprocal feedback in infancy may serve as a precursor to the role-playing behaviors apparent in the make-believe activities of later childhood during which the child must empathize and enact the behaviors of another. Mutual regulation during dyadic interaction may also predict the child's later development of social play behavior with peers. Failure may result in frustration during play with peers, and the preschooler who has not acquired the skills of mutual sharing may retreat into solitary play behaviors, further isolating himself from others and perpetuating feelings of alienation. Thus, the caregiver's ability to stimulate the infant through play and previewing to establish reciprocal responsiveness during the first two years of life is vital.

The reciprocal and predictive quality that imbues play sequences during the first year of life has been variously described. Trevarthen (1985) characterizes such interaction within the dyad as *turn-taking,* in which one partner solicits the other's attention while the other partner responds with gaze behavior or vocalization, giving the initiating partner, once again, an opportunity to respond. Such interactions are typified by a give-and-take flavor in which infant and caregiver repeatedly exchange communications between themselves. It is important to note how such interaction may go awry. As observed earlier, by the fourth month, the infant can represent the caregiver's facial expressions, vocalizations and body movements, and consequently, can predict specific interactional sequences with the caregiver. But if the caregiver fails to respond adequately to the infant's signals, the infant will eventually withdraw or emit signs of distress. In such situations, the infant may be torn between his need to elicit stimulation from the caregiver and his desire to avoid the caregiver's negativity or nonresponsive attitude. If this pattern is repeated, the caregiver's nonresponsiveness may exert detrimental developmental effects upon the infant who depends upon the caregiver for his initial exposure to contingency-related concepts (Trevarthen and Hubley, 1979).

The infant's budding awareness of contingency relationships, which comes to fruition by approximately the third month of life, also plays a role in enhancing the capacity for play. According to Lewis, Wolan-Sullivan and Brooks-Gunn (1985), the caregiver's contingent responses to the infant provide the infant with feelings of *efficacy* and *control* during play interaction. This sense of mastery is vital in motivating the infant to devise ways of further maintaining the dyadic interaction. From as early as three months of age, infants begin to respond to stimuli contingent upon the responses received and to learn to expect specific responses from their caregivers. These expectancies serve as the foundation from which the infant will eventually devise predictions about the future. Failure to elicit such responses from the parent may result in the infant experiencing feelings of lack of control which, in turn, may be generalized by the infant to feelings about his own development. The infant's failure to experience contingent learning from his caregiver may predict future deficits during play situations and, as a result, cognitive and affective deficits may ensue. Failure to experience contingency also prevents the infant from experimenting with his burgeoning predictive skills and ultimately from gaining knowledge during previewing exercises.

While Trevarthen coined the phrase of "turn-taking" to describe the reciprocal quality suffusing dyadic play during the first few months of life, Tronick, Cohn and Shea (1986) define early infant-caregiver interaction in terms of a *mutual regulation* model. They note that the infant employs gaze behaviors, emotional expressions and vocalizations in order to control social exchange with the caregiver. When the infant transmits expressions to the caregiver, for example, he meets with either success or failure; if the caregiver responds effectively to the infant, success has been achieved, but if the caregiver either misattunes, thereby creating the experience of noncontingency, or ignores the infant, thereby creating the experience of neglect, feeling of failure, which suffuses the entire dyad may be created. Under this scenario, the infant's predictive capacities will be stifled. For Tronick, Cohn and Shea, parental failure to respond adequately to the infant depends on factors outside the immediate play environment. For example, the caregiver's own socioemotional history will have a significant impact on how she responds to the infant, and the kind of affect displayed by the caregiver will, in turn, influence infant response.

To learn to observe himself in an objectified manner, the infant first needs to adopt the perspective of the other. This requires an understanding that the other, most frequently the caregiver, has feelings and perceptions that are different from those of the infant. Researchers have labeled this understanding as *intersubjectivity*. Related to the quality of intersubjectivity is the quality of *subjectivity* which refers to the infant's capacity to realize that he has feelings and perceptions that may be separate and distinct from those of the caregiver. Once the infant recognizes his separateness, he eventually comes to understand that he is an independent actor who responds to the behaviors of the caregiver, as well as an autonomous initiator of behaviors of his own. But this sense of separateness also motivates the infant to seek ways of continuing the dyadic rapport in order to acquire greater mastery and control over the environment.

Moreover, just as the infant forms representations of the other, so too does he gradually develop representations of his own activities. During play, the infant begins to experiment with these representations, envisioning actions and emotional responses, and attributing them to himself. Throughout this activity the infant is experimenting with the notion that he is simultaneously creating these play interactions and developing behavioral sequences for himself. Thus, he is capable of bifurcating his perception of himself into "self" and "other." As a result of this bifurcation, the infant comes to recognize that the image he envisions in his fantasies is not himself as much as it is a *symbol* of himself. In this way, the process of representational thought, which began to emerge as early as the third month of life when the infant experienced inculcating schemes of discrepancy and contingency, ultimately culminates in the ability to represent symbolically.

Conclusion

As this discussion indicates, play behavior during the first year of life permits the infant to enter an arena teeming with activity within which he can experiment with his ability to predict caregiver behaviors and to design his own behaviors for eliciting a particular caregiver response. Even more significantly, however, it is within this arena that the relationship between caregiver and infant is cemented and fortified. As the infant's partner, the caregiver must gradually stimulate the infant to expand his abilities to both explore the environment around him, and subsequently, to return to the secure base that the caregiver represents to reassess and exercise his new acquisitions. Through such activities, the infant acquires an awareness that the environment is a predictable domain with the potential of being mastered and controlled.

Although play behavior inevitably becomes more sophisticated and more evident during the second year of life, it is from the contours of play in the first months of life that clues to the nature of previewing can best be ascertained. Thus, when treating caregiver-infant pairs in which the infant is under two years of age, the therapist must observe patterns of stimulus-response, the degree of contingency associations provided and the facility with which the caregiver is able to introduce discrepancy into the infant's experience. Significantly, the therapist should monitor the degree to which the interaction is imbued with both play and previewing activity, because from these skills the infant's sense of self emerges in a consolidated and integrated fashion. Moreover, it is important to focus on how the infant uses play to experiment with previewing behaviors and to generate predictable responses. By being alerted to these phenomena, diagnostic assessment and treatment will be dramatically facilitated.

CHAPTER 6

Language: A Paradigm for Tracing Previewing Behaviors

Introduction

As discussed in earlier chapters, recent studies reveal that even from the first days of life behaviors that resemble previewing manifestations may be used by the caregiver to stimulate the infant's future developmental acquisition. Interactions that incorporate previewing behaviors are designed to not only assist the infant in surviving in the alien and sometimes treacherous world outside of the womb, but also to guide the infant in the cumulative mastery of adaptational skills that are increasingly more complex and intricate. Clinical evidence gathered from observing dyadic interactions suggests that both the intuitive behaviors of the caregiver and the constitutional endowment of the infant play a key role in determining the outcome of the infant's developmental destiny. As a result, by focusing on the interactional environment the pathway of development becomes predictable to the outward observer and, as the infant becomes attuned to the external milieu, eventually becomes predictable to the infant as well.

An illustration may serve to better explain the predictable nature of developmental phenomena. Several researchers have focused on the infant's acquisition of language skills during the first two years of life. It has been noted, for example, that within a few weeks of birth, infants can distinguish between different sounds. By four months, infants are capable of recognizing the sound of their mother's voice and prefer the maternal voice over other human voices. Within a few more months, infants begin imitating sounds, reference certain sounds by such gestures as pointing, and show intention through gaze alternation. Towards the end of the first year, a phenomenon referred to as *canonical babbling* has been reported. Canonical babbling involves connecting a consonant and vowel sound, such as "ma" to form precursory words.

Researchers speculate that the next step in the linguistics process is the infant's ability to recognize that specific words or sounds represent specific objects. Shortly thereafter, intersubjectivity, the capacity to comprehend that others are individuals with representational abilities separate and distinct from the infant's representations, evolves. Ultimately, the infant acquires the ability to think and communicate in a symbolic fashion and to use words literally as well as metaphorically.

From this brief sketch of the developmental attainment of language, one can see a gradual sophistication and coalescence of both the infant's representational and predictive abilities. From observing language development it is also apparent that, as the infant develops, his ability to represent increasingly complex patterns and his need to experience more previewing behaviors intensifies. Indeed, it may be argued that previewing is an organizing principle of development, which allows the infant to anticipate the implications of social interaction, and to exert mastery and control over these interactions. As a result, when considered in its entirety, the developmental process represents for the infant a perpetual previewing of experiences.

This chapter will use the example of language acquisition to explore how previewing stimulates the infant's innate capacities, and in particular, the infant's ability to exert mastery over future social interactions. Moreover, the caregiver's participation in this process, as an auxiliary supporter of the infant's acquisitions, will also be discussed. Throughout this chapter, the example of language acquisition will be used to give the reader an understanding of the orderly and hierarchical process of development. Linguistic skills are used here for several reasons. First, virtually all infants, regardless of whether they come from a supportive environment or from the deprivations that attend institutionalization, learn to speak by the end of the second year of life. This fact suggests that although language acquisition may be enhanced by an enriched environment, it is largely propelled by constitutional capacities inherent in the infant from birth. Thus, even infants from deprived backgrounds learn to make some predictions about the world and to use their predictive skill in learning to speak. Second, language itself is an ideal example of a skill that helps the infant anticipate social events. The ability to express our thoughts verbally presupposes our ability to conceive of ideas before they become objectified in the external world. Similarly, as the infant learns to speak, he is also honing his skills in the area of anticipatory representation. Thus, the following discussion will rely heavily on the work of researchers in the area of linguistics in order to provide an analogue for understanding how previewing allows the infant to develop the capacity to anticipate and predict the world around him.

The Relation of Dyadic Regulation to Language Expression

Antenatal Regulation

Clinical evidence indicates that speech acquisition and predictive abilities are part of the global, all-encompassing process of coordinating maturational capacities that is apparent from the first days of life. Condon and

Sander (1974a,b) explored this theme by examining the degree of synchronization between neonatal movement and adult speech. The researchers found that as early as the first day of life, the human neonate moves in a precise and sustained fashion that appears to be synchronous with the structure articulated in adult speech. Condon and Sander found that all of the infant's body parts that moved (including brows, eyes and mouth) displayed synchrony to adult vocalization. Microanalysis of sound films was used to detect key gestures, postures, and configurations of infant movement that accompanied adult speech. When these methods were applied to the study of the interaction between neonate and caregiver, a synchronization of infant movement with the articulatory aspects of adult speech was found. From these findings we may surmise that the infant begins to formulate predictions about stimuli from the first days of life onwards.

This study suggests that from the first days of life the infant moves in rhythm with the organization of the caregiver's interactions, and that he begins to represent speech through complex, sociobiological entrainment in numerous repetitions of linguistic forms. This process appears to begin long before the infant actually uses these forms in direct speaking and communicating. By the time the infant begins to speak, then, he may have already internally represented the form and structure of the language system of his culture. According to the researchers, this would encompass a multiplicity of linguistic elements, including rhythmic and syntactic hierarchies, segmenting features, and paralinguistic nuances, not to mention body motion styles and rhythms. Each of these elements is transformed by the infant into a representation that reflects how each of the speech elements is experienced. The Condon and Sandler study, then, highlights the significance of exposure to adult vocalization cues, in the form of baby talk, early in life. Such cues likely play a key role in stimulating the infant and reinforcing predictable patterns.

Observing the synchrony between adult speech and neonatal body movement raises issues about the nature of communication, and particularly about the role of the auditory function in development. It may be that the infant's early attraction to adult speech stems from the fact that speech stimulates representational skills, a key prerequisite for predicting interactional patterns with the caregiver.

While we have outlined the developmental capacities that seem to be largely inherent to the infant, the caregiver's role in encouraging the infant to predict communication, in terms of generating, imitating and reinforcing affective expression and cognitive maturation through dyadic interaction, is crucial.

One innovative study, conducted by DeCasper and Spence (1986), demonstrates that infants are so predisposed to the development of the predictive capacities of language that they may be capable of recognizing the maternal voice prenatally. Infants demonstrate this by displaying a *preference* for the maternal voice, which assists them in their acquisition of language skills. Moreover, a preference for female voices over male voices in general and a preference for intrauterine heartbeat sounds over male voices has also been shown (Brazelton, 1978; DeCasper and Fifer, 1980). DeCasper and Spence reported that neonates do *not* respond like passive and neutral listeners to vocalizations. Instead, they display a distinct preference to their own mother's voice over the voices of other females.

In the study examined here, it was confirmed that third-trimester fetuses may either "hear" or at least exhibit a behavioral responsiveness to particular kinds of sounds. Based on their experiemnt, DeCasper and Spence concluded that prenatal experience with maternal speech sounds causes some characteristics of the sounds to be *differentially* reinforcing after birth because the infant remembers, represents, and thereby responds to the sound when it is repeated. The researchers hypothesize that speech sounds provide exposure to at least two kinds of discrimination. First, speech cues foster awareness of the discrimination of sounds that is relevant to language per se. Second, hearing the sounds of the mother's voice prenatally conditions the infant to begin predicting after birth the identity of the speaker and the source of the sounds. Discrimination of this type suggests that some rudimentary predictive capacity may be stimulated in utero.

In the DeCasper and Spence investigation, thirty-three healthy women who were approximately seven-and-a-half months pregnant were recruited. All were experiencing uncomplicated pregnancies. After becoming familiar with three short children's stories, the expectant women taped all the stories. Each woman was then assigned one target story. The women were instructed to read their target story aloud twice each day in a quiet place, so that their voice would be the only sound the baby would hear. After the infants were born, sixteen of them were reexposed to the target story. Response was based on the incidence of sucking bursts displayed by the infant. In comparison to a control group, it was found that infants who were exposed to the story prenatally by their caregivers displayed a heightened response that indicated the capacity to recognize and predict the caregiver's voice.

The researchers reported that several implications may be derived from their findings. First, exposed infants found the target story more reinforcing than exposure to a novel story because the target story reconfirmed an earlier representation. Second, the researchers found that the target story had reinforcing potential for infants who appeared incapable of distinguishing between the two stories. DeCasper and Spence concluded that fetuses are therefore capable of learning and predicting something about acoustic cues. In particular, after birth these infants responded to such subtleties as syllable beat, consonants and harmonic structure.

In a later study, the same research team (Spence and DeCasper, 1987), demonstrated that infants who had experienced antenatal exposure to their caregiver's voices, learned to recognize contingency sequences far more rapidly than infants who had not been exposed. This finding suggests that predictive capacities may proliferate once the infant learns to recognize stimuli and becomes conditioned to them. The researchers also replicated their previous findings in addition to ascertaining that previously exposed infants would "learn" particular contingencies more rapidly.

Postnatal Regulation

These last two studies demonstrate persuasively the effects of the potent combination of both the infant's inherent developmental capacities for predicting and the caregiver's stimulation of the infant through exposure to contingencies. Moreover, these research findings underscore the significance of an attentive caregiver who provides adequate stimulation for the infant. Both factors operate to spur on the inevitable unfolding of development of more enhanced infant predictive abilities, which results in heightened control and mastery over the environment.

Further evidence of the infant's acute capacity for recognizing and predicting the nuances of language was provided by Fernald and Kuhl (1987) who examined the acoustical determinants of infant preference for *motherese speech*. Earlier studies had demonstrated that when speaking to infants and young children, adults modify their speech patterns dramatically (Snow, 1977). Researchers have reported that adults characteristically employ a more simplified syntax and vocabulary, consisting of one and two syllable words, interspersed with special phrases of affection, when addressing infants (Ferguson, 1964). Also typical are the higher pitches, larger pauses, shorter utterances, and greater instances of repetition, as well as more intonation and prosody (Menn and Boyce, 1982; Stern, Spieker, Barnett, and MacKain, 1983; Fernald and Simon, 1984). Considered individually, it becomes clear how each of these phenomena gradually reinforce the infant's representational and predictive capacities. In addition, adaptive caregivers tend to manifest these qualities frequently when engaging in vocal cuing during previewing episodes with their infants.

In conducting their investigation, Fernald and Kuhl used three experiments to explore the acoustic determinations of infant listening preference for this type of motherese speech. To examine whether the intonation of such speech was sufficient to elicit a preference, the researchers isolated three acoustic correlates of intonation, including the fundamental frequency or pitch of speech, the amplitude or loudness of speech, and the duration of speech. A group of twenty four-month-olds were tested while listening to prerecorded tapes of their mothers' voices. It was found that the infants displayed a marked preference for the patterns of motherese speech, but not for the amplitude or duration of motherese. This preference for patterns is significant because it suggests that infants may become conditioned more readily to repeated configurations of speech that are continually reinforced by the caregiver. When repeated speech sequences are combined with appropriate affective cues from the caregiver, the infant may come to recognize and represent such speech as a contingent experience and will be motivated to devise behaviors that will elicit this pattern of speech from the caregiver.

The researchers concluded that it is the fundamental frequency of infant-directed speech that accounts for the infant's acoustic preference for motherese. Frequency, it should be remembered, enhances the infants capacity to discern recognizable and predictable sequences. In this context, frequency reinforces a contingency experience. In interpreting these findings, it is important to keep the limitations of the study in mind. Specifically, the study segmented various aspects of motherese to create verbal cues that are not generally encountered in daily experience. In the familiar speech adults direct to infants, the exaggerated modulation of fundamental frequency is inevitably mingled with distinctive patterns of intensity and rhythm. Furthermore, mothers typically coordinate facial expression and other gestures with their vocalizations during affective interactions with their infants, (Stern 1974, 1985). While exaggerated pitch may be a particularly compelling acoustic characteristic of motherese speech, its effectiveness is undoubtedly enhanced by the dynamic mix of vocal and visual behaviors that are coordinated with acoustic quality. This study, then, provides some qualified evidence of the infant's inherent abilities to predict, recognize and express a preference for the speech of the mother within the first months of life.

The distinct infant preference for motherese speech has several implications. First, this preference suggests that the infant has come to recognize patterns or contingencies that occur during an episode of maternal speech and seeks to reexperience these contingencies by cuing the caregiver to continue the interaction. Second, since human conversation generally occurs in an interactive framework, exposure to motherese reinforces the notion that in order to experience such contingencies one must seek the attention of another. Lastly, the infant's proclivity for motherese indicates that the infant has begun to represent interactive sequences predictive of certain speech patterns and correlating behaviors.

Indeed, the Fernald and Kuhl study suggests that two significant factors play a role in fostering these skills. The first involves the inherent constitutional component that establishes a predisposition for recognizing and responding to human verbal sounds. This predisposition to human rhythmic noises may stem from the fact that the first sounds to which the infant is exposed occur in utero in the form of the mother's heartbeat and other physiological sounds. The second factor that contributes to infant acquisition of language skill is the caregiver's encouragement of the infant's innate responsiveness to human sounds. Such encouragement occurs from the first days of life onwards in the form of characteristic moth-erese, and continues well into the second year as the caregiver continues to preview inchoate conversation to the infant.

Trevarthen (1980, 1985) has provided ample evidence of how the infant begins to engage in the discriminatory behavior indicative of predictive abilities. By examining infants from two months on during exchange with their caregivers, Trevarthen was able to trace the evolution of an intact communicative network which is notable not only because it provides insights into how the infant ultimately learns to communicate, but also because it indicates that developmental processes are motivated in part by ability to predict maternal behavior. According to Trevarthen, such interactions allow the infant to generalize his experience across other sit-uations in the external world.

In observations of six-week-old infants, Trevarthen witnessed a pattern of interaction with the caregiver in which infants displayed a pleasurable affect during periods of sustained eye contact. Also during these inter-vals, the infant would periodically evince lip and tongue movements cou-pled with hand gestures. Trevarthen labeled this form of communicative behavior *prespeech,* observing that it appears to represent a rudimentary form of articulation that several months later will eventually evolve into the form of phonetic vocalizations known as babbling. Significantly, mothers are reported to be able to interpret and attribute meaning to this interactive behavior. As a result, such prespeech may be among the care-giver's initial efforts to expose the infant to mature forms of language through previewing.

By three months, according to Trevarthen, more sophistication in the communicative network can be observed during microanalytic assess-ments of the infant-caregiver exchange. For example, communication ap-pears to follow an almost rehearsed *turn-taking pattern,* whereby both partners begin sending recurring messages. As the mother calls the infant, the infant orients to the sound of her voice and focuses strongly on the mother's face, giving preferential treatment to the eye area. Trevarthen also reported that at approximately this developmental period caregivers begin imitating the infant's facial expression and that the infant mirrors back this expression. Each of the infant's behaviors in Trevarthen's ex-ample indicates a kind of *intentionality,* as if the infant purposefully wishes to engage in more sophisticated interpersonal sequences and to continue to predict the caregiver's behaviors. From these observations of three-month-olds and their caregivers during episodes of interaction, Trevarthen concluded that the expressive manifestations of the dyad are governed by principles of internal coordination. Both infant and caregiver regulate their relationship with a system of coactivation, turn-taking, re-ciprocation and contingency response that suffuses all of their engage-ments. The rhythm inherent in these interactions suggests that each dy-adic member has learned to predict the behaviors of the other.

Jaffe, Stern and Peery (1973) have contributed to the understanding of this dynamic by observing that the mother generally assists the infant in regulating mood states. One aspect of this regulatory assistance is apparent by patterns of eye contact between caregiver and infant. Bloom (1989) for example, has explored the nature of early infant vocal sounds, and has noted that well in advance of the infant's first words inchoate dialogues, characterized by turn-taking, occur between adults and infants that rely upon vocalization. Moreover, this researcher confirms the findings of others that the quality of the adult's vocal input, as defined by timing and verbal quality, has an effect on the quality of the infant's prelinguistic responses. In particular, verbal input that included turn-taking had been found to facilitate the production of syllabic sounds in three-month-old infants. To explain why this phenomenon occurs, Bloom (1988) has suggested that the neuromuscular turn-taking, combined with verbal turn-taking, may have a soothing effect, and the quiet state that occurs during pauses might give infants the enhanced respiratory and neuromotor control necessary for the production of vocalizations of a longer duration.

In Bloom's study, the duration of all nondistress, nonvegetative vocalizations was measured. It was hypothesized that syllabic sounds would be longer than vocalic sounds and that verbal turn-taking would increase the duration of all sounds. Syllabic sounds were defined as those which had greater oral resonance and pitch contour, sounded more relaxed and were produced toward the front of the mouth with the mouth open and moving frequently. In contrast, all other cooing sounds were classified as vocalic, and they generally had more nasal resonance, were more often produced toward the back of the mouth, were more uniform in pitch, and seemed more effortful. In analyzing the duration of sounds, syllabic and vocalic sounds were the dependent variables and adult turn-taking and vocal social input were considered the independent variables.

The researcher pointed out that between the second and fourth month of life developmental increases in duration may have profound effects on the quality of vocal sounds. Increased duration of vocalization is a medium for the maturation and modulation of sound quality. The basis for the development of increased duration of phonation has been well documented and increased duration in the third month of life remains partly a function of change in the infant's physiology, including the position of the rib cage, the descent of the larynx and the release from obligate nasal breathing. Paralleling these physiological developments is the increased quantity of vocalizations by these infants, as reported by Bloom and others. Thus, although the advent of language itself signifies a significant turning point in the infant's maturation, even by the third month of life, which is well prior to the onset of discernable speech, an incipient ommunication network is evident during interaction between adaptive mothers and their infants.

From this incipient system, the infant begins to anticipate the caregiver's verbalizations and to formulate representations of the caregiver's interactional behavior. This form of prediction arises because the infant is being increasingly exposed to contingent experiences on the part of the caregiver (Watson, 1977). Trevarthen explains that contingency may be understood as a stimulus-response manifestation. The earliest form of contingency occurs when the caregiver manifests a particular behavior in response to an infant cue. When repeated frequently, this sequence is transformed into a predictable cause-effect sequence by the infant. Stern and Gibbon (1980) have suggested that infants appear inherently stimulated by contingencies, which may be one reason why infants are more attracted to partners who interact with them by using a range of expressions and gestures. This attraction to contingency sequences during vocalization may be understood, in part, as an aspect of the infant's proclivity to seize upon any environmental phenomena that promotes predictive abilities.

Trevarthen's comments on the infant's evolving capacity to communicate are noteworthy, because this theory attempts to explain the processes whereby the infant comes to comprehend that the other, generally the caregiver, is distinct from the self of the infant. In developing this concept, Trevarthen noted that some of the nonverbal components of conversation may even be integrated into the infant's cognitive capacities prenatally. According to Trevarthen, even from the first weeks of life it appears that the infant is motivated to discern patterns in the world around him. Although it is up to the caregiver to provide the requisite stimulation, the motivation to be stimulated by predictable behaviors and contingent patterns, from which previewing behavior derives, is inherent in the infant.

In an effort to further identify the factors instrumental in motivating infants to engage in speech, several researchers have focused on *analogous* forms of communication between infants and their caregivers. Most notably, researchers have examined patterns of affective exchange that are common among dyads. Tronick, Cohn, and Shea (1986) proposed a mutual regulation model of early infant-caregiver social interchange that characterizes the adaptive dyadic system as one in which emotional messages are exchanged between the partners. Within this model, one partner achieves his or her goals during coordination or turn-taking with those of the other partner. The infant's behavior in this context meets the criteria usually advanced for goal directedness: persistence, use of multiple means to the same state, and appropriateness of actions. The main goal of this affective exchange is a shared positive emotional state.

According to Tronick et al., the ability of the caregiver and infant to mutually regulate the nature of the interaction has a fundamental effect on how the infant feels about himself, and in particular, on the child's feeling of effectance, the sense of what he can or cannot accomplish in the world. But this model applies to the caregiver as well. When the interaction flounders, the mother will experience a sense of failure. Moreover, because of the difference in their level of development, the infant's reactions are largely influenced by the immediate external and internal stimuli. The mother, however, is obviously more developed but is also affected by other factors impacting on her self-esteem.

Based on their observations of three-month-old infants interacting with their caregivers, Tronick et al. found a complex system of emotional communication which encompassed such diverse affective states as happiness, sadness, wariness, and protest. Mothers who were more emotionally sensitive to their infants had infants whose emotional repertoire was more comprehensive and who were adept at conveying messages back to the caregiver. This skill may be a prerequisite for later behaviors designed to elicit previewing from the caregiver.

Trevarthen (1979) has noted that for an infant to share emotional and cognitive awareness with another he must have two skills. First, he must be able to exhibit at least the rudimentary manifestations of self-consciousness and intentionality. Trevarthen refers to this attribute as *subjectivity*. In order to communicate, according to Trevarthen, infants must also be able to adapt or fit this subjective control to the subjective state of the other, meaning that they must be able to demonstrate empathy or awareness of the perceptions of another. This skill is referred to as *intersubjectivity*. Trevarthen has shown that emotional responsiveness is a form of communication that, in many respects, prefigures the advent of language.

Kopp (1989) has delineated the hypothetical pathway whereby the infant progresses from a system of emotional regulation that is dominated by affective states to emotional regulation that is dominated by the use of language. *Emotional regulation* is a term that Kopp uses to describe the process of coping with heightened emotions including joy, pleasure, distress, anger, fear. In Kopp's view, emotional regulation emerges like an orderly structure during the early years of life and is manifested in various behaviors engaged in by the infant. These behaviors involve manipulating a body part, vocalizations, play with an object and facial expression. At the same time, Kopp postulates that another form of emotional regulation, which the researcher refer to as *elemental cognitive*, develops in a parallel fashion to emotional maturation. The elemental cognitive mechanism combines perceptual discriminations of an event, memory of past experiences in similar situations and learned associations of contingencies.

In Kopp's model of development, the infant's emotional repertoire emerges within the first three months of life. At this point, the infant begins to develop a system for using emotions to predict cognition. By five months, infants show behaviors demonstrating communicative competence, suggesting that they expect their manifestations to be responded to by a supportive partner. As a result, a rudimentary communicative network has evolved whereby the infant has learned to use his emotions and the affective displays of the caregiver to predict future behaviors. Most likely, by engaging in previewing behavior adaptive caregivers reinforce this predictive ability in the infant.

At some point, however, communication via emotional display becomes insufficient for the infant who seeks a more sophisticated method for conveying his needs and reinforcing predictions about the future. Kopp theorizes that language fills this role by enabling children not only to experience emotions directly, but also to reflect upon and regulate them. Thus, by Kopp's reasoning, language skills begin to emerge in full force because the child has become adept at the use of emotions to predict behaviors and strives for a more complex way to regulate emotions in the future.

To elaborate upon the notions of motivation and stimulation mentioned earlier, Trevarthen posited an artificial dichotomy between the infant's motivational urge to know and predict the physical world and the infant's proclivity to explore and communicate with other people. He labeled the former tendency *subjectivity* and the latter tendency *intersubjectivity*. Within the category of subjective motivations, Trevarthen included the infant's desire:

1.) to seek unambiguous sensory information in a single field which unifies all modalities of sense;
2.) to gain comprehension of small objects perceived by virtue of independent a motion or by a boundary of high perceptual capacity, and to develop a facility in knowing and using objects by exploring their characteristics;
3.) to increase awareness by learning to attend to novel events and places, internally recording predictable patterns of response; and
4.) to maintain a coherent state of equilibrium while carrying out these activities.

In the category of intersubjective behavior, Trevarthen addressed such Manifestations as:

1.) coordinating closely with the holding, feeding and cleaning movements of the mother and encouraging her presence in threatening circumstances through the expression of distress. Learning to distinguish the mother from others is a prerequisite of this capacity;
2.) seeking proximity and face-to-face interaction with others to reinforce predictable patterns, while experiencing the sensory dimensions of expressions, such as the movements of the hands, facial configuration and tone of voice;
3.) responding with positive affect, demonstrated through lip and tongue movements, vocalizations and gestures, all of which reinforce an anticipated response for both the infant and the caregiver;

4.) exhibiting emotions that correlate with one's cognitive manifestations, in order to communicate one's state of mind to the other;

5.) engaging in the reciprocal give-and-take of communication that complements the psychological state of the other; and

6.) expressing coherent signals of confusion or distress, if the behaviors of the partner become incomprehensible or threatening.

As can be seen from each of Trevarthen's examples, during the first few months of life the infant appears motivated to learn these communicative skills and to sustain the interaction with the caregiver as he matures in the direction of greater levels of predictive accuracy. Somewhat less obvious is that each of these tendencies also suggests that the infant is enhancing his ability to derive predictions about the current status of interaction with the caregiver and to use these predictions to developffurther representations about imminent developmental events. The infant is, in other words, beginning to anticipate previewing experiences with the caregiver. Indeed, each quality described by Trevarthen requires that the infant predict certain behaviors—either his own or those of his caregiver—and use these myriad predictions in formulating and coordinating new responses to guide the interaction with the caregiver. We may hypothesize, then, that just as the infant may be born with an inherent capacity to motivate the interaction with the caregiver, so too does the infant appear to possess a complementary ability to encode the experience during interactive sequences. Eventually such experiences are recalled and used as a prototype for drawing comparisons with the current sequence in order to verify the contingency between the experience the infant has anticipated and the actual interaction that transpired.

Murray and Trevarthen (1986) have confirmed that the infant exerts a strong influence on the nature of the interaction with the mother, even from the first weeks of life. In particular, these researchers verified that certain features of infant behavior, such as constitutional traits or state-related behavior, affect the interaction. Thus, an accurate portrait of infant-mother interaction discloses a cluster of purposeful interventions, such as responsiveness between two partners, suggesting that even from the beginning of the relationship the infant is using his predictive capacities to anticipate responses and to begin manipulating and guiding the direction of the interaction in some fashion.

Winnicott (1965) and Ainsworth, Bell and Stayton (1974) have reported that in circumstances of attuned, harmonious interaction, maternal speech and behavior is child-, rather than mother-centered. Adaptive caregivers have been found to "tune in" to the infant and absorb infant cues in a kind of feedback mode, which generally allows for a more sophisticated level of communication, even with very young infants. Within this interactive arena the caregiver's skill in engaging in previewing exercises emerges.

To verify the participatory role played by the infant during early dyadic interaction, Murray and Trevarthen selected eight mothers and their full-term infants, five boys and three girls, aged two months. Mother and infant were placed in separate rooms, positioned in front of a video recorder. The mother's speech was recorded during video presentations of her infant in two live and two replay sequences. Mothers were told that the researchers were interested in the social development of the infants and were requested to chat as naturally as possible with the infant. The infant was positioned in an adjoining room in front of the video image of his mother. From their observations, Murray and Trevarthen noted that the infant plays a more active communicative role in early dyadic interaction than previously imagined and that characteristics of the mother's baby talk represent at least some accommodation to the infant's need to verify his predictions. This interactive quality indicates that the infant's participation is influenced by his ability to anticipate or predict what is "coming up next" during the interpersonal exchange and by his related skill in manifesting an appropriate behavior designed to elicit a particular predictable response from the caregiver.

As these manifestations are occurring, the mother regulates her behavior in highly intuitive ways, according to Trevarthen, speaking slowly and rhythmically, moving at a regular pace, with repeated head movements which attract the attention and interest of the baby. The mother also observes closely how her advances are received and interpreted by the infant. The infant gazes at the mother's face responsively, particularly in the eye area; later, the mouth and hands become key points of observation. The infant shows signs of recognition by softening his face and smiling. From a reading of such maternal facial expressions, the infant is excited or animated and begins to signal by using limb movements and vocalizing. Often the infant will call out in the form of excited coos or shouts, while his head is held back and will gaze directly at the mother. Each of these behaviors indicates that the infant has learned to predict a particular caregiver response and is signaling to the caregiver in a certain manner in order to evoke predictable behaviors. The infant's exquisite degree of observation, focusing on minute details of caregiver activity, suggests an effort to formulate representations of interaction with the caregiver and to use such representations to validate predictions about future interpersonal outcomes.

The Relation of Affect and Cognition to Intentional Behavior

Harding (1982) has observed that infants using goal-directed behaviors are, in fact, already exhibiting intention and it is this intention which organizes the behavior that is then communicated to the caregiver. The researcher explains that there are numerous components of intention, each of which may have distinct developmental courses determined by the cognitive capacities necessary for their occurrence. The evolution of these components may adhere to a sequence similar to the model of intentional behavior developed by T. A. Ryan (1970). According to Ryan's model, there are four elements of intention, including:

1.) an initial arousal or tension that occurs when the individual perceives a situation and becomes aware of a goal;
2.) the formation of a representation for achieving the goal;
3.) an attitude of necessity leading to the formation of alternative representations, if necessary; and
4.) persistence of behavior in striving to achieve the goal.

Among those investigators who have hypothesized about the development of intention are Piaget (1952) and Bruner (1973). For Piaget, clear-cut intentional behavior is not observed until at least the third stage of sensorimotor development (at about four-ten months). At that juncture, the infant begins to coordinate behaviors in sequences which appear directed towards predicting a particular goal. Piaget refers to these sequences as *secondary circular reactions.* In contrast, Bruner concluded that intentions are formed earlier, when the infant demonstrates preferences for particular stimuli. According to Bruner, the infant is able to coordinate motor activity with the intention of reaching a goal. Piaget and Bruner differ in identifying the factors motivating the emergence of intention. For Bruner, the emergence of intention is fueled by an affective component; it is only necessary that the infant be sufficiently aroused to achieve an intended future behavior. In Piaget's view, however, the ability to formulate an intention involves cognitive processing. The infant must devise a representation of a series of behaviors leading to the successful achievement of the goal. In fact, however, it is likely that both affective and cognitive development are concurrent, and that coordination in both domains is necessary before manifestations of intentionality emerge.

Facial expression is associated with a particular meaning and this meaning is used to evaluate future behavior and predict a course of action. Stern also reports on an affective phenomenon, which he labels *interaffectivity,* that represents the affective correlate of Trevarthen's notion of intersubjectivity. The latter quality appears to be a cognitive developmental characteristic. Interaffectivity, according to Stern, indicates that infants of approximately nine months begin to notice congruence between their own affective state and the affective expression observed in a significant other, such as the caregiver. If the infant is sad and upset by several minutes of separation from the caregiver, as soon as a reunion episode occurs the infant will stop being upset, but will remain solemn. If then, immediately following the reunion, when he is still sad, the infant is shown a happy face and a sad face, he will display a preference for the sad face. This does not happen, however, if the infant either is made to laugh first or had not been separated from the caregiver in the first place. From these data, Stern concludes that the infant somehow matches the feeling state as experienced within and as seen "on" or "in" another. He refers to this matching-up process as interaffectivity, and notes that interaffectivity may be the first, most pervasive and most immediately important form of sharing subjective emotional experiences. Interaffectivity may also be viewed as a form of communication that involves representing and matching expressions with which the infant is familiar. Moreover, what Stern refers to as matching may actually encompass a broader series of skills that are embraced by the infant's predictive abilities.

Bloom and Capatides (1987) have suggested that the child's capacity to learn communication through language is tied to a *reflective state*. In turn, this reflective state facilitates other cognitive functions, such as the infant's capacity to represent, the capacity to develop expectations about upcoming events and eventually the capacity to display behaviors intentionally. Moreover, according to Bloom and Capatides, affective expression and language development may share an inverse relationship, in the sense that affective regulation may hinder the emergence of language. The researchers studied twelve infants ranging in age from nine months to two years. First words and spurts in vocabulary were identified in the infant's transition from prespeech vocalizing to the emergence of full-fledged speech. Expressions of affect were coded for properties of intensity and valence, including positive, negative, neutral, and mixed. It was found that the more time the infant spent displaying neutral affect, the earlier the onset of language acquisition. The researchers concluded that neutral affective displays may support the infant's early transition to language by facilitating the reflective stance required for the development of the representational and predictive abilities that are a prerequisite for learning to speak. This reflective stance is first observed during the quiet-alert states that support cognitive processes of early infancy and that occur during early turn-taking episodes.

This study raises several questions. First, do affect and cognition evolve along separate and noncoordinating lines of development? Second, if affect and cognition evolve in parallel fashion, does early affective expression substitute for cognitive forms of communication, such as language? Finally, if affective expression effectively communicates the infant's desires, why does language eventually supersede affect as the prime mode of communication?

Bloom, Beckwith and Capatides (1988) have provided new insights into how affective capacities may sometimes develop with cognitive capacities, while in other circumstances affective capacities may overshadow cognition. These researchers studied infants between the ages of nine and twenty-one months and found that at nine months of age, all of the infants displayed identical skill with respect to the frequency and range of their emotional expression and the relative amount of time they spent displaying neutral and positive affect. As the cohort was followed, an increase in affective expression was noted. However, it was discovered that one group of infants increased their frequency of verbal expression relatively early, while in the other group, frequency of emotional expression heightened early and linguistic skill emerged later.

The researchers commented that all of the infants studied acquired language skills within normal age limits. Nevertheless, when the infants exhibited more neutral affective expressions, language skills developed earlier. According to the investigators, one explanation for the finding may be that more diverse cognitive activities are required for learning words than are required for the expression of emotion. Learning linguistic units, such as words and sentences, requires attention to the acoustic signal and to some aspect of the context, and mandates comparison of these contents with prior representations recalled from memory. In contrast, the expression of affect entails an evaluation of representations and predictions involved in one's immediate position, a subjective feeling and neurophysiological state. Bloom et al. suggest that the experiences and processes that contribute to emotional expression may compete for the cognitive resources required for language learning. In distinction, neutral affective expression, which the researchers characterized as the continuation of the quiet-alert states of early infancy, would engender the reflexive, contemplative stance that is mandatory for learning words. Affective expression may influence the development of representations, which, in turn, are a prerequisite for developing predictive abilities designed to elicit a particular response from the environment.

What is noteworthy about this study is not that the two groups of infants developed the ability to express themselves through language at different times. Rather it is fascinating that both groups developed language skills within the normative period, although one group displayed a greater precocity in language abilities. Thus, Bloom et al. may be correct in positing that there is some degree of divergence between the cognitive and affective pathways of development. While both contribute to the infant's development of predictive capacities it appears, nevertheless, that at a particular juncture before the end of the second year of life, these pathways converge, so that the infant is able to manifest communicative skills coordinating both of these domains to a degree sufficient to create and sustain a network of predictive abilities. In addition, it should be remembered that previewing behaviors tend to foster the development of both affective and cognitive capacities. So long as the infant has begun to represent phenomena, he can begin to engage in predictions and to convert these predictions into behaviors designed to elicit a previewing response from the caregiver. Moreover, the caregiver will be attuned to infant response in order to devise appropriate previewing exercises for the infant.

Kaye (1982), has defined *representation* as the process whereby knowledge becomes accessible to thought through the images one generates from past experiences. According to Kaye, one of the prerequisites of representational capacity is the capacity to encode information in memory. What is encoded can be represented in different ways at different times, depending upon the situation and purpose, and can be retrieved from memory. As Kaye explains, memory is a name for the process whereby acquired information is stored over time. Moreover, what is represented will often, and perhaps always, be substantially different from any event that was originally encoded, because the reconstruction process combines elements from many encodings. As a result, representation does not refer to memory alone. Instead representation involves the purposeful process of retrieving information from memory and restoring it to a format that resembles the original experience that has been perceived.

All three aspects of knowledge-the encoding process, the representational process, and the information accumulated in memory-develop gradually. When we speak of the ability to formulate representations from the images encountered in the external world, we should bear in mind each of these three features. A theory of development that stresses the infant's constitutional endowment would posit that any one, two or all three aspects need to develop before predictions become possible. Despite such innate proclivities, specific developmental refinements occur during the first year of life that indicate the acquisition of speech is a gradual and painstaking process (Aslin, Pisoni and Juscy, 1983; Baldwin and Markham, 1989; Grieser and Kuhl, 1989). For example, infants learn through experience to become attuned to and to predict coarticulation cues. Fluent speakers do not pronounce the phonemes of their language like separate building blocks, one at a time. Each time a speaker begins a new syllable, he is preparing his mouth for the vowel and consonant that follows. As a consequence of such coarticulation cues, therefore, the "b" in "boat" is pronounced differently from the "b" in "bee." Fluent listeners rely on such coarticulation phenomena, anticipating the identity of a the next word or syllable solely on the basis of slight differences in pronunciation at or before the initial phoneme. However, because the use of coarticulation cues depends on experience with word and syllable structures, this aspect of speech perception has to be learned and requires that the infant engage in representations of individual units of speech and subsequent predictions about specific words.

The theory of previewing posits that encoding perceptions and the the process of representing such perceptions signifies that infants have internalized and thus inculcated how to predict the communications emitted by their caregivers. Assimilation of information by the infant leads to accommodations on the stage of internal representation, which Piaget (1952) referred to as *schemas*. By virtue of such accommodations, the infant begins to acquire significations, the learned relations between signs and events in the world, and uses these learned relations to develop predictions. Gradually, these signs are transformed into symbols. Thus, the infant's constitutional motivation to formulate expectations and the environmentally induced expectations that emerge from the dyadic interaction are complimentary. While the infant may possess inherent representation and predicitve capacities, it is the caregiver who, through nurturing skills and previewing exercises, encourages the infant to demonstrate and continually refine these capacities.

Several researchers have postulated that the fundamental aspects of speech perception *cannot* be learned but are inherent and emerge hierarchically along the spectrum of development (Bates, O'Connell, and Shore, 1987; Eilers and Minifie, 1975; Lieberman, 1970, 1973). Eimas (1985), among others, has proposed that human beings are born with an innate, species-specific perceptual system that evolved to pick up the unique constellations of sound that human beings make during verbal communication. However, this theory fails to account for why caregivers preview speech to the infant in the form of baby talk.

Another way of approaching the infant's developmental acquisition of speech is to focus on the kinds of sounds the infant emits as he progresses toward full-fledged language. Bates, O' Connell and Shore (1987) report that during the first two to three weeks of life, infant sounds are restricted to "vegetative noises," primarily in the nature of crying and cooing. Genuine laughing and gurgling commence at approximately two to three months, and systematic play with speech sounds is a phenomenon reported at approximately three months, when infants also begin to engage in games of reciprocal imitation, which have been referred to as "vocal tennis" by Uzgiris and Hunt (1975). The systematic production of consonant sounds generally appears by six months, and when such consonants do surface there is reason to believe that the infant is attempting to stimulate his prediction of an environmental sound target.

As the infant progresses, Bates et al. report a distinctive drift in the direction of language-specific sounds at four to seven months, almost immediately preceding the point at which consonant sounds begin to appear with frequency. By six to ten months, the infant may be expected to engage in what has been referred to as canonical babbling, the systematic production of consonant-vowel sequences (e.g., "ma" or "da"), that are easily recognized by most caregivers (Koopmans-van-Beinum and van der Selt, 1985). Such babbling seems to indicate that children are cognizant of language in a new and explicit fashion. It is as if the infant is experimenting with his newfound capacity to anticipate a specific behavior on the part of the caregiver when a particular sound is emitted. Evidence of language comprehension occurs soon thereafter, followed by changes in the organization of babbling that is linked to reorganizations in the representations and production of meaningful speech. Significantly, such babbling has not been reported among institutionalized infant's deprived of exposure to maternal baby talk, suggesting that this form of caregiver manifestation plays a fundamental role in helping the infant to predict speech and to begin using language at an early age.

It appears that many of the infant's developmental capacities contribute to the development of language acquisition in a proliferative fashion as well. Oller and Eilers (1988) explored this hypothesis by focusing on one perceptual ability-audition-in the development of the infant's speech. The researchers examined how the capacity to hear contributes to the onset of infant "babbling," believed by many to be a precursor of speech. Oller and Eilers explained that previous literature on child development reflects a widespread belief that deaf infants "babble" in the same fashion that hearing infants do, although the deaf have been thought to vocalize less during the second half year of life than hearing infants (Van der Zanden, 1981). Oller and Eilers have dispelled this notion, however, noting that well-formed syllable production is manifested in the first ten months of life by hearing infants, but not by deaf infants, indicating that audition plays an important role in the development of language. Distinctions between infant babbling in deaf and hearing infants are evident when infant vocal sounds are microanalyzed.

Oller and Eiler's study involved twenty-one normally hearing infants who participated in longitudinal trials of vocal development. The age of onset of canonical babbling was determined for all the infants. For eleven of the twenty-one infants, sufficient data allowed a more detailed analysis of the number of canonical syllables per utterance at five, six, and eleven months. Data for the vocalizations of nine hearing-impaired infants were also obtained. The researchers found that in deaf infants—even those who have been intensively stimulated and provided with auditory amplification—a substantial delay occurred with respect to the onset of canonical babbling. This finding led the researchers to ask how the deaf infants ever produced babbling sounds at all. They hypothesized that regardless of how heavily impaired the children were, they did have a means of perceiving the sounds of speech, either visually, through amplified hearing, or through the perception of vibrations. The diminished quality or quantity of their perceptions appears to have hampered the development of babbling, although it did not prohibit it altogether. This study demonstrates that audition plays a significant role in the development of speech and in particular, in the development of precursory skills, such as canonical babbling, which appear to signify a precursory form of speech and contribute to stimulating speech.

Other studies have focused on developmentally impaired infants to demonstrate how such children display maturational patterns that are different from those of developmentally normal child. For example, Mundy,

Sigman, Kasari and Yirmiya (1988), studied the nonverbal communication skills in Down Syndrome children. The researchers concentrated on the nonverbal communication competence of eighteen Down Syndrome infants of forty-eight months of age. The results of the investigation indicated that Down infants displayed both strengths and weaknesses in nonverbal communication skills. Normal children involved in the study displayed a significantly enhanced ability to communicate nonverbal requests for objects or assistance with objects as compared with the Down Syndrome children. This may be due to the fact that such children begin to represent earlier, and use their representational skills to engage in *analogic* forms of communication. Nonverbal skills for requesting objects correlated significantly with expressive language in the Down Syndrome children. From these findings the researchers concluded that in Down Syndrome children a deficit in expressive language correlates with a deficit in earlier developing nonverbal skills.

The nonverbal communication behaviors examined by the researchers fell into three categories: social interaction, indicating, and requesting. When rating social interaction, the researchers evaluated the child's capacity to elicit attention or physical contact from the experiment and to engage in turn-taking with the experimenter. When assessing indicating behavior, the researchers charted behaviors used to direct attention to an object or event, which resulted in a common focus of attention between the child and experimenter. Finally, in the requesting category an emphasis was placed upon behaviors used to request aid in obtaining objects and events. Except for the first category of social interaction, all of these behaviors involved objects in the interaction and the capacity to engage in predictions about those objects. The findings of the study indicate that, although Down Syndrome children are comparable to normals in their ability to engage in social interactions, the deficits exhibited by such children (like indicating and requesting) may impede the subsequent development of expressive language skills in such children. Moreover, this study implies that an interactive partner, who provides stimulation of predictive abilities, is essential in the development of representation capacities in general.

Each of these studies suggests that prior to the emergence of full-fledged language skills as the dominant mode of communication in young children, infants evolve a series of capacities that help them first to communicate with the external world and second, to engage in predictions about future events. These skills are given further stimulation by the presence of an active and involved caregiver who supports their effort through repeated, predictable sequences of interaction (Ruddy and Bornstein 1982, Tamis-LeMonda and Bornstein 1989; Taylor and Gelman 1989; Trad 1989). Nevertheless, for most normal infants, developmental phenomena will occur even if the caregiver is providing less than optimal stimulation.

Witelson (1987) reviewed the neurobiological aspects of language acquisition in young children and found that most theorists now concur that the infant is endowed from birth with an impressive cognitive capacity. Indeed, Witelson reported that it is likely cerebral dominance for both hemispheres is present from birth, in the sense that the essential processing difference between the two hemispheres of the brain exists at birth and does not alter dramatically with development. What does increase and develop, however, is the amount of cognition available for mediation by the hemispheres. In other words, as the infant is stimulated, greater and greater amounts of data are stored in memory and converted into internal representations. These representations are, in turn, used by the infant to formulate cause-effect relationships and to develop representations of contingency sequences. As contingency relationships become ingrained, the infant comes to expect and anticipate certain forms of behavioral response. Each time such a response is forthcoming, contingencies are reinforced. Once predictive capacities emerge, the infant will become upset if certain behaviors do not occur and will strive to elicit those behaviors by manipulating the environment in some fashion. Gesturing is one such form of manipulating, as is the use of language, which signifies perhaps the most sophisticated use of developmental capacities to control events in the external universe.

Around the time when canonical babbling emerges, infants begin to display signs of intersubjectivity. This concept, defined by Trevarthen and referred to earlier, involves the infant's capacity to understand that significant others, such as caregivers, have their own representations which are separate and distinct from those of the infant. Trevarthen explains that in order for infants to share their mental experience with others, they must possess two skills. First, they must be able to exhibit at least the basic components of individual awareness and intentionality. These qualities are referred to by Trevarthen as subjectivity and imply an incipient awareness of a sense of self and of boundary demarcation. Next, in order to communicate, infants must also be able to adapt their subjectivity to the subjectivity of others. They must, in other words, demonstrate intersubjectivity. Other researchers have referred to intersubjectivity as the capacity to share meaning with another person, so that both individuals experience the same representation of some object, event, or symbol. Although not yet fully understood, it is clear that infants begin to display this capacity for shared meaning by the end of the first year of life, provided that an interactive partner has provided the infant with a consistent level of adequate stimulation. Once the separateness of the caregiver is acknowledged, moreover, the infant begins to predict his response to this phenomenon by manifesting particular cues.

For Kaye, the onset of intersubjectivity marks the commencement of the infant's capacity to symbolize. Kaye notes that in order to experience a shared meaning with another, two prerequisites are involved. The first is *intentional signification,* the external representation of some class of things or events, or relations among them, using a sign that remains distinguished from the thing signified. This sign, or gesture, may assume the form of a manual or facial expression, according to Kaye, but may also take the form of words or melodies. Gestures designate something without being equivalent to it. Thus, the intention of the sign is crucial to whether it is differentiated from what it signifies. The second prerequisite is that the meaning attributed to the thing is by convention only. That is, a signal is a sign for a particular thing only because the members of a group (e.g., speakers of a specific language) have arbitrarily designated that meaning to it. Moreover, gestures are distinctly human; no nonhuman has ever been shown to have produced a sign with the intention of signifying an event that was remote in time or space, so that the sign designates an event without being the equivalent to it. Finally, Kaye emphasizes that the development of *symbolic thought* should be regarded as a social process that can emerge only from extensive interaction with others and the full-fledged emergence of predictive capacities. The researcher observes that while symbols may have a mental process accompanying them, the symbolic process is distinct from the gesture itself, which reflects an interpersonal act. The mind can represent a symbol, just as it can represent nonsignifying objects, and this form of representation heralds the most sophisticated of the infant's acquisitions in the realm of language development (Werner and Kaplan, 1963). Not only is the infant now capable of predicting maternal speech, but he can communicate intentions to the caregiver using his own language.

One fascinating issue that arises from these studies involves how researchers are capable of deducing the kinds of developmental events are occurring within the infant during this period of time. For example, how are investigators able to surmise the nature of the infant's experience? One answer is provided by the fact that although infancy is a period when *digital* forms of communication (such as language which relies upon arbitrary symbols such as words), are not the primary vehicle for conveying information, *analogic* modes of communication are frequent and common. Among the most prevalent forms of analogic communication used by the infant are primitive vocal sounds and gestures. These behaviors are classic analogic signals, because the message being conveyed is actually reenacted and predicted in the form of a gesture, the emblem of an analogic message.

For Bates et al., analogic modes are actually precursors of digital forms of communication. These researchers highlight three forms of prelinguistic communication: intentionality, convention and reference. With respect to *intentional* communications, Bates et al. note that the infant communicates to the caregiver from the first moments of life by emitting positive and negative signals that have a predictive effect. Three specific types of intentionality are described. The first is gaze alterations. As described by the researchers, if an adult and an object goal (e.g., a toy) are not in the same line of vision, a seven-month-old will look directly at the object and reach for it without turning back to the adult. By nine months, the infant will alternate gaze between the object and the adult, to communicate that he wishes the adult to obtain the object for him. Assuming that the infant's initial gesture has failed to stimulate the intended response, he will repeat or substitute signals until the goal is achieved. This phenomenon is the ability to repair failed messages. Gaze alternation is significant since it is remininscent of the patterns of visual cuing engaged in by adaptive dyads. Once this routine has been repeated several times, the infant may develop a shorthand signal. For example, the sound ''mmm'' may convey a meaning or carry a social significance to the caregiver. This cluster of analogic communications enables the infant to convey intention to the caregiver and strongly suggests that the infant is capable of predicting an upcoming event and engaging in behavior designed to elicit a particular response from the caregiver.

Conventions play a key role with respect to the development of language, Bates et al. explain. With the exception of a few words, there are no natural or intuitive associations between words and their meanings. Words stand for their unique meanings only because the society has consensually decided that they will. For the child to learn how to speak his native language, he must, therefore, understand the completely arbitrary relationships between sounds or signs and their socially imposed meanings.

It is likely that two distinct learning processes are involved in the acquisition of cultural conventions, including the conventions of language. These are imitation (the ability to reproduce an arbitrary sound or movement, whether the child understands it cognitively or not) and ritualization (the ability to produce streamlined versions of a sound or movement at predictable points in a social context). Both of these skills are fueled by caregiver stimulation, which during episodes of baby talk, provides examples of both imitation and ritualization. But the infant would not be engaging in this form of imitation unless he derived some kind of pleasure from it. Pleasure in acquiring language is likely to derive from two sources. First, repetition of words and sounds by the caregiver enables the infant to experience contingencies which are preserved in representational form; second, these activities occur in the exchange with the caregiver, a relationship generally rewarding to the infant. Moreover, since speech incorporates an arbitrary component it is likely that another developmental phenomenon is at work, the infant's predictive capacities referred to earlier.

The classic example of a *reference* communication is pointing. Bates et al. note that pointing is the quintessential act of reference, because it represents the way that one human being singles out an object of contemplation and offers it to another for consideration. The giving and showing gestures of the nine-month-old may be interpreted as a form of this referencing ability. By soliciting the adult's acknowledgment of an interesting toy or object, the infant becomes an active partner in establishing a shared object-world and predicting shared meaning with the caregiver. Such pointing behaviors may actually be facilitate predictive capacities (Werner and Kaplan, 1963), because, as the infant begins to explore the world and fixate on particular objects of interest, the index finger used in pointing helps in some fashion to clarify the distinction between subject and object.

Other aspects of pointing have also been discussed in the developmental literature. For example, it has been observed that pointing is one aspect of communication where production appears to occur ahead of comprehension. Research on the comprehension of pointing reveals that one-year-olds are incapable of locating a visual target on the basis of an adult pointing gesture (Messer, 1978). One fascinating finding is that under eighteen months of age there is a virtual absence of pointing to the self. In fact, pointing to the self does not appear systematically until the child begins explicitly to refer to himself in speech using the pronouns "I" and "me," indicating that the infant has not yet fully represented to himself that he is a separate entity. Indeed, the consolidation of a sense of self is estimated to occur by approximately two years of age (Emde, 1984).

Stern (1985) has provided insight into how the infant's affective and cognitive skills may unfold in a parallel fashion. By posing the question of whether infants can attribute shared affective states to their social partners, Stern finds evidence of such attributes in the phenomenon of *social referencing* described by Emde and Sorce (1983), and Klinnert et al. (1983). These researchers tested for social referencing by means of "the visual cliff" experiment. The visual cliff involves one-year-old infants who are placed in a setting that will likely generate uncertainty between approach and withdrawal. The infant is lured with an attractive stimulus across a visual cliff, an apparent optical drop-off, which is mildly frightening at the age of one year. Often, the infant may be approached by a relatively unusual but highly stimulating object, such as a bleeping mechanical robot toy. When the infant encounters one of these situations and gives evidence of uncertainty, he looks in the direction of the mother to read her face for its affective content. Essentially, the infant is looking at the caregiver to get an appraisal that will help resolve the uncertainty and to formulate some prediction of what the caregiver is experiencing. If the mother shows pleasure by smiling, the infant will most likely cross the visual cliff. In contrast, if the caregiver shows fear, the infant will run back from the cliff and perhaps become upset. Similarly, if the caregiver displays no fear and smiles at the robot, the infant will smile as well. If the caregiver displays fear, however, the infant will stop his movements and display wariness. According to Stern, infants would not check with the caregiver in this fashion unless they attributed to her the capacity to signal an affect that had relevance to their own actual or potential emotional state. Moreover, such cuing suggests that analogic communication is transpiring within the dyad, whereby the infant uses caregiver communications to predict his own response to an uncertain stimulus or a stimulus with which he is unfamiliar.

The Relationship Between Infant Predictive Abilities and Caregiver Interaction

In discussing the development of infant communicative and predictive skills, one cannot ignore the primary domain in which these skills first emerge and flourish-the domain of interaction with the caregiver.

Given the studies referred to earlier, it is relatively easy to understand how the infant's predictive capacities can be fostered by adaptive and intuitive caregiver behaviors aimed at stimulating the infant. Moreover, upon reflection it is also apparent that particular kinds of caregiver behaviors operate not only to bolster the infant's predictive capacities, but also to stimulate language development. In this context it should be remembered that language is a form of communication, perhaps the most sophisticated kind of communication that human beings can use. Therefore, since the caregiver's goal is to enhance communication with the infant and, similarly, the infant's goal is to fortify and perpetuate the interaction with the caregiver, it is not unusual that both members will strive to learn the most effective and efficient means for communicating with one another.

Among the most obvious caregiver behaviors that enhance the infant's predictive capacities is vocal cuing, which begins within the first days of life and continues well into the second year. By engaging in this form of stimulation, the caregiver is actually previewing conversational dialogue for the infant in a manner that conveys to the infant what the communicative speech will be like. In addition, because vocal cuing is often accompanied by other forms of caregiver-initiated behavior, such as body contact and gestures, the infant soon comes to grasp the notion that the physical sounds of speech are associated with other objects and actions as well. In other words, speech becomes linked contingently to other things and the infant's representations of speech are in turn associated with these things.

As a result, speech becomes an active behavior which, from the point of view of the infant, seems to encompass the infinite variations associated with other behaviors. Eventually, as the caregiver's repeats particular phrases in conjunction with particular acts the infant comes to predict that particular behaviors will occur when he hears particular words being spoken. In this fashion, words and actions become associated, facilitating the infant's subsequent capacity to attribute meaning to particular words that are associated with the objects or the intentional behaviors.

The infant's ability to engage in game playing with others is an accomplishment requiring the coordination of multiple developmental skills. Game playing mandates the mutual involvement of two players who develop and repeat game roles and alternate turns as they play (Goldman and Ross, 1978; Ross, 1982). Although initially infants serve as an enthralled audience in games with adults, eventually by the end of the first year the infant's predictive capacities emerge, allowing them to assume an increasingly more active role during play episodes (Hodapp, Goldfield and Boyatzis, 1984). According to Ross and Lollis (1987), most infant games have simple rules, often based on contingency or cause-effect relationships.

Ross and Lollis focused on how such communication skills emerge within the context of an activity that most infants are exposed to in their everyday lives, namely, game playing with the caregiver. The researchers examined the evolving capacity of infants for requesting that a partner participate in social games. Ross and Lollis explored how the infants responded when game playing was interrupted by the failure of the adult partner to take a turn. Subjects included nineteen children aged nine, twelve, fifteen, and eighteen months. Subjects came to the laboratory with their caregivers and, after a brief interview, the game session was initiated. The caregiver was instructed to begin a series of games with the child and, after the completion of several turn-taking episodes, to fail to take a turn. During these interruption periods, the adult was instructed to watch the infant with a relaxed, neutral expression.

It was found that during interruption periods infants increased their communicative behavior, as if to convey they were protesting the adults' lack of involvement. Such behavior indicated that from as early as nine months, infants are capable of cognitively mastering and predicting the content of games, can engage in object-person interaction, and participate in the regulation of games by requesting that their partners participate. Beyond the findings voiced by the study, we may also note that such infants were displaying strong predictive abilities and were apparently distressed when an expected contingency—the participation of the caregiver—did not occur.

Bruner (1983) has proposed that games facilitate language acquisition by offering a repeating-action format for early communication that reinforces representations. Moreover, games and language share certain formal properties such as semantic rules and structures. Moreover, games also instill nonlinguistic forms of communication, such as prolonged waiting after one's own turn, glancing from partner to object, showing, offering or giving the game toy, repeating one's turn, waiting for the partner and vocalizing. These patterns indicate how games reinforce contingency relationships and predictions that are represented by the infant.

The work of Acredolo and Goodwyn (1988) who found that infant communication develops along a *spectrum* and that symbolizing and gesturing (analogic modes) precede the emergence of verbal speech (digital communication). Acredolo and Goodwyn examined how infants use nonverbal gestures to symbolically represent objects, needs, states, and qualities. A group of sixteen infants were followed between the ages of eleven to twenty-four months. It was found that symbolic gestures and language skills tend to develop in a parallel fashion, that girls tend to rely more heavily on such gestures than boys, and that structured parent-child interactions are significant to the development of such gestures. Gradually, according to the researchers, the infant relinquishes gestures in favor of verbal communication. As the infant's social world expands, he wishes to communicate with more than just the caregiver. Furthermore, the motivation to expand the nature and degree of predictive abilities in order to exert control over the environment is also important, propelling the infant in the direction of language development.

Conclusion

This chapter has selected one particular developmental acquisition that emerges during the first two years of life-language-and has used it as a paradigm from which to derive principles about the incremental developmental events that the infant undergoes prior to exhibiting the milestone in its full-fledged form. The development of language has been used here principally because it demonstrates how the infant's incremental developmental gains smooth the way for predicting or anticipating future development.

For example, the discussion of linearity, invariance and coarticulation cues indicted that infants learn to speak primarily because they are engaged in the internal process of *anticipating* the sound of syllables and eventually words and their structure in sentences. Beginning with the vegetative noises characteristic of newborns, the infant begins to imitate the caregiver. A distinctive preference for motherese sounds has been reported at four months and eventually language specific sounds emerge by the sixth month. In fact, researchers have demonstrated that the infant can distinguish the mother's voice even antenatally. These recognitions of language coalesce and provide the infant an opportunity to form representations of contingent events. Next, canonical babbling occurs, whereby the infant begins to systematically produce consonant-vowel sequences. This form of infant speech is readily identified by parents, who encourage it by repeating particular speech patterns to the infant. During this phase, representations are transformed into predictions. Once again, with the evolution of such sounds, one is able to see how infant speech is propelled forward via external cues that continually help the infant to predict the next phase of language acquisition.

The development of language in infants has also been analyzed as an internal process, involving the evolution of representational skills, as well as skills in subjective awareness, intentionality, intersubjectivity, and symbolism. From careful examination of the development of such intellectually oriented skills, one can see how the ability to predict or anticipate is seminal to such developmental phenomena as intentionality, subjectivity, and intersubjectivity, as well as to the capacity to engage in symbolic thought. Some might even say that symbolic thought is itself a way of predicting imminent events and attempting to exert control ever them.

We have also seen that while the infant's developmental capacity in the area of language acquisition appears to be due to largely innate, external factors such as caregiver encouragement of the infant's developmental progress, other external factors, such as the interaction with the caregiver are significantly implicated as well. From this discussion, then, it becomes apparent that the infant appears to possess an innate proclivity for predictive capacities. The general skill of anticipating upcoming developmental change and of incrementally exercising behaviors are self-perpetuating and hierarchically organized in the sense that they promote future developmental acquisition.

CHAPTER 7

Previewing as a Principle for Motivating Interpersonal Communication

Introduction

Most practitioners would concur that working with caregivers and their infants is rewarding in a way that is dramatically different from the treatment of other adult patients. This experience of professional satisfaction arises for several reasons. First, in contrast to the treatment of adult psychopathology, if psychopathology threatens the interaction between the caregiver and infant, it is, more often than not, susceptible to intervention. This is primarily because the relationship between caregiver and infant is relatively fresh, and aberrant patterns have not yet had an opportunity to become entrenched. Therefore the potential for instilling adaptive patterns of interaction is enhanced.

Second, dyadic interaction is composed of the most pristine elements of human communication. The exchanges between caregiver and infant are laden with various types of perceptions, including the *somatic, affective, cognitive,* and *motivational* signals that emerge during interaction. Consider, for example, the caregiver who is rocking her infant to sleep while singing a lullaby. We are initially entranced by the ritual like atmosphere of this interaction and its soothing effect on the infant. Yet, on closer analysis it becomes clear that the caregiver is matching her behavior to that of the infant by engaging in a series of well-orchestrated responses. In addition, the cradling gestures the caregiver creates with her arms convey an aura of security and support. Each of these distinct interactive nuances blends to communicate a compelling unitary message.

From this context we can infer yet a third reason why caregiver-infant therapy is so uniquely fulfilling. Such therapy involves the observation of *intuitive behaviors.* Every sequence of caregiver-infant behavior seems to be imbued with an intuitive force that promotes adaptive maturation in a predictable fashion. This force enables the caregiver to respond readily to the infant in an appropriate and consistent manner. Intuition, used in this context, refers to the caregiver's capacity to reflect, represent and respond to the infant's somatic, affective, cognitive, and motivational signals in an integrated fashion.This level of perception allows the caregiver to acquire an exquisite sensitivity and rhythm that enables her to virtually "feel" the infant without touching him and to "know" that the infant will need attention even before any outward manifestation becomes evident. To an outward observer, this intense communion, which integrates virtually every perception within the dyadic relationship, acquires an almost mystical quality.

But intuition is not really mystical. The caregiver's capacity to be intuitive with the infant simply means that the caregiver is highly attuned to the infant and can predict the infant's needs. Researchers who have analyzed caregivers and their infants by means of microanalytic procedures have discovered that intuition allows caregivers to attend to a wide variety of cues being emitted by the infant. Intuition allows caregivers to perceive the infant from many different perspectives and to integrate these perceptions into a coherent framework, in order not only to sustain, but also to enhance discrete periods of interaction. The precision of such intuitive behaviors is based in the caregiver's ability to assemble seemingly scattered cues and to coordinate them into a response that motivates both dyadic members to maintain the interaction. The degree of complexity of the caregiver's responses should be appreciated. These responses represent numerous intricate signals that are communicated to the infant somatically, affectively, cognitively, and motivationally, and are ultimately combined to help the infant coordinate his responses and predict further interactive sequences. From this interplay of infant and caregiver exchange, the capacity to predict and adapt to imminent developmental changes emerges.

When the caregiver is using her intuitive capacities to their full potential, both dyadic members engage in a harmonious flow of predictable communicative exchange. For both dyadic members, communication converges into a communion of responses. Intuitive responses serve to perpetuate these sequences of dyadic exchange. Interactive patterns gradually recede and resurface in a well-paced, cyclical fashion. This orchestration enables caregiver and infant to share the rewards of anticipating mutual goals. Among adaptive dyads, such rhythms of interaction become more sophisticated and intricate as the period of infancy progresses, because the dyad has now become acclimated to an increasing number of predictable sequences.

The first task of the practitioner working with caregivers and infants is to *observe* and *dissect* the contours of this intuitive behavior with precision. The therapist's second task involves *pinpointing* elements of the interaction between the caregiver and infant. Sharpening the boundaries between consonant and nonconsonant sets of behaviors is vital because even dyads whose exchange is disturbed or maladaptive may nevertheless display episodes during which sequences of intuitive behavior emerge. It is important to recognize these adaptive behaviors, so that the therapist can begin to instruct the caregiver in how to *assess* and to *assert* adaptive and predictable behavior with the infant.

Initially confronted with these challenges in my work with new mothers, as well as in direct treatment of infants and preschool children, I approached such patients using traditional models and techniques which have proven to be effective with adult patients. My experience revealed, however, that the application of such models was inadequate for modifying interactive problems in the dyadic context. As I gained more experience in treating caregivers and their infants, I began to recognize the unique form of communication that transpires between the members of the dyad. Although not reliant upon language, this form of communication nevertheless represents a compelling process for the exchange of a full array of information.

I have labelled this phenomenon previewing (Trad 1989a, 1989b). In essence, previewing alerts the infant to the specific behaviors and skills on the next developmental horizon. It is important to emphasize that previewing is a phenomenon inherent in the dyadic process and, indeed, may be the organizing principle which propels development toward the cumulative acquisition of adaptive skills on the part of both the caregiver and child. In essence, previewing encompasses all of the behavioral ministrations of the caregiver that serve to introduce and acquaint the infant to upcoming developmental acquisitions. Previewing is engaged in, to varying degrees, by all caregivers whether the caregiver shares an adaptive, growth-enhancing relationship with the infant or whether the caregiver's relationship with the infant is troubled by emotional conflict.

But previewing entails more than the outward behaviors that indicate an acknowledgment of the infant's developmental progress. Such behaviors signify merely the "tip of the iceberg" where the previewing process is concerned. In fact, previewing includes the caregiver's diverse representations of the infant's future development and the interpersonal implications that such development will have for the dyad. As an all-embracing concept, previewing embodies the full texture of the caregiver's ability to convey predictions to the infant in a supportive fashion as both members of the dyad traverse the developmental journey which begins at birth. Through previewing, the caregiver and infant are, in a sense, united in an effort to sustain a dynamic partnership. This partnership captures the rich complexity of human interaction and enables the dyadic members to share an immediate sense of the gratification of mutual needs, as well as a more long-ranging sense of the sustentation of the relationship. Moreover, this form of communication facilitates the consensual validation of developmental achievement and of the interpersonal implications that result from such achievement.

For the purposes of this discussion, we will define previewing as consisting of three elements. First, previewing involves the caregiver's capacity to *reflect and represent* the contours of infant development on the stage of active consciousness. This awareness encompasses not only the caregiver's knowledge of the infant's current status, but also her capacity to anticipate and predict imminent developmental acquisitions in a adaptive fashion. The second aspect of previewing refers to the caregiver as an *auxiliary and supportive partner* for the infant during previewing episodes. In adopting this stance, the caregiver conveys to the infant that she will be there to encourage and guide the infant as he traverses developmental pathways and exercises developmental skills that are still unfamiliar to him. Finally, the third aspect of previewing encompasses all of the *physical ministrations* the caregiver uses to introduce the infant to imminent developmental milestones.

Beyond its capacity to decipher the behavioral interplay between caregiver and infant, however, previewing also provides the practitioner with an innovative approach to conducting dyadic therapy. In contrast to virtually all other forms of psychotherapy, previewing focuses attention on the attitudes and events that will transpire in the future. Previewing, in other words, orients the therapist and patient towards upcoming events, rather than merely highlighting earlier unresolved conflicts. This *forward-looking* approach can alert the therapist to the potential emergence of conflict in the caregiver. Although the roots of the unresolved conflict may lie in the past, this conflict may surface in some fashion in the caregiver's relationship with the infant. In fact, by observing the relationship between caregiver and infant, and by being attuned to evidence of previewing in this relationship, the therapist may acquire more insight into the caregiver's conflict than would be obtained through traditional retrospective techniques. While psychoanalytically oriented psychotherapy relies upon a verbal report of past events, previewing focuses on encouraging the caregiver to engage in representational exercises from which to preview developmental events. In so doing, the therapist experiences the flow of the caregiver's interpersonal exchange with the infant directly. This technique helps the practitioner detect distortions in the way the caregiver conveys predictions about upcoming development to the infant. This is not to suggest that because previewing is prospective, rather than retrospective, it will, in and of itself, prevent repressed material from intruding into the dyadic relationship. In fact, by asking a caregiver to express her representations about the infant's future development or to engage in previewing exercises, contaminants from previous experiences and relationships will intrude into the mother's representations and behaviors. Nevertheless, because previewing orients the caregiver towards future events, it provides the therapist with a kind of window into how maladaptive patterns may emerge and insinuate themselves into the dyadic relationship. Thus, asking the caregiver to engage in previewing exercises allows the practitioner to detect affects and attributional impressions that deviate from the model of adaptive caregiving. Treatment strategies may then be designed for helping the mother surmount these negative or debilitating behaviors before they are acted out in actual exchanges with the infant. The following discussion will further acquaint the reader with the concept of previewing, and with the ways in which this phenomenon of interpersonal prediction can be used by the therapist to diagnose and treat maladaptive patterns of exchange among caregivers, their infants and young children.

When maladaptive patterns prevail over adaptive ones in the dyad, the therapist must devise a series of strategies aimed at guiding the caregiver in devising methods for *assessing* and *asserting adaptive* patterns of response into the daily routine of the infant. By enhancing or learning these patterns of intuitive exchange, the caregiver will eventually become adept at previewing upcoming development to the infant. This chapter strives to present the therapist with such information and to stimulate creative therapeutic efforts for eradicating maladaptive patterns, while enhancing interactional sequences in which exchange is adaptive.

Previewing as a Dynamic Process

The role played by the caregiver in the development of the infant is of immense significance. The caregiver will need to know the expectations of the infant and to fulfill these expectations by engaging in specific behaviors. As a result, the caregiver is expected to teach the infant how to assess upcoming developmental trends and to adaptively guide the infant in the eventual assertion of these emerging skills.

What is Previewing?

My recognition of the phenomenon of previewing first occurred when I was conducting group and individual sessions for new mothers and their infants. The mothers I treated in the group format had been motivated to attend sessions primarily in order to share experiences with other new mothers and to learn more about the practical aspects of raising an infant. In general, these mothers were competent, well educated and lacked any history of abnormal psychiatric behavior. In contrast, those mothers who attended individual sessions tended to have psychiatric histories, generally involving affective disorders, schizophrenia, substance abuse or borderline personality organization, and had been recommended for treatment because their primary therapist wanted to ensure that the relationship the mother was establishing with the infant was adaptive. Both groups of caregivers were notable for their diversity. Parents ranged in age from twelve to their early thirties. Many of them had been highly successful in their professional lives and were seeking a forum to help them adapt to their new role as full-time caregivers. I am convinced that this very diversity in the backgrounds of the caregivers made any contrasts drawn from their interactions with their infants all the more prominent and highlighted my recognition of previewing. At first, virtually all of the caregivers seemed to describe their infants in purely somatic terms, emphasizing bodily functions such as feeding, sleeping, or elimination patterns, or highlighting motor skills such as inchoate sitting motions.

Eventually, however, these descriptions began to assume a more complex and intricate character. Although the descriptions were markedly different for each individual caregiver, each new parent was asked to engage in a form of speculation or prediction about the infant's growth and about what kinds of developmental skills the infant would next manifest. When this question was asked, there was, an almost innate proclivity to begin predicting the broad direction of infant development, not merely in terms of the *behavioral* manifestations the infant would exhibit, but also with respect to the infant's *subjective* experience. These mothers were, in other words, able to endow their infants' future experience with meaning. Such descriptions were provided not only by the competent parents, but also by the parents who had psychiatric disturbances.

The full nature of these descriptions indicated that each of these caregivers shared particular psychological qualities that emerged in the interaction with the infant. When parsed, three such distinctive qualities were evident. First, virtually all the new mothers appeared to possess an innate knowledge of the normative rhythms of development. It was as if these mothers could visualize or represent future growth on an internal panorama. Depending upon the psychological health of the parent, this "map" would be either extraordinary detailed or would be only a vague sketch with shadowy roads. Nevertheless, each of the caregivers appeared to harbor in varying degrees this type of awareness of the progressive and relentless trends of development.

Second, each caregiver displayed a proclivity to represent the infant's *previous, current,* and *future* developmental status. Representation refers to a reflective state during which knowledge becomes accessible to thought processes through the images perceived in the environment or encountered in the past.

Third, and perhaps most significant, each caregiver demonstrated a spontaneity in *predicting* the future course of infant development and in using these predictions to attribute meaning to the infant's experience. In fact, the most compelling aspect of the interaction of these mothers with their babies was their continual interest in the future and in the imminent external behavior and internal capacities they anticipated their infants would experience. The mothers also displayed facility in adopting the infant's perspective when describing these phenomena. For example, it was not unusual for a mother to imagine how the baby would feel and what the baby would be thinking as these developmental events occurred.

When considered together, these three qualities-an innate knowledge of developmental trends, the ability to represent the infant without the constraints of time, the ability to predict future development and to attribute meaning to it-suggest remarkable abilities of new mothers. Indeed, one is compelled to ask how new caregivers acquire skills that are displayed with such spontaneity. The answer to this question remains unclear, although several researchers, such as Papousek and Papousek (1975, 1977), have suggested the role that *intuition* may play with regard to these phenomena. As discussed in Chapter 2, Papousek and Papousek use the term intuition to refer to qualities and skills which are manifested in an almost reflexive or instinctive fashion, and yet, because of their intricacy, implicate more than an instinctive response. It appears that intuitive behaviors surface as a consequence of the extraordinary intimacy between caregiver and infant.

The concept of previewing which has evolved from clinical observations of caregiver and infant interaction incorporates some of these features of intuition. On a variety of occasions, a mother would offer a prediction about her infant's future development and would then automatically rehearse this prediction through activity with the infant. As an illustration, one of the caregivers arrived for a session in an especially exuberant mood. She initiated the discussion by reporting that her six-month-old son would soon begin to crawl. She knew this, she said, because the infant had begun kicking his legs in a "certain way" that appeared to herald the onset of this skill. "I'm helping him along," she added. Then, she positioned herself on the floor near the infant. She placed a toy, one of the infant's favorites, a couple of feet away from him, but within his direct line of vision. The caregiver waited for several seconds, and then, as the infant began to make kicking gestures with his feet and arms, she held his body and began to slowly move it in the direction of the toy, simulating genuine crawling behavior. After engaging in this activity for several minutes while providing verbal encouragement in the form of several "good boy" comments, the caregiver began to cease her motions and gradually stopped altogether. "He gets tired if we do it for too long," she informed me. This sequence captures the three prerequisites of previewing behavior. The caregiver had observed certain behaviors in the infant and from these manifestations she had represented or envisioned that her son would soon begin crawling; next, she had devised specific behaviors designed to accommodate to his skills and motivate his incipient crawling; finally, she had engaged in this skill in a supportive fashion that exposed the infant to the sensation of crawling, but allowed him to resume his current developmental status when he was ready.

Although there are numerous instances of such activities, this example captures in part the rich flavor of previewing as it is manifested during the interaction. Here the caregiver is required to recognize the behavioral manifestations of the infant that suggest the onset of an imminent developmental achievement, such as crawling, walking, talking, grasping a small object etc. Once the caregiver has predicted that precursory manifestations will result in the ultimate attainment of a developmental skill, she devises behaviors that help introduce the infant to the interpersonal context in which the developmental acquisition will flourish. In the example above the caregiver knew the infant would soon begin crawling on his own; in the interim, she facilitated the advent of this achievement by engaging in behaviors designed to acquaint the infant with what crawling would be like. Her verbal encouragement conveyed an attitude conducive to competence and mastery, while her sensitivity to the infant's need to discontinue the behavior suggested that this caregiver was instilling the infant with the requisite level of motivation for continuing the previewing episode in the future. Thus, the three seminal features of previewing-the ability to represent future development, the ability to devise appropriate behaviors for introducing the infant to the imminent developmental milestone, and the ability to serve as an auxiliary and supportive partner as the infant is introduced to imminent milestones-were all present in the above example.

The concept of previewing, then, encompasses a wide range of phenomena that are exhibited by caregivers. In general, the indicia of previewing may be divided into three categories. In the first category are those psychological phenomena which are experienced by the caregiver in relation to the infant. The caregiver appears to harbor an exquisitely fine-tuned awareness of overall developmental trends and is able to reflect and thus represent these trends on the stage of active consciousness. My experience with both adaptive mothers and mothers with a psychiatric history indicates that virtually all caregivers speculate about imminent developmental change, although in varying degrees. The practitioner can "tap" into the caregiver's level of awareness by asking her to describe her perceptions about imminent change. For those who are unable to provide such descriptions, the therapist can begin by offering some examples of what he or she notices about the infant's changing developmental status. In addition, caregivers should be encouraged to share this knowledge with their infants through interactive sequences.

Beyond these qualities of psychological previewing, new caregivers also appear to engage in a unique form of behavioral exchange with the infant that gradually acquaints the infant with imminent developmental achievement. These adaptive interactional manifestations convey to the infant a sense of what future developmental acquisitions will actually feel like, protecting the infant from experiencing somatic, affective, cognitive or motivational deficits that stem from not being able to coordinate developmental precursors on his own. Developmental precursors refer to those behavioral manifestations that signal that the infant is on the verge of exhibiting a milestone in its full-fledged form. For example, the infant who attempts to grasp for a utensil but misses because his motor skills are still too gross and unrefined is exhibiting a precusory form of grasping behavior. Similarly, the infant who begins to kick his legs as if to simulate crawling but cannot propel his body forward or coordinate arm and leg movements is also displaying a form of precursory behavior. Another example is inchoate language behavior, whereby the infant engages in babbling manifestations that occur almost immediately after the caregiver verbalizes to the infant.

Developmental precursors are significant for a variety of reasons. First, they provide indications that the infant's development is progressing normally and that milestones will occur at an adaptive pace. As such, the emergence of precursors enables the therapist to rule out deficits in the infant. The therapist should also be aware of the possibility that an infant who fails to exhibit precursory behavior may be withdrawing from a caregiver who has failed repeatedly to encourage such infant manifestations. Second, developmental precursors represent a means by which the infant can signal the caregiver. The therapist should analyze how the caregiver interprets and responds to these signals. For example, is the caregiver cognizant of the precursory behavior and does she view it as a prelude to the manifestation of a milestone? Caregivers who recognize their infant's precursory behaviors and are enthusiastic about them are likely to communicate positive affect to the infant who, in turn, will continue to engage in the behavior in order to perpetuate the positive feeling shared with the caregiver. Finally, precursory manifestations should stimulate the caregiver to begin engaging in previewing exercises that will expose the infant to the sensation of what the achievement of the full-fledged milestone will be like and to the implications that these manifestations will provoke in the interpersonal arena. This kind of caregiver response fosters the infant's predictive abilities and creates an infant system for monitoring and correcting acts in relation to the goal of execution (Bernstein, 1967; Bodin, 1972). Moreover, caregiver feedback supplies perception of the consequences of acts, providing contingent information used en route to a goal.

Kaye (1982) has commented on the role of the caregiver during interaction with the infant, referring to the infant as an "apprentice" whose development is supervised by the caregiver. According to Kaye, the caregiver devises manageable subtasks for the infant to perform. Eventually, as the infant begins to display some degree of mastery and competence, the caregiver relinquishes control, thereby enhancing the infant's sense of achievement to an even greater degree.

The concept of the "zone of proximal development" proposed by Vygotsky (1978) bears some relation to Kaye's notion that the infant functions as an apprentice to the caregiver. Vygotsky explains that the zone of proximal development is the distance between the actual developmental level of the infant and the infant's potential developmental level. The infant's actual developmental level is the status of the infant's cognitive and affective functioning based on already completed developmental cycles. The level of potential development is determined through problem solving under adult guidance or in collaboration with more capable peers.

The zone of proximal development, according to Vygotsky, defines those functions that have not yet matured but are in the process of maturation, those functions that will mature imminently, but are currently in an embryonic state. In essence, the caregiver fills in the gap between actual and potential development. The concept of "holding" proposed by Winnicott (1965) also bears some relation to the two previous concepts. According to Winnicott, holding is the phase during which the "ego" changes from an unintegrated state too structured, integrated state. For Winnicott, the completion of the holding phase correlates with the emergence of symbolic functioning.

While these concepts-the infant as apprentice, the zone of proximal development, and the holding phase-provide some insight into how the caregiver participates in the acquisition of developmental skills, none of these concepts captures the mechanism of how the caregiver is initially motivated to engage in such behaviors or how the dyadic relationship becomes more sophisticated because of the cumulative effects of such interactions. The concept of previewing, however, begins to offer answers to some of these questions. Caregiver previewing necessitates first that the caregiver intuitively represent the infant's future development and then enact future sequences of interaction with the infant by devising specific exercises. Unlike Kaye's concept of the infant as an apprentice, previewing focuses on the patterns that the caregiver seeks to predict and instill in the infant. Previewing highlights the process whereby caregiver and infant share the experience of a future skill or developmental acquisition. Through previewing, the caregiver's highest goal is to promote adaptation through continuous contingent experiences. This relationship will be self-perpetuating and will manifest in the form of an enhanced wish to learn and master the challenges posed by development and the environment through the security and intimacy provided by the caregiver's support.

Indeed, the interpersonal component that is inherent in the previewing experience cannot be underscored enough. Previewing serves not only as a mechanism for introducing the infant to imminent development, but also as a means of reinforcing the sense of intimacy and security that is derived from an adaptive relationship with the caregiver. Several researchers have indicated that this social component is essential in order for the infant to develop a coherent and stable sense of identity. Lacan is among these observers (others are Muller and Richardson, 1982). Lacan's (1977) principal thesis is that the neonate initially experiences his incompetence in the world as a kind of developmental chaos. Motor skills are undeveloped, movement is turbulent and the external world is perceived as being fragmentary and noncontingent. To rectify this image of an uncontrollable and unmanageable world, the infant must experience some form of unity and coherence. For Lacan, this unity is promoted by the infant's reflection of himself. This self-reflection generally occurs between six and eighteen months. With the knowledge of an inchoate identity, the infant is able to represent himself as capable in some fashion of guiding his own developmental destiny. Lacan has observed that there is an "identification between the infant and [his] reflection in the most profound sense; namely, the transformation that takes place in the subject when he assumes an image" (p. 294). Lacan views this recognition on the part of the infant as being decisive in the formulation of a stable ego.

It appears that Lacan is describing not only the infant's realization of "self," but also, the infant's capacity to represent images in the external world, including, most significantly, his own image. Thus, Lacan's primary thesis is that the infant's realization of his own image or, as the researcher refers to it, "the image of one's own body" propels development forward, leading to the formation of the "I."

If we accept Lacan's thesis, however, we must ask how the infant arrives at the perception of self and evolves the capacity to represent images of both himself and the external world. One answer is provided by examining the role of previewing. When the infant is first born, his sense of the internal/external world is primitive. Nevertheless, it is likely that among the infant's first perceptions is the sensation of uncontrollability he experiences with respect to bodily functioning. The infant urinates and defecates as a result of forces which he is incapable of resisting. Pangs of hunger and the need to sleep also appear to surface spontaneously. As a result of these physiological drives, the infant experiences his body as an uncontrollable and unpredictable domain.

The caregiver makes her presence known to the infant by alleviating both the discomfort and the insecurity that are aroused by the seemingly uncontrollable forces of the body; the caregiver ministers to the infant's needs. As these behaviors are repeated day after day, the infant comes to recognize that there is in fact a means of exerting control over the chaos of his body. This control is found in the interaction with the caregiver. As long as the interaction is sustained, the infant will experience both the fulfillment of his immediate needs and will be able to stave off the anxiety and insecurity that attend uncontrollability.

The pattern of interaction between infant and caregiver eventually becomes routine and ingrained. The infant has come to rely upon the caregiver to fulfill his needs; the caregiver responds by assuaging discomfort and providing security. Soon, however, the infant's burgeoning developmental skills begin to emerge. Moreover, each emerging developmental precursor tends to resurrect earlier feelings of insecurity in the infant. As before, he will rely upon the caregiver to quell these feelings by providing him with the continuous guidance and direction essential for controlling his body. In this fashion, the interaction between infant and caregiver and the perpetuation of their relationship become the dyad's prime motivation. It is from this seminal interaction that we may trace Lacan's emphasis on the social component of personality.

During this early period of interaction, the caregiver's ministrations have not merely served to provide the infant with a sense of comfort and security. Instead, it is likely that the infant has begun to use his incipient cognitive processes to begin accumulating representations of experiences during these sequences of interaction. From such sequences, the infant can predict caregiver responses as he manifests a particular behavior and can similarly anticipate how to respond to certain behaviors initiated by the caregiver. According to Lacan's thesis, it is from the cumulative effect of these representations that the infant comes to formulate an image of himself which is capable of both initiating and responding to the caregiver's behavior.

Given this scenario, we can also understand how previewing contributes to reinforcing the infant's sense of self. As noted earlier, caregiver previewing tends to emerge as soon as the infant manifests precursory behaviors indicative of upcoming developmental milestones. In essence, these precursory behaviors signify an inchoate form of the milestone and as they emerge, the infant is reminded once again of the fact that his body is unpredictable and, at times, uncontrollable. If the caregiver is aware of these precursory manifestations, however, she may use them to guide the infant through previewing exercises in the direction of the full-fledged milestone. The infant's insecurity will thereby be assuaged and his representation of himself as a competent actor will be enhanced. As a result, it appears that, in addition to its other functions, previewing interactions on the part of the caregiver also act as a deterrent to the experience of somatic, affective, cognitive, or motivational deficits.

Beyond introducing the infant to specific developmental skills, previewing strives to enhance the infant's capacity to *anticipate, assess, predict and assert* the alterations that are inherent in the developmental process itself. By acquainting the infant with an imminent developmental milestone and by responding to the infant's somatic, affective, cognitive and motivational cues, the caregiver manages to convey control and security to the infant. This control, however, does not merely extend to the infant's mastery of that particular developmental acquisition. Instead, the infant experiences a sense of control over the interactional process itself. In this fashion, previewing provides the infant with insight of how he is incorporating—beyond specific discrete tasks—control over the interpersonal relationship with the caregiver.

A recent study supports these observations. Isabella, Belsky, and von Eye (1989) discerned the origins of infant-mother attachment patterns as manifested in one-year-old infants by examining the degree of interactional synchrony and attunement exhibited during dyadic exchange. The researchers focused in particular on fourteen individual behavior categories. Maternal vocalization, contingent exchange, infant vocalization, direct maternal response to infant vocalization, infant exploratory behavior, and infant gaze at the caregiver are some of these behaviors. Researcher evaluated the incidence of these behaviors in fifty-one dyads who were observed at one, three, and nine months, and who were administered the Ainsworth Strange Situation Paradigm in order to assess the type of attachment manifested by the infant at one year of age. It was found that when maternal sensitivity, as manifested by contingent stimulation and appropriate response to infant signals, was high, the attachment within the dyad tended to be "secure." Conversely, when this kind of optimal stimulation was absent at one, three, and nine months, making dyadic interaction asynchronic, the infant displayed an "insecure" attachment to the caregiver at one year of age. The researchers concluded by noting that synchronous interaction was a good predictor of secure attachment, while asynchronous interaction tended to foreshadow insecure attachment.

Previewing has a further advantage of demonstrating to the therapist how psychopathological responses can insinuate themselves into the dyadic relationship, impeding both the caregiver-infant interaction and the acquisition of specific developmental skills. This is because, through previewing, the caregiver has the opportunity to share her predictions about development with the infant. If such predictions are maladaptive or designed to thwart, rather than foster, development, the infant may begin to display these patterns himself. In addition, as suggested by the discussion above, maladaptive previewing may foster feelings of insecurity and uncontrollability, an experience that motivates the dyad to master maladaptive interactions instead of being able to overcome them. Thus, the concept of previewing helps to explain in a manner not previously proposed a wide variety of phenomena that affect the dyadic adaptation.

The Psychological Residue of Previewing

Because the potential implications of previewing emerge most clearly in the verbal descriptions the caregiver provides to the therapist, as well as during caregiver initiated episodes of interaction with the infant, therapists must understand the ramifications that this phenomenon will exert upon the infant as an individual in the throes of developmental change. While the infant, unlike the caregiver, cannot give verbal expression to the impact of previewing, it is clear from observations that infants who are exposed to previewing by their caregivers will display enhanced developmental progress and an ease in negotiating the challenges of the external world.

Previewing, then, appears to bolster the infant's burgeoning developmental capacity in a wide variety of ways. Four specific ways in which previewing operates to enhance development are worthy of mention here.

Previewing Facilitates the Infant's Predictive Abilities

As noted, one of the most distinctive features about the phenomenon of previewing is that it orients both caregiver and infant toward impending and future development. It is especially important for the infant to be exposed to previewing experiences, because all developmental capacities are dependent upon the infant's ability to formulate reliable expectations about the future.

In particular, researchers have found that even newborns can detect discrepancies in their environment (McCall and McGhee, 1977), and three-month-old infants can discern contingencies (i.e., cause-effect relationships) among environmental stimuli and among environmental events (Watson, 1966, 1972; Stern and Gibbon, 1978). Once the infant is habituated to a particular contingency, repetition of that specific contingency or of a slightly varied contingency at a later date will result in a display of pleasure. This manifestation of positive affect is believed to derive from the gratification the infant experiences in the recognition of similar patterns which trigger a sense of security in a world that is often strange and unfamiliar. Furthermore, DeCasper and Carstens (1981) have demonstrated that even neonates can learn and retain contingency relationships for relatively long periods. Contingency relationships, then, offer the infant a means for predicting and recognizing sequences, thereby enabling the infant to exert control and mastery over the environment. Indeed, evidence of contingency awareness suggests that by three months the infant possesses a rudimentary capacity to represent developmental sequences.

In essence, previewing exercises reinforce the experience of contingency for the infant, but on a grander, more elaborate scale. When the caregiver lends support to the infant's crawling motions or imitates the infant's vocalizations to simulate a conversation between the two, she is conveying to the infant the message that such incipient manifestations will eventually result in the consolidation of full-fledged developmental milestones that will assist the infant in mastering the challenges posed by the interpersonal milieu. Previewing as a form of prediction thus enables the infant to perceive the response that is appropriate to the behavioral manifestations that stimulate his development.

Previewing Enhances the Infant's Ability to Integrate Multi-Modal Perceptions

Previewing behaviors consolidate the infant's perceptual capacities in a unique fashion. Gradually, as development progresses, the infant begins to attain an awareness of his separateness from the caregiver. As this awareness crystallizes, the infant comes to recognize that his reality (i.e., *the subjective self*) is different and apart from the reality of the external environment and the caregiver (i.e., *the objective world*). Until the realization of a full demarcation between subjective and objective comes to fruition, it poses a potential obstacle to infant development.

In addition to this duality of subjective and objective domains, the infant will also be challenged to begin integrating the diverse modes of functioning he possesses. For example, somatic responses must be coordinated with appropriate affective displays, which, in turn, must be processed by particular cognitive processes. in order to propel motivational forces that ultimately determine whether or not to continue the interaction. In order for the infant to give meaning to the world, a coherence among the multitude of skills possessed by the infant needs to be acquired. Finally, as discussed in previous chapters, the infant must learn to integrate and regulate perceptions from different sensory domains. The integration of all of these multimodal phenomena will eventually occur as inevitable sequelae of development. Infants who are continuously previewed in an auxiliary fashion by their caregivers will be able to engage in this form of multimodal integration earlier and will achieve a smoother developmental course.

Previewing facilitates multimodal coordination because predictive manifestations stimulate several domains of perception to function simultaneously. During the performance of virtually all previewing behaviors, for example, caregivers will provide verbal orientation and cues to the infant, which are perceived as cognitive messages. In addition, caregivers will generally imbue the previewing behaviors with a particular affective and/or tactile tone which is conveyed to the infant. As a result, the infant will combine tactile, auditory and visual messages into one comprehensive representation. Thus, previewing helps the infant integrate emerging dimensions simultaneously.

Previewing Objectifies Present and Future Reality

Researchers such as De Gramont (1987) and Goldberg (1989) have contributed to the literature by theorizing about the role of language in enhancing the individual's awareness of himself as a creator of *meaning*. De Gramont has suggested that language, of all human skills, is unique, because it is the vehicle whereby our subjective impressions of the world are converted into an objective message that can be conveyed to and understood by another. Language is, in other words, a unifying medium that enables us to share our perceptions with one another. It is through language, according to De Gramont, that we escape our subjectivity and predict a shared reality, capable of being mutually validated with another.

Among the functions played by language that have been enumerated by De Gramont are: (1) its ability to transform the seemingly uncontrollable environment around us into a discrete domain that is capable of being predicted and mastered; (2) its ability to provide us with the skill to predict upcoming events; (3) its ability to offer us an elastic and flexible mode of expressing perceptions; and (4) its ability to facilitate the resolution of conflict by providing a means of working through emotional conflicts.

The way in which language enables us to perform these complex functions is highly unique and distinguishes it from all other forms of communication. The distinctiveness of language lies in the fact that it is a *symbolic* means of communication. Language is symbolic because the medium used, i.e., letters, words, etc., capture the content of what is being expressed in a particular code. Phrased another way, the components of language (letters, words) have no inherent meaning in and of themselves; rather, a particular meaning is attributed to them. This attribution refers to an object or concept in the objective world to which all those who speak the language have consensually designated a particular meaning. Language, therefore, divorces the concept, known in linguistics as the referent, from the symbol, which is the code that will stand for that thing or concept. Because of language's reliance on symbols, Watzlawick, Beavin, and Jackson (1967) have called this form of communication the *digital* mode.

There is, however, another form of communication, referred to as the *analogic mode,* which is less sophisticated than language. Most forms of nonverbal communication fall within the analogic mode, including our posture, our gestures, our tone, and I submit, some of the physical manifestations associated with previewing behaviors. In particular, previewing behaviors that attempt to simulate upcoming developmental milestones are analogic because the behavior demonstrated represents or stands for identical behavior that will occur in the future. Analogic communication is different from digital communication in that the medium of communication attempts to duplicate or serve as an analogy to the content of what we are communicating.

This distinction is important not only because it suggests the hierarchy whereby human beings eventually learn to communicate complex thought processes and emotions through language but also because it provides another milestone for enhancing predictive abilities. Beyond the distinction between analogic and digital communication, however, I propose that previewing experiences may serve as an intermediary mode between these forms of communication. During previewing exercises messages are communicated using the analogic mode (e.g., such intuitive behaviors as visual cuing, feeding, vocal cuing, and holding the infant in a particular fashion that simulates the experience of walking or crawling are the essence of analogic forms of communication), and the digital mode (e.g., previewing exchanges themselves symbolize for the infant future developments and convey the message that such imminent growth will be predictable). Indeed, it may be argued that by introducing the infant to future changes via previewing, the caregiver is, in essence, enhancing the infant's ability for symbolic representation. While the caregiver is helping the infant to accommodate the future by providing a pretend-like situation symbolic of future change, she is also providing an analogue of future social exchange. For this reason, previewing is among the most complex and significant experience to which the young infant is exposed during the first two years of life.

Previewing Supports the Infant's Emerging Sense of Control and Mastery Over the Interaction

Previewing accomplishes, quite literally, the task of introducing the infant to future development, allowing the infant to coordinate representations of his current proprioceptive experience with the resulting behaviors. By being exposed to future developmental skills, the infant will be able to predict what such development will be like. The caregiver who is using previewing in a well-paced fashion, will acquaint the infant with upcoming developmental trends in a manner that is both supportive and encouraging. Every gesture that the caregiver uses will be firm enough to convey to the infant that he is being guided by a supportive partner, and yet will be gentle and flexible enough so that the infant is given sufficient latitude to explore and experiment with his own resources without feeling overwhelmed. Because previewing is geared to the pacing of the infant's development, when done properly and appropriately, such exercises tend to give a keen edge to the infant's curiosity about the future, motivating the onset of future growth.

Previewing, then, whets the infant's somatic, affective, cognitive, and motivational appetites. Moreover, because previewing generally occurs with a supportive caregiver, whatever hesitations the infant may harbor about future development are quelled, because the caregiver conveys the message that she will be available to guide the infant back to an already mastered developmental plateau when challenges posed by these new behaviors become overwhelming or taxing for the infant. The qualities that are embedded within previewing exercises enable the infant to experience a quality of prediction about his environment. Such predictions trigger control and mastery which, in turn, generate feelings of security that serve to fuel the desire to achieve even greater levels of competence. As feelings of security are enhanced and reinforced, the infant becomes increasingly more convinced that he is capable of exerting control and mastery over his environment. Thus, previewing has a self-perpetuating and proliferating aspect, in the sense that the greater the infant's ability to predict events in the environment, the more stimulated he will be to achieve even greater control over future developmental acquisitions.

Previewing Provides the Infant with the Ability to Compensate for Developmental Deficits

The discussion so far has focused upon the benefits previewing can instill in the infant in an optimal situation in which the caregiver is administering these behaviors adaptively, in harmony with the rhythms of the infant's adaptational status. It should be noted, however, that even in situations where the interaction between caregiver and infant is less than optimal, instances of previewing can still, to some extent, serve to promote the infant's development, since previewing orients the infant toward the future skills that will develop over time. As one example of this type of interaction, one mother I was treating rarely engaged in vocal exchanges with her infant. When I asked her to explain why this was the case she shrugged her shoulders, indicating that she just did not have the inclination to speak to her son. In addition, this caregiver was also hesitant when I asked her to predict her infant's upcoming developments. Despite these deficits, the caregiver appeared to enjoy holding her infant while she stood near the window and both mother and child gazed out. At these times, she would often guide her infant's hand as he grasped for moving toys that revolved on a mobile suspended from the window shade. These behaviors seemed to stimulate the infant's motor skills. As a consequence, even if the infant is not receiving adequate stimulation from the caregiver, the presence of some modicum of previewing will serve to encourage the onset of impending development and to foster the acquisition of new skills. Indeed, in a situation in which the infant is not receiving adequate stimulation in other areas, previewing behaviors, even if administered only intermittently (e.g., by alternate caregivers), may serve to motivate the infant to practice greater predictive skill leading to enhanced development.

Some prime examples of how previewing can serve as a mechanism spurring on future skill are encountered in the case histories of the infants of parents who are developmentally disabled. For such infants and young children, previewing not only acts as an introduction to burgeoning developmental skills, but also indicates that there are alternative methods for cementing and reinforcing predictive communications within the dyadic interaction. In these cases, previewing can compensate for the lack of stimulation an infant or young child might receive in a particular domain of functioning.

Previewing behaviors can also play a role in another situation. Assuming that the caregiver lacks sufficient skill to stimulate the infant adequately, the infant's natural proclivities will propel him in the direction of development, in any event, and he may seize upon any form of behavior that will serve to coordinate the ability to use burgeoning skills to their fullest potential. Thus, the infant may seize upon the advantages offered by previewing as an opportunity to extricate himself from an interaction with the caregiver that is less than fulfilling. In such a scenario, behaviors displayed by the caregiver (e.g., lack of reciprocity) may accelerate the pace of development and lead to a form of precocity that is not entirely advantageous. Nevertheless, previewing in this context may help the infant surmount the deficits inherent in the maladaptive interaction with the caregiver.

Given this description of what caregiver previewing is and how these psychological and behavioral manifestations affect the rhythms of infant development, we may turn in the next chapter to an examination of previewing from the perspective of the adaptive and maladaptive caregiver.

Conclusion

This chapter has focused on the concept of previewing as the epitome of the interpersonal communication between mother and infant during the first few years of life. As discussed, previewing appears to emerge in varying degrees in virtually all new mothers. Although previewing encompasses numerous behaviors and perceptions, three main components of this phenomenon have been highlighted here. These components are the caregiver's ability to represent various facets of the infant's development and to recognize the precursory behaviors that signify the advent of full-fledged developmental milestones; the caregiver's capacity to devise specific behaviors and exercises that can be engaged in with the infant in order to introduce him to upcoming developmental achievement; and, the caregiver's capacity to help the infant return to the developmental status he was exhibiting prior to the previewing exercises in a supportive fashion.

The significance of previewing extends beyond the specific behaviors engaged in by the caregiver, however. As has been described, through previewing the infant attains the recognition that the seemingly uncontrollable forces of his own physiology can not only be controlled, but may also be predicted. This capacity to predict and control, with the help of a supportive caregiver, motivates the infant to devise ways of maintaining the gratifying relationship with the caregiver. In addition, the predictive notions embedded in previewing exercises enable the infant to surmount any of the debilitating feelings aroused by the unpredictability of burgeoning development. Previewing also enables the infant to engage in a fairly sophisticated form of communication with the caregiver. Such communication has analogic aspects, in that the previewing behaviors themselves represent paradigms of what of future development will be like while simultaneously representing digital forms of communication symbolizing future interactions for the infant.

CHAPTER 8

Previewing as a Principle for Intervention

Introduction

As discussed in the preceding chapter, previewing may represent one of the most dynamic aspects of the caregiver-infant relationship. Now that the concept has been defined, it is relatively easy to begin identifying instances of previewing-or the lack thereof-in virtually any dyad that is observed. Indeed, because previewing behavior is such an omnipresent factor in the interaction between caregiver and infant, it is a valuable instrument for diagnosing both adaptive and maladaptive aspects of the relationship. Beyond this diagnostic benefit, previewing may also be used as an innovative treatment technique for modifying the dyadic exchange in a fashion that promotes the infant's maturation, while enhancing the intimacy between mother and infant.

There are three main reasons why previewing as a therapeutic technique is beneficial in the treatment of caregivers and their infants. The first reason involves the orientation of previewing manifestations toward future development acquisition. Unlike traditional forms of treatment which strive to unearth conflict by focusing on a retrospective analysis of events, memories and dreams, previewing is unique because it is *prospective,* focusing on the future. Rather than attempting to unravel the past, previewing propels the patient-here the caregiver-to proceed toward upcoming developmental events. As many researchers have observed, because unresolved conflict from an earlier stage of development will be replicated in contemporaneous relationships and interactions, previewing provides the therapist with an unparalleled opportunity for both observing the way in which conflict will operate and for devising strategies for overcoming the effects of such conflict. By examining the caregiver's expectations through previewing the therapist circumvents the process of having to delve into the caregiver's past to unearth conflict before restoration of an adaptive interaction can be established.

When previewing manifestations are used by the therapist in this fashion they exert an effect similar to a Rorschach test. The caregiver is asked to represent or envision future interaction with the infant. In formulating this representation, the caregiver will not only rely upon her expectations about the infant's future developmental course, but will also include aspects of her own behavioral style, including most significantly, the way in which she establishes affective bonds with others. Thus, when the therapist asks the caregiver to describe what she believes the infant's next developmental achievement will be and how she envisions future interaction, the caregiver will generally provide insights into how she relates to others. From the mother's comments, the therapist can then ascertain the nature of the dyadic relationship. In this sense, by asking the mother to envision the future relationship through representational exercises, the therapist can predict upcoming patterns of interaction and can devise interventive strategies if these anticipated patterns are maladaptive.

A second reason why previewing is an optimal psychotherapeutic strategy for mother-infant dyads lies in the fact that therapy can be immediately applied to modify the interaction between the pair. In contrast to individual therapy, which focuses on the seminal relationship between therapist and patient, dyadic therapy involving a caregiver and infant or toddler brings two overlapping relationships into the treatment setting simultaneously. The therapist can observe interaction within the dyad, discuss the interaction with the caregiver and subsequently either instruct the caregiver on methods for enhancing the exchange with the infant or actually model and demonstrate adaptive interactions with the infant directly. The mother can then be instructed to imitate these patterns. In addition, the infant's innate proclivities to learn and predict interactive behaviors are accentuated in this form of therapeutic exchange, because treatment focuses on establishing a relationship that is a source of continual gratification and fulfillment for the dyad.

Finally, previewing is an efficacious treatment technique because it adheres to the natural pace of development that is inherent in the caregiver-infant relationship. Since the infant will develop in any event, when used as a therapeutic tool, previewing merely enhances a naturally occurring phenomena. In other words, previewing takes advantage of developmental phenomena that the infant is already experiencing and enhances the mother's ability to recognize and promote maturational trends, while encouraging an affective and cognitive bond within the dyad.

The Adaptive Caregiver

Before we can understand how previewing may be used to help mothers who are exhibiting maladaptive patterns with their infants, it is worthwhile to examine how adaptive caregivers enhance the infant's development by integrating previewing manifestations into their daily routine.

The adaptive caregiver, whose actions are based on intuition, is relatively easy to recognize. The interaction between such caregivers and their infants is pleasurable to observe because one senses an easygoing rhythm in all behavioral responses, coupled with a continuous sense of fulfilled expectations between the members of the pair.

If the mood created by such caregivers were to be described, one might say that they are able to foreshadow or preview not only developmental capacities but also the social implications that such change will bring for their infants. This kind of harmonious exchange was evident in one such caregiver and her four-month-old infant who attended group sessions at my clinic. The caregiver often held the infant in a reclining position and gradually raised his torso, so that he was sitting up. Having attained this erect posture, the infant would mouth a stuffed animal, all the while glancing back and forth at the caregiver as she maintained a continually secure, yet gentle grasp upon the upper portion of his body. Eventually, the mother would ease the infant back into a reclining position and present him with a bottle which he then accepted with a welcoming grasp. The developmental milestone of sitting momentarily without support occurs at approximately five months; the fact that this caregiver was engaging in the behavior when the infant was four months old indicated that her behavior was a prime example of previewing an imminent developmental skill. This sequence evolved very smoothly, and the contours between the infant's changing motivations were so graceful, that it was almost as if the dyad had previously rehearsed the scene. When I asked the caregiver to describe the experience of holding the infant in this fashion, she noted that she had known intuitively, perhaps from the gestures of his upper body, that he wanted to experience the sensation of sitting up on his own and that she was also able to tell when he wished to be returned to his earlier position. She indicated that the times she held the baby in this manner she felt as if they were communicating through touch. "It's as if our bodies become one," she said, "and I can sense what he wants."

Careful observation of such previewing episodes discloses that the adaptive caregiver is, in fact, aware of the infant's precursory movements and is engaging in a form of rehearsal with the infant. By being acutely aware of the infant's current developmental status and any signs of incipient maturation, the caregiver is able to both detect and respond to infinitesimal forms of progression which gradually emerge. Such caregivers are able to perceive even the most incremental change in their infants—whether the change is embodied in gestures, vocalizations or eye contact—and to predict how this change will be crystallized into yet a further developmental milestone. These milestones are then previewed for the infant, as the caregiver supports and coordinates the infant's efforts, efforts which can only barely be perceived by an outward observer, but of which the caregiver is fully cognizant. This form of support is impressive because the caregiver is offering a form of *auxiliary coordination* that helps the infant coordinate on a variety of levels. These levels include the somatic, affective, cognitive impressions and perpetuate the infant's motivation to assess and explore the environment. In this sense, the adaptive caregiver functions as a supportive partner who helps the infant to gradually synthesize novel developmental accomplishments and to smooth transitions between new and previous levels of functioning.

Another example will further reinforce the atmosphere of adaptation and rhythmicity created by a previewing exercise. Most caregivers patiently await the day when the infant will take his first steps. Adaptive caregivers are capable of representing and predicting, and thus previewing intuitively virtually any developmental milestone, forecasting its occurrence by looking for early signs of manifestations in the infant. Such caregivers sense how the infant begins to demonstrate an ability for erect posture, for example. In time, they will assist the infant by holding his arms as he takes his first steps. Yet, such caregivers are also attuned to cues that reveal that the infant is exhausted or wishes to stop the previewing routine to which he has been newly exposed. When the caregiver begins to sense that this point has been reached, she will slowly place the infant on the floor once again. Previewing the milestone of walking for the infant is repeated whenever the caregiver intuitively anticipates the infant's inclination to engage in such rehearsals of imminent development. But adaptive caregivers do not hinder development either by applying unsolicited pressures or by ignoring the infant's cues; rather they stand poised ready to observe and respond to the infant's cues and signs of precursory development, supporting the infant's expectations at all times. Moreover, they provide the infant with a smooth passage from the incipient demonstrations of any given milestone to the infant's currently mastered functional status.

From these descriptions it is clear that adaptive caregivers are distinguished in two important respects. First, adaptive caregivers are able to represent, predict and subsequently preview or foreshadow forthcoming developmental milestones for the infant. Very simply, they can sense what is on the developmental horizon for the infant, what new skill or developmental acquisition is on the verge of being manifested. Second, the adaptive caregiver motivates the infant to practice the milestone appropriately by engaging in previewing exercises. During such exercises the caregiver will gradually support the infant in simulating the physical gestures and signs of the full-fledged milestone. Such a caregiver will not attempt to freeze the infant in his or her current state of development, nor will she press the infant to precociously demonstrate a milestone when the baby is not yet ready to articulate such maturational skills. Thus, such caregivers are so attuned to the developmental status of their infants that they are able to function as *auxiliary coordinators,* making the transitions between developmental stages relatively effortless and decidedly pleasurable. As a result, the transitions between the different levels of functioning are very smooth, as the infant gradually practices and masters each new skill.

But adaptive caregivers are distinctive in yet a third way that is not so readily apparent from direct observation. Adaptive caregivers are, in actuality, *synthesizing* a variety of perceptions that derive from an awareness that the infant is functioning on a *multidimensional* level. This includes the dimensions of somatic affective and cognitive awareness, as well as the overall psychological motivation behind the infant's behaviors. If we further analyze one of the examples cited above, it becomes clear how this sensitivity to multidimensional functioning operates. The illustration of the caregiver singing a lullaby to the infant represents an ideal paradigm for exploring this phenomenon of multidimensional synthesis. In the gentleness of her tone of voice and the cradling gestures of her embrace, the caregiver conveys a particular feeling state or affect to the infant during such episodes. By singing specific words to the infant, such as "hush little baby, don't you cry. Mama's going to sing you a lullaby," the caregiver manages to consolidate affective, cognitive and somatic cues. Specific motions and gestures of the caregiver as she rocks the infant reflect how she is representing the infant's state of mind and how she is beginning to coordinate *content* with *process* while interacting with the infant. Lastly, all of these elements blend into *bidirectional* motivational cues that flow from the caregiver to the infant and vice versa. By coordinating her gestures while singing (process) with the underlying meaning (content) of the lullaby, the caregiver is providing a supportive atmosphere that assists the infant in making smooth transitions and in engaging in the integration of different sensory perceptions.

Each of these four elements of an adaptive response is interwoven during previewing exercises. Perception and communication of the *affective dimension* enables the infant to validate his own emotional state through that of the caregiver, who in turn validates and reinforces the particular feeling experienced by the infant. If during the interaction such cues are shared repeatedly, the infant eventually comes to perceive that both he and the caregiver possess a full spectrum of emotions that can be predicted, shared and regulated. This sharing of emotions allows the infant to gradually attain the capacity for self-regulation.

An example of how the cognitive dimension becomes predictable through previewing is provided by the emergence of language cues that stimulate the development of language. Virtually all infant researchers are familiar with the phenomenon of "baby talk," the semi-playful type of vocalization that adults engage in with infants. But this ostensibly innocent banter actually serves a more complex function than that of entertaining the infant or capturing his attention. In fact, caregivers engaged in this type of activity are actually rehearsing a dialogue in front of the infant in order to convey the notion of how actual conversation occurs. By repeating words to the infant, and by varying the tone, pitch, and pacing of these words, the caregiver is rehearsing the fundamental constituent elements of a dialogue. Moreover, the adaptive caregiver will not overtax the infant's capacities by prolonging this dialogue beyond the point where the infant is capable of paying attention.

Adaptive caregivers are also attuned to the somatic capacities of their infants. Perceiving and communicating the *somatic dimension* in this context refers to the caregiver's consideration and awareness of the infant's overall constitutional endowment. This constitutional dimension includes a sensitivity to body temperature, muscular ability, stamina, appetite, etc. Caregivers who are adaptive will display their sensitivity by, for example, offering the infant a cup or spoon at the appropriate time developmentally when behaviors that are precursory to full-fledged grasping have begun to be manifested. Such sensitivity to motor ability enables the caregiver to perceive when the infant is ready to be placed in an erect sitting posture or when the infant is developmentally equipped to take his first supported steps.

The final component of response that adaptive caregivers coordinate into their repertoire of responses involves *motivation*. During all exchanges between infant and caregiver, motivational cues are conveyed. These cues refer to the stimulation and enthusiasm with which the caregiver imbues her responses. Such cues serve to arouse the infant's curiosity, propelling him to engage in behaviors that will sustain the interaction. Adaptive caregivers tend to convey motivational cues that are appropriate to the infant's developmental status. For instance, the caregiver who is singing a lullaby knows that the infant is tired and ready to sleep. Such motivational messages communicate security and a soothing affect that will help the infant make the transition into a sleepy state. If the infant wishes to play, however, the adaptive caregiver will actively participate by creating an atmosphere for exploration. Depending upon the circumstance and the cues being emitted by the infant, therefore, adaptive caregivers will adjust their behavior accordingly in order to maintain appropriate levels of motivational messages for the infant.

In assessing the caregiver's level of adaptability, the therapist must be attuned to the full spectrum of phenomena mentioned above. Primarily, the therapist must assess whether the caregiver is foreshadowing or previewing developmental milestones for the infant, how she conveys the advent of these developmental achievements and how she supports the infant's efforts in negotiating transitions between currently mastered developmental states, precursors of imminent milestones and full-fledged developmental achievements. Therapists should always ask themselves whether the caregiver is demonstrating an extreme response, by either neglecting to predict future development and thereby "freezing" the infant at his current developmental level or, conversely, whether the caregiver has a tendency to "press" the infant into exhibiting developmental achievements before the infant is entirely ready or maturationally equipped to do so. One way of gauging if the caregiver's interactional behavior falls at an appropriate point on this spectrum of previewing behavior involves assessing the infant's multidimensional responses. If the infant appears apathetic and listless, for example, the caregiver may be providing minimal stimulation or may be overtaxing and exhausting the infant. In contrast, infants who become upset and manifest signs of distress after brief periods of interaction with the caregiver may be communicating that the caregiver is pressing too hard to elicit a developmental response the infant is not yet capable of generating. The therapist must, therefore, observe how the caregiver assists the infant in negotiating developmental states and analyze the fluidity with which these transitions are facilitated. It is also important to evaluate how sensitive the caregiver is in her response to the infant's more subtle cues.

In addition, the therapist should be alert to the four components outlined above, the infant's somatic, affective, cognitive and motivational states. For each sequence of interaction observed, an analysis of these individual components needs to be performed. If the caregiver is playing with the infant in the therapist's presence, for instance, the therapist should observe whether an appropriate affective tone is infusing the interaction. This factor can be assessed by observing whether the infant appears to be experiencing an emotional response appropriate to the situation and whether the caregiver's emotional expression matches that of the infant. Does the caregiver strive to reinforce the affect for the infant, thereby validating the infant's experience or is she oblivious to the infant's emotional status? Does an atmosphere of affect attunement suffuse the dyadic exchange?

The caregiver's facility in conveying appropriate cognitive and somatic responses can also be evaluated via observation. The therapist must observe the interplay of vocal cuing, along with the caregiver's ability as an auxiliary coordinator to help the infant exercise muscles supportively. Is the caregiver sensitive to other aspects of the infant's psychomotor status, such as body temperature? One method for gauging this somatic sensitivity is by scrutinizing how the infant is clothed and whether the caregiver removes outer clothing in warm weather and vice versa. In addition, the somatic dimension incorporates the caregiver's capacity to identify the infant's temperamental status and to regulate her responses to that status.

With this in mind, the therapist should attend to the overall ambience the caregiver generates during episodes of interaction. Does the caregiver provide an atmosphere that facilitates the emergence of predictive capacities, enabling the infant to explore and experiment, while at the same time offering the infant a sense of security and support? In essence, when evaluating these components, the therapist should focus on how skillfully the caregiver *represents,* and subsequently supports the upcoming consolidation of developmental milestones through previewing behaviors. Adaptive caregivers permit the infant to incrementally attain a sense of familiarity with upcoming developmental milestones, without foisting such behaviors on the infant. At the same time, however, in the course of acquisition such caregivers gradually allow this new behavior to re-cede, so that the infant has an opportunity to savor the taste of what the new developmental achievement will ultimately be like without feeling incompetent by his inability to exhibit the milestone independently. Such caregivers convey a resonance of the upcoming developmental acquisi-tion, while supporting the attainment of control over new functions at the infant's own pace. If the motivational cues conveyed by the caregiver are appropriate, then the infant's developmental progress will be both *hierarchical*—in the sense that each achievement will generate a further achievement—and *coordinated*—in the sense that skills will be integrated smoothly without distress or deficits.

Once this evaluation has been completed, the therapist will be ready to diagnose the overall developmental status of the dyad, as well as to iden-tify specific areas of the dyad's interaction. It is important to remember that if the dyad is functioning in an adaptive fashion, an overall tone of rhythmicity and attunement will characterize dyadic exchange. The thera-pist can then begin to devise a treatment strategy designed to cope with the unique problems encountered in a particular caregiver and infant dyad.

The Maladaptive Caregiver

Just as the adaptive caregiver was distinctive because of certain patterns that could be observed during dyadic interaction, so too is the maladap-tive caregiver, who is far less adept at managing behavioral displays and who tends to overlook infant signals altogether or to exhibit inappropriate responses to infant cues. It is important to keep in mind, however, that the purpose of accurate diagnosis is not so much to label the overall dy-adic interaction but rather to gain insight into specific and discrete mal-adaptive patterns that are susceptible to modification. In fact, when working with caregivers and their infants it is not unusual for certain as-pects of interaction to be adaptive, while other aspects are impaired.

Essentially, maladaptive caregivers should be assessed in the same fashion as adaptive ones. The four dimensions discussed above for evalu-ating the caregiver's sensitivity-somatic affective, cognitive, and motiva-tional-emerge during maladaptive sequences in a specific fashion that is readily observable by the therapist. Familiarity with these deviant mani-festations helps the therapist during the evaluation. For example, in as-sessing the communication of affective dimensions, some caregivers will exert virtually no control over emotional states. That is, either the care-giver superimposes her emotional state upon the infant in a smothering or overwhelming fashion, or the infant appears to display a full range of emotions indiscriminately, while the caregiver seems nonresponsive and unconcerned. During such maladaptive interactions, both infant and care-giver miss opportunities for *joint attention* (e.g., both members fail to derive fulfillment and satisfaction) as the object upon whom to direct their emotional displays. In addition, these displays tend to be unpredictable and disconnected. For example, while the infant is crying, he is not sustaining visual contact with the caregiver. On the other hand, the caregiver does not attempt to join her attentive skills with the cues of the infant; instead, it is as if the caregiver's gaze is aimed at a different target. This type of interaction prevents the infant from predicting discrete emotions and coordinating them within the context of a specific interpersonal situation. Moreover, such a noninteractive style precludes the infant from the experience of *affective validation,* a process that allows each emotion to be reinforced for the infant by the caregiver, so that the infant gradually acquires skill in displaying a variety of affects that are situation specific.

Communication of the cognitive dimension also emerges differently during maladaptive interaction. The most telling signal to the therapist that caregiver and infant lack cognitive rapport is reflected by a lack of synchronicity or a discrepancy between the caregiver's affect content, process and cognition. Unlike adaptive caregivers who display and simulate the signs of a full-fledged dialogue through modulations in voice tone and pitch, maladaptive interaction is distinctive because vocal exchanges with the infant occur in a monotone fashion and often the caregiver maintains minimal eye contact during such sequences. Because of this, the infant is unable to determine if the caregiver is engaging in dialogue or to comprehend that the caregiver is anticipating a response. Moreover, a flat monologue prevents the infant from deriving any predictions about this form of behavior. This type of distinctive monotonal style precludes the infant from comprehending that particular discrete affects can be associated with specific thought patterns or cognitions. As a result, development is stifled because the infant is denied an opportunity to coordinate different cognitions and affects. Nor is the infant allowed to engage in reality-testing exercises to validate and share his experience with a supportive "other" who guides his developmental course. In effect, such infants remain stuck in a developmental impasse because they lack the differentiated stimulation that would provide them with the capacity to predict the meaning of cognitive and affective messages, as well as the motivation to do so.

In portraying how maladaptive caregivers respond to their infants' development, I am reminded of a young caregiver I was seeing in treatment during individual sessions with her infant. The caregiver was a recovering drug addict, who would sit in a chair opposite me, while the infant remained in his carriage. Despite the fact that these sessions took place in the summer when the weather was humid and the infant incessantly stirred in an effort to cast off his blanket, the caregiver remained oblivious to his state. Each time the infant thrust off the blanket, the caregiver would abruptly hover over him again, as if she had not the faintest clue as to why he was gesturing in this manner.

Eventually, as the session progressed, the caregiver would remove the infant from the carriage and prop him on her lap, while she faced the infant's back. During such sequences she rarely gazed at the infant face-to-face, nor did she check his facial expressions. Instead, as if she were responding to some invisible clock, she would periodically remove a bottle of milk from her bag and automatically stick it into the infant's mouth. Although she would occasionally gaze in the infant's direction, she appeared oblivious to his hand or mouth gestures. The nipple would either be forced into the baby's mouth or removed, seemingly at whim. Nor was this caregiver adept at creating a cradle with her arms to fully support neck and the upper portion of the infant's body.

When she wasn't feeding the baby, this caregiver would often position the infant in an awkwardly erect posture on both legs and bounce him up and down as he faced me. She tended to engage in this behavior when the infant began to display signs of distress. I got the impression that she was almost trying to shake the baby up in an effort to quell his cries.

This example vividly captures the behaviors of a caregiver whose perceptive abilities are minimal. Fortunately, therapists will generally not encounter behavior that is so blatantly inappropriate and insensitive to the infant's developmental needs. Nevertheless, this case illustrates the myriad of ways in which a caregiver can demonstrate lack of attunement to the infant's physiological and psychological capacities and can, in fact, frustrate these capacities to the point where the developmental process becomes stagnant. Because the assumption is that virtually every new mother will be skilled at such seemingly "natural" functions as feeding and holding the infant appropriately, skills that support such physiological functions often tend to be overlooked by therapists in their assessments. Nevertheless, as illustrated by the above example, there are numerous ways in which the caregiver's ability to manage the infant in an appropriate fashion can go awry. Therapists should, therefore, be alert to these behaviors, because caregiver deficits in the area of somatic sensitivity can devastate development if permitted to continue.

Another reason for emphasizing the importance of observing caregiver skills in the domain of somatic functions is that maladaptive behavior in this area is often readily susceptible to treatment. Caregivers can be taught to recognize and predict the infant's physiological status, as well as to improve their intuitive sensitivity to the infant's physiological needs. Moreover, once such sensitivity is achieved, caregiver skills in other domains, such as the affective and cognitive realms, are likely to improve as well. Most caregivers will be able to learn how to appraise the infant's temperature, for example. If these basic skills are learned, the caregiver's perception of the infant's signals in general is likely to dramatically improve, and this improvement will be demonstrated by an invigorated attitude towards representing the infant's imminent developmental trends, generating predictions about the infant's responses, devising appropriated behaviors to acquaint the infant with these new skills, and finally easing the infant back to his previous level of development. In essence, then, the caregiver can be guided through the steps of previewing.

The caregiver's failure to imbue interaction with an appropriate motivational atmosphere will be revealed in the lack of support provided for the infant. Maladaptive caregivers may fall prey to overwhelming feelings of helplessness because they find the infant's behaviors unpredictable. In turn, this emotion prevents the caregiver from adequately providing support during periods of transition between developmental milestones. As a consequence, the infant will either become overly distressed in an effort to evoke a response from the caregiver or may lapse into a despondent state, because developmental achievement then becomes an unattainable feat. Such infants may begin to experience the developmental phenomena as unpredictable and beyond their control, because there is no supportive caregiver present to convert maturation into a predictable experience for the infant. The symptoms displayed by these dyads resemble a state of learned helplessness in which lack of control about attaining any mastery over the relationship with the infant dominates all behavior.

In summary, caregivers may display maladaptation in a variety of forms during interaction with the infant. It is the therapist's task to isolate as precisely as possible the source of disturbance in the dyad. To do this, keen observational skills must be exercised during episodes of interaction between the infant and the caregiver. Subsequently, the therapist must dissect these interactive sequences with respect to each of the four dimensions discussed. After this has been done, an appropriate treatment strategy can be prescribed based on the principles described below.

Previewing and the Adaptive Caregiver

A sense of wonder at the diversity of the world is captured by the adaptive caregiver who represents the infant's developmental progress and communicates this progress to the infant through previewing behaviors. By use of distinctive gestures and vocalizations, such caregivers gradually and gently introduce the infant to future developmental changes and to the effect of those changes on future social exchanges.

Nevertheless, even with adaptive caregivers whose use of previewing is exquisitely attuned to the pace of the infant's developmental potential conflict may arise. Indeed, for such caregivers conflict may emerge by virtue of the very experience of previewing itself. Through previewing both caregiver and infant are provided with a kind of window, an unparalleled opportunity to predict the way in which future development will unfold. Precisely for this reason adaptive caregivers may be more sensitive than other mothers to the separation that inevitably awaits the dyad once the infant has acquired the developmental skill to become increasingly more autonomous. In fact, for the adaptive caregiver such separation, a natural outgrowth of development, may come to signify a dramatic change in the experience of mutual intimacy and fulfillment that has been shared within the dyad. As a consequence, adaptive caregivers may, at some point in the relationship with the infant, begin to thwart the occurrence of further previewing episodes, in an effort to hold the infant back from the natural pace of developmental growth and to retain the intimacy shared within the dyadic relationship. This trend can stifle development and sent confusing and contradictory messages to the infant.

In one such case that I treated, a caregiver with a seven-month-old infant girl had demonstrated highly adaptive behavior for the five months during which she attended a new mothers' group. Throughout that time the caregiver had shown a strong proclivity for engaging in a diverse array of previewing behaviors, both in the conversations about the infant she shared with the group and in the behavioral manifestations demonstrated towards the infant during the sessions. However, at one session, the caregiver arrived appearing highly subdued. Upon being questioned, she confessed to the group that she was experiencing depression about her decision to begin weaning the infant from breastfeeding. During the previous week she reported that the infant had turned from her breast and sought a bottle. This behavior had continued over the next several days, indicating to the caregiver that the infant had begun the process of weaning spontaneously. The caregiver particularly emphasized the fact that she felt the infant had "rejected" her by this action.

The advent of weaning in this case was particularly ironic, because the caregiver herself had predicted that the infant would begin weaning at approximately that age and had even previewed how she would feel with the onset of this behavior. However, when it became apparent that the infant had chosen to pursue weaning independent of her ministrations, the caregiver became upset.

Treatment in this instance focused on reinforcing the positive benefits that could be gained from previewing exercises. For example, since this caregiver had such a fine-tuned sense of the infant's development, she was encouraged to begin predicting future experiences that would occur after the weaning, experiences that would restore the sense of intimacy that had previously been shared during earlier dyadic interaction. Gradually, as the caregiver began to focus on the future and to recognize that her relationship with the infant would not end and that she could continue to share with the infant enthusiasm about developmental growth, the ambivalence and depression that arose with the advent of the weaning process began to abate. This caregiver was eventually able to resume her adaptive ministrations and previewing exercises with the infant.

Previewing and the Maladaptive Caregiver

Previewing behaviors and the capacity to predict the infant's imminent development are signs of an adaptive relationship within the dyad. Thus, when the therapist encounters a dyad in which these behaviors are either absent or appear only in sporadic fashion, there is probably some form of interactional failure permeating the exchange between caregiver and infant.

If this is the case, the caregiver can still be instructed in the techniques of previewing to better enhance the relationship within the dyad. In one such dyad I was treating, intuitive behaviors were absent from the caregiver's behavior towards the infant. Rarely did the caregiver verbalize her feelings while interacting with the infant, engage in direct eye contact or exhibit holding behaviors designed to soothe the infant's discomfort. The intuitive behaviors ordinarily encountered in adaptive caregivers were, in other words, absent from this dyadic relationship. When asked about the infant's future developmental course, the caregiver tended to express ignorance by shrugging her shoulders, coupled with an indifferent attitude.

Treatment techniques here focused upon encouraging the caregiver to observe infant behavior each week and report on developmental progress. This technique was designed to help the caregiver represent the infant's development. Initially, the caregiver was reticent about this technique, but gradually, she began to express her perceptions about the infant-at first describing only the infant in a gross somatic state-"I know when he wants to eat apple sauce, because he moves his hands in a certain way"-and later beginning to become more sophisticated in her attunement to the infant's perceptions. During this period, the caregiver was encouraged to represent or envision what the infant's future developmental course would be like and how these developmental changes would affect the dyadic relationship. The caregiver began, for example, to spontaneously attribute emotional states to her infant, such as "he's curious about new toys, especially the wind-up kind" and "he gets tired if I bounce him up and down on my lap for too long. I think he becomes distressed. So I try not to do it too much." Throughout this period of time the caregiver was continually encouraged to begin engaging in predictions about the infant's upcoming development.

Another strategy used with this caregiver involved modeling. On occasions when the therapist sensed that the caregiver was not responsive to the infant, the therapist would interact with the baby. This technique served two purposes. First, the caregiver was provided with a paradigm of adaptive behavior, which she could then imitate. Second, by interacting with the infant in this fashion, the therapist was given an opportunity to experience the perceptions being conveyed by the infant firsthand and could respond to them.

Once a diagnosis of maladaptation has been made, therefore, the therapist's task should be channeled towards encouraging the caregiver to engage in the kinds of intuitive behaviors that more adaptive caregivers engage in with their infants. Such behaviors include visual and vocal cuing, appropriate holding behavior and the provision of adequate stimulation. In addition, time should be devoted to helping the caregiver represent the infant's developmental course. As such representations become more sophisticated, the caregiver will most likely experience enhanced competence during interaction and, with some supportive guidance, can soon begin initiating previewing behaviors with the infant.

Previewing During Treatment

Since previewing is a normally occurring developmental phenomenon, it may also have value as a technique for conducting direct psychotherapeutic interventions with caregivers. I am not suggesting here that previewing be used to usurp or replace other types of intervention that have been found appropriate during the psychotherapeutic process; rather, a knowledge of the advantages of previewing and how this phenomenon can be applied to caregivers may supplement the therapist's techniques for exploring the etiology of conflict experienced by the caregiver, especially during interaction with the infant.

In particular, previewing can overcome some of the communication deficits inherent in techniques that rely primarily on language and on the caregiver's retelling of events that have already occurred. As De Gramont (1987) has explained, language enables the speaker to structure reality in a fashion that may generate the gaps or "repressions" that are the focus of the psychotherapy inquiry. As will be discussed below, encouraging the caregiver to represent events and experiences and then to formulate previewing exercises with the infant lowers the caregiver's latitude for selectively organizing reality. As a result, during previewing an abundance of unrepressed material often emerges. Stated conversely, during previewing, unrepressed material tends to fuel the narrative, because defensive operations have not been called upon to disguise the "truth" and, therefore, narrative information surfaces in a spontaneous, unrehearsed fashion, as the caregiver reflects on the infant's development and makes predictions about the future.

The unrehearsed nature of the material that emerges from previewing techniques offers yet a further advantage for the therapist. While more traditional inquiry techniques direct the caregiver towards uncovering her past history, previewing orients the caregiver towards the future. The tendency of the caregiver to bias her utterances and to selectively embellish the "truth" in order to be understood and appreciated by the therapist is therefore diminished, because with previewing the caregiver is forced to deal with events and experiences that are in process or have not yet actually occurred. In this sense, previewing functions as a kind of instantaneous Rorschach test, giving the therapist access to previously unavailable or repressed material.

Previewing episodes, then, facilitate the detection of emergent conflict because the caregiver has not yet had the opportunity to either engage in defensive operations around potential conflict or to embellish the true nature of events, thereby creating distortions in her narrative. Previewing also enhances the therapist's ability to *predict* the kind of conflict each individual caregiver is likely to encounter in the future during dyadic exchange. This is because, when the caregiver is asked to preview as part of the psychotherapeutic inquiry, areas of conflict or of potential conflict may be embedded in her descriptions. The caregiver will, in essence, be describing how she establishes a relational bond with another. The conflict generally encountered by the caregiver in all her significant relationships emerges in its raw form, devoid of the protective sheath of defensive operations, and exposed in a fashion analogous to a surgeon's exposure of the palpitating heart. By having the caregiver engage in several previewing exercises that rely on perceptions of the infant's imminent development, the therapist can thus extrapolate a pattern and decipher the typical configurations of conflict that are operating in that particular dyadic relationship. The ability to predict how conflict may arise for the caregiver in future interactions with the infant is thereby enhanced.

Moreover, previewing heightens the therapist's understanding of how the caregiver integrates somatic, affective, cognitive, and motivational perceptions, while she communicates predictions about these phenomena to the infant. This knowledge permits the therapist to guide the inquiry toward determining whether the genesis of the interactional conflict is rooted in a maternal deficit, such as a deficiency in nurturing skills, or in the baby's constitutional endowment, such as an idiosyncratic disposition. As will be seen with the following examples of caregivers and infants, previewing techniques enable the therapist to probe beyond the conflict itself to the actual evolution of the conflict before it is acted out within the dyadic relationship.

Exploring the caregiver's ability to preview can further instill a sense of the *predictability* of social interactions. As the caregiver begins to articulate the trends of developmental change, she will experience a sense of mastery and control in the dyad. In essence, previewing is a developmental phenomenon that facilitates the infant's capacities for predicting future events and experiences. When such events and experiences subsequently occur, the infant's sense of self and of belief in the predictable and thus controllable nature of the interpersonal relationship is thereby validated. For infants whose caregivers do not expose them to previewing or who experience primarily negative previewing, the therapist must instruct the caregiver in how to display positive previewing behaviors to the infant. These techniques bolster the caregiver's representational abilities, while improving the infant's ability to master and control challenges posed by the environment as he is exposed to imminent developmental skills.

The following discussion focuses on each of these aspects of previewing in greater detail.

Previewing as a Means for Accessing Repressed Material

Language represents a potent mode of communication because it liberates both speaker and listener from their functional ties to a particular setting and summarizes reality in a commonly shared representation which is used as a referent in the absence of the reality itself. Despite its compelling potency, however, language can also be used to distort reality (Spence, 1982, De Gramont, 1987). This distortion occurs, de Gramont points out, in the form of *capturing*. A capture occurs when some highly personal material, such as an affective memory, is triggered by a particular setting that disrupts the verbal context normally evoked by that setting. One example of capturing and the way in which it distorts language is exemplified by Burham (1970), who reported that a schizophrenic patient had responded to the phrase "Santa Claus" with the comment, "Sainted claws, hands that have never masturbated." Affective capturing thus creates a schism between the ordinary definition of the words and the more idiosyncratic meaning trapped in a primitive analog created by the patient. Another example of the susceptibility of language to capturing is provided by Bateson and Jackson (1964). These researchers observe that the symptoms of hysteria occur when an analogic meaning was translated into a digital meaning and subsequently retranslated back into an analogic meaning. Following this model, the hysteric may use a headache as a conventional excuse for avoiding a task and then actually experience a literal headache.

Taking these examples into consideration it appears that the internal scaffolding we construct with language is susceptible to capturing, which distorts meaning and blocks the process of symbolic realization. In De Gramont's terminology, capturing resembles the more traditional notion of *cathexis*, which refers to investment of the psychic energy of a drive in a conscious or unconscious representation. It is these captures or instances of cathexis which, most likely, create the narrative gaps that eventually become the main focus of the psychotherapeutic inquiry. The prime explanation for why language emerges in distorted fashion when the underlying experience has been subject to capture is that defensive operations have been called upon by the patient to disguise the true nature of the conflict the experience has evoked. These defensive operations shield the conflict from the patient's consciousness. Nevertheless, since the defensive operations are merely accommodations to the conflict that disguises it from the consciousness of the patient, rather than resolutions of the conflict itself, some residual evidence of the conflict will likely break through, surfacing in the form of either a symptom or a distorted perception, and both of these phenomena are conveyed to the analyst through language in which the ordinary definition of the words has been somehow divorced from the meaning the patient attributes to the words.

It is not, then, language per se as a communicative vehicle that impedes the therapist's ability to delineate the nature of the patient's conflict. Rather, it is precisely because language is such a compelling and flexible tool that it can be used to convey conflict, although the description of the conflict may surface in a distorted fashion which must be subjected to inquiry. With previewing, however, many of these distortions are precluded, because the patient is being requested to engage in representing some future event which has not yet been experienced and thus the representation of the event is unlikely to have been distorted or contaminated by the defensive operations.

Traditional psychoanalysis offers the patient a safe haven within which to express a discrete symptom. Often the analysis begins with retrospective inquiries that seek to tease out the contours of the conflict that are embedded in the symptom. In order to diagnose the conflict, the therapist is, in a sense, at the mercy of the defensive operations the patient has used, much like an elaborate internal fortress, to disguise the nature of the conflict. Such defensive operations, conveyed to the therapist through the patient's narrative, can not only camouflage conflict, but may also create false impressions that lead the therapist away from, rather than toward, the conflict itself. The therapist is thereby forced to navigate a labyrinth of numerous deceptive pathways. In contrast, having the patient preview some imminent developmental event or seminal experience enables the therapist to delineate the scope of inquiry from the outset and provides the therapist with greater control over the direction of the treatment. Indeed, a key advantage of previewing as a treatment technique is that issues of control between patient and therapist are avoided. Previewing frees the therapist from the constraints and false leads that surface with retrospective inquiry, because the patient will be asked to focus on a predictive fantasy of unrehearsed events and experiences that have not yet been subjected to the defensive operations.

In a similar fashion, asking the caregiver to represent the infant's imminent developmental events or to envision what the relationship with the infant will be like in several months can provide the therapist with a relatively uncontaminated view of the kinds of conflict likely to surface in the dyad. This is because the caregiver is essentially being asked to engage in predictions about the future and, in so doing, she will be relying on her own past experiences in the context of other significant relationships to forecast how the infant's development will unfold. Thus, the therapist will be able to see where conflict is likely to emerge, because the caregiver is freely associating and projecting images onto the imaginary stage of future experience. As one illustration, a caregiver who has difficulty imagining her infant walking may be conveying anxiety that the advent of this milestone will signal a separation between mother and child. In another case, the inability of a caregiver to attribute a full spectrum of emotions to the infant-such as laughter, sadness, curiosity-may signify that the caregiver herself has difficulty in conveying emotions to her child. When used skillfully, then, the material emerging from previewing episodes offers unprecedented insight into the way in which the dyadic relationship will most probably unfold, and is a valuable tool for the therapist.

Previewing as a Means of Obtaining an Unbiased Report

In addition to the defensive operations, previewing neutralizes other factors that play a role in the patient's ability to distort versions of events, thereby disguise the true nature of the conflict. Spence (1982) has highlighted some of these factors in his discussion of the distinction between narrative truth and historical truth. Historical truth involves a reportage of the facts in objective fashion; it is like a fragment of history detailing events that actually transpired. Narrative truth on the other hand, focuses attention upon the way in which the speaker has chosen to select or reconstruct events. In psychoanalysis, the facts alone are not sufficient. It is how the facts are presented which allows their full significance to be appreciated by the listener. In other words, if one of the goals of therapy is to discover the underlying conflict or motif embedded in the patient's story, the therapist must be attuned to the sequences, coherence and the transformations of language used by the patient. Spence reminds us that if we assume the patient is under the influence of the narrative tradition, then we should be wary of the contaminating effect introduced into the report as a result of the patient's wish to be understood and appreciated by the analyst.

Problems similar to those articulated by Spence had previously been voiced by Walsh (1958) when he posited the difference between plain and significant narrative. Plain narrative, according to Walsh, is a straightforward description of what has occurred, whereas significant narrative involves an account of the facts which brings out their connections. Thus, as Walsh explains, the validity of significant narrative cannot be checked by appealing to the known facts, because the connections between events drawn by the patient are not open for inspection in the same way events themselves are.

The problems raised by both Spence and Walsh are, however, largely eradicated when the therapist relies upon the caregiver's ability to preview imminent developmental events and experiences, rather than only relying upon a retrospective inquiry. Because previewing requires the patient to construct a narrative in a spontaneous way, the possibility that associations will be reconstructed from earlier memories can be more directly addressed, as can the patient's ability to monitor or selectively control the consequences involved in the reconstructions of past events. As a result, the therapist obtains a more accurate view of the patient's actual perceptions and of how these perceptions are connected and interpreted by the patient.

Previewing as a Means of Predicting Conflict

Perhaps the most advantageous role previewing plays in the therapeutic process is its ability to identify conflict far more rapidly than other techniques, as well as its ability to predict future areas of conflict in the dyadic relationship. As noted earlier, because previewing requires the patient to focus on future, yet-to-be-realized events and experiences, whatever potential for conflict these events and experiences trigger has not yet generated any behavioral consequences or defensive operations in the dyad. The therapist can therefore explore the core of the patient's conflict and, through further previewing, can begin to assess whether the conflict is derived from deficiencies of maternal nature or from developmental deficits in the child.

An illustration is warranted here. A resident under my supervision reported on a case involving a twenty-three-year-old caregiver and her ten-and-a-half-month-old son. The resident reported that over the past several weeks the caregiver had seemed anxious and upset, but that she had been unable to isolate the problem through inquiry. When I looked at the chart, I noticed that the infant had not only not yet begun to walk, but also that various developmental precursors for this milestone were not evident with this infant. As a result, I suggested that the resident help the caregiver preview walking behavior.

The resident followed my suggestion and at the next session asked the caregiver how she thought she would feel when the infant began walking. For the first time, the caregiver was able to focus on her anxiety directly, by divulging material pertaining to her personal associations of walking behavior with the infant's autonomy.

Caregiver: (Seems to be in deep thought). I suddenly remember a funny incident when I was a kid.

Therapist: Can you tell me about it?

Caregiver: I remember, I guess I was only four years old or . . . maybe even younger . . . you know my mother used to tell me I was three . . . and she said I was always wandering off . . . and I got lost.

Therapist: What do you mean?

Caregiver: My mother had taken me shopping to a department store and I remember getting lost. I must have wandered away. The security guard found me. I was very frightened.

Therapist: Anything else?

Caregiver: Um . . . yes, yes . . . when my mother found me first she was crying, then she started yelling. I'll never forget it.

Therapist: What do you mean?

Caregiver: She started screaming at the top of her lungs 'Don't you ever walk away from me!'

Therapist: What do you think that means with reference to your attitude toward your son?

Caregiver: I'm not sure yet . . . I suppose . . . I seem to get so upset when he starts to walk . . . maybe there is a connection.

Therapist: What do you think will happen when he walks?

Caregiver: (Spontaneously) He will get lost, just the way I did . . . and I won't be able to find him. Maybe there is a connection, because I always feel nervous when he starts walking so I take him in my lap.

Therapist: But it's important that he start to walk on his own.

Caregiver: I know, I know.

By virtue of this dialogue, the therapist was able to formulate some insights about the nature of the caregiver's conflict. From this disclosure, it appeared that the caregiver was having difficulty in negotiating her relationship with her mother as she confronted her infant's independence. Her son's developmental acquisitions were now evoking earlier conflict and contaminating the dyadic exchange. The infant's normal development appeared to arouse anxiety. Stifling her son's independence was one way of insuring that he did not get lost. This therapeutic dialogue offers a choice example of how previewing obliterates barriers of past memories and future anticipations. Here the caregiver has focused on a present problem, triggering an earlier memory, which was used to resolve a potential future conflict.

In order to help the caregiver overcome this conflict so she could begin engaging in more positive previewing exercises with her son, the therapist encouraged her to discuss further associations stemming from this childhood incident. Gradually, the caregiver was able to understand how she had inappropriately identified her own childhood trauma with her son and how this conflict was preventing her from sharing developmental experiences with the child. Once the caregiver was able to make this connection, the caregiver was urged by the therapist to envision how and when the infant would begin walking and how she would feel when he began manifesting this behavior. At first, the caregiver's representations resulted in anxiety; gradually, however, these anxious feelings abated and the caregiver was able to view her infant's attainment of motor skills more positive. Next, the caregiver was asked to devise somefwalking exercises that she could engage in with the infant. When the caregiver was reluctant to do this, the therapist used modeling behaviors to demonstrate the infant's eagerness to experiment with his burgeoning mobility. Soon the caregiver was able to imitate these behaviors and was participating with pleasure in her infant's new developmental acquisition.

Although purely retrospective inquiry may have eventually elicited similar kinds of information, in this case, by beginning the inquiry with a focus on imminent developmental events the therapist was able to tap the core of the conflict almost immediately. Indeed, the therapist was able to begin assessing the conflict once the caregiver began returning the dialogue to the theme that had initially led to treatment: her nervousness about her son. In contrast, during retrospective inquiry the therapist's energies may be devoted to circumventing the defensive operations that disguise the core of the conflict.

Previewing as a Means of Facilitating Multimodal Integration

The infant's capacity to integrate a coherent reality through the process of multimodal perception has been described by Stern (1985). Multimodal perception is defined as a general innate capacity to take information received in one perceptual modality and to somehow translate it into another perceptual modality. For example, the capacity to understand that an object's color (visual) and an object's sound (auditory) are both properties of the same object is an example of multimodal functioning. Language fits into the infant's existing ability to discern the multidimensional qualities of the world through multimodal perception. Language enables us to perceive various dimensions of an experience and to subsequently anchor our perceptions in a particular modality.

As a mode of communication, previewing also exposes the individual to multimodal functioning, while still permitting the previewer to anchor perceptions in one dimension. In this discussion, we have referred to four dimensions that are commonly viewed as developmental milestones: somatic, cognition, affect, and motivational status. Inquiring about each of these dimensions during a previewing episode allows the therapist to attain further insight into the nature and source of the caregiver's conflict. In addition, by asking the caregiver to focus on each of these dimensions, skill in integrating all of the infant's perceptions are enhanced.

Previewing as a Means of Instilling Mastery and Control

As noted earlier, previewing first emerges from the interactions between caregiver and infant, and represents a method for acquainting the infant with imminent developmental achievement. If performed in an adaptive fashion, previewing presents the infant with a paradigm of what the developmental acquisition will actually "feel like," in terms of somatic, affect-ive, cognitive and motivational awareness. Subsequently, when the infant matures sufficiently to engage in the developmental task independently, he will experience feelings of mastery over an event that was previewed earlier. In contrast, infants who have been deprived of adequate preview-ing experiences or infants who have been exposed to negative previewing by their caregivers, will be more prone to feel uncertain or anxious about coping with maturational change in an interpersonal relationship. This un-certainty arises because such infants have not been shown by an adaptive caregiver how to master a particular developmental skill. As a conse-quence, infants who have not undergone previewing episodes may be more likely to experience the external world, as well as their own internal perceptions and burgeoning developmental skills, as unpredictable and, hence, uncontrollable phenomena. This uncontrollability may later pre-cipitate a lack of motivation.

On the other hand, the use of previewing during the therapeutic process may instill feelings of mastery and control in the caregiver. If previewing is used repeatedly to help the mother anticipate upcoming events and to develop strategies for dealing effectively with these events, she will likely experience a sense of mastery and competence once the event actually occurs. In turn, this sense of mastery will be conveyed to the infant dur-ing previewing exercises. In this fashion, the therapist's observations of previewing exchanges during the therapeutic process serves the same goal as previewing does during the caregiver-infant interaction; the thera-pist functions as the supportive partner, guiding the caregiver's expecta-tions regarding the imminent event.

Conclusion

This chapter elaborates upon the concept of previewing as a principle organizing development that emerges from the nature of interaction be-tween the caregiver and infant. Since previewing combines the caregiv-er's capacity to articulate goals and express them in the form of language, and to subsequently devise physical behaviors that convey this message to the infant, it is a phenomenon that relies on both the digital and the analogic modes of communication. Indeed, previewing was earlier re-ferred to as a hybrid mode of communication that helps to explain how the infant eventually grows from an understanding of physical behaviors with direct referents to an understanding of language itself which relies on symbolic reasoning.

In exploring how the previewing phenomenon evolves within the care-giver-infant relationship, it becomes clear that previewing enhances the infant's capacity for predicting events and experiences that will be encountered, for integrating experiences in a multi-modal fashion, and for attaining a sense of mastery and control both over stimuli from the external world and internal perceptions.

Given the potent effects of previewing on the infant's early development, it is not unusual to find that the introduction of these techniques into the therapeutic process may often provide insights that are less attainable with traditional methods.Previewing techniques may overcome some of the communication deficits inherent in techniques that rely only on retrospective inquiry. This is because previewing adopts a prospective orientation that guides the patient's narrative towards predicting events and experiences that have not yet been encountered. As a result, through previewing, the therapist more readily accesses large amounts of repressed material that have not yet been felt in dyadic exchanges or subjected to the shielding effect of defensive operations. Previewing also circumvents the patient's proclivity to selectively bias reports of past events. Thus, the therapist acquires insight into the core of the patient's conflict far more rapidly and the related ability to predict future areas of conflict is also enhanced. The therapist can probe the nature of the conflict in greater detail through previewing as well, because in the ongoing child-caring context inquiries pertaining to affect, cognition, somatic state and motivational status help narrow the zone of conflict, permitting the therapist to better grasp the etiology of the conflict. Moreover, since previewing can be used to predict behavior that will eventually occur, the therapist can subsequently validate the insights into dyad once the developmental milestone has been achieved. Finally, just as previewing promotes the infant's sense of mastery and control over both external and internal forces, so too can previewing instill these feelings of competence in caregivers. Although the full advantages of previewing as a therapeutic technique have yet to be explored, this discussion has attempted to highlight some of the benefits obtained with this approach.

This chapter has focused upon a unique and remarkable phenomenon that appears, in varying degrees, in virtually every caregiver-infant dyad. Previewing presents the therapist with a distinctive new paradigm for organizing the interpersonal experience of the infant's development in a coherent fashion. As a diagnostic aid, previewing allows the therapist to detect previously imperceptible areas of disharmony within the interaction and to evaluate where and when conflict may erupt. Above all, previewing enables the therapist to orient the caregiver toward the predictive and adaptive development of the infant. But previewing also offers the therapist more than an exciting new vista from which to view caregiver-infant interaction; it is therapeutic instrument that can be used not only to treat maladaptive caregivers, but to enhance the exchange between adaptive caregivers and their infants as well.

CHAPTER 9

Using Previewing to Stimulate Optimal Development

Introduction

Several years ago, I had the occasion to interview the mother of an eight-month-old infant who cried incessantly. The infant had been examined repeatedly by a pediatrician who discerned no organic abnormality that could be responsible for the episodes of crying. In fact, this physician had attempted to reassure the caregiver by telling her that the baby was "colicky", a catch-all phrase used to describe infants who are irritable for a variety of reasons during the first few months of life. In most instances, this irritability gradually subsides by the second year of life. But the caregiver refused to accept these reassurances. Instead, she was convinced that the infant's behavior was her fault, that she was lacking some key quality as a caregiver. Somehow her skills in soothing the infant were inadequate, and the fact that the infant wailed uncontrollably for four hours each day was attributable to some failure of nurturance on her part. "Sometimes I get so angry at him," she said in frustration, "But then I realize he's only a baby and it can't be his fault." This last comment was punctuated by cuddling the infant in her arms, as if to eradicate any ambivalence she may have felt toward her son. Then the mother sighed and said, "My neighbor tells me to use mother's intuition when the baby gets upset, but I don't know what she means. Sometimes I wonder if there is such a thing as 'intuition' when it comes to being a mother."

This anecdote illustrates how often new caregivers lack an awareness of the processes of development and of the role they play in facilitating the infant's maturation. Normal development progresses from a state of undifferentiation and nonintegration to one that is more differentiated and integrated. For example, a neonate will respond globally and diffusely to a bright light or pinprick by gesturing with his whole body. In other words, the physiological mechanisms of the neonate evince one orchestrated response. But after several months, a more sophisticated response is observable, as the infant begins to differentiate functions and to exhibit the most economical and efficient reaction. In observing such consolidation, the majority of caregivers experience gratification at their infant's development.

This gratification convinces the caregiver that the infant is capable of learning new skills and that development will proceed in a fairly regular and predictable fashion. In order to encourage such development, most caregivers will begin to intuitively preview upcoming maturational trends to their infants. Initially, such previewing behaviors will consist of the fundamental intuitive manifestations discussed earlier, including frequent eye contact, vocalizations and touching behaviors. As time goes on and the infant develops more sophisticated skills, the caregiver will strive to engage in previewing behaviors that challenge and stimulate the infant in even more complex ways. For example, with the advent of motor skills, the caregiver will begin to preview crawling and walking behaviors; similarly, the baby talk vocalizations exhibited during the first months of life by the caregiver will eventually yield to more complex verbalizations that preview genuine speech patterns and conversation by the end of the first year of life. In this fashion, the caregiver's level of previewing behavior keeps pace with the infant's maturational rhythms.

In some cases, however, this caregiver proclivity to stimulate the infant by engaging in ever more complex previewing behaviors may not emerge. The reasons why such previewing will be absent or only intermittent are varied and include such factors as caregiver depression, caregiver temperament that is incompatible with the infant's temperament or other psychological factors originating with the caregiver that preclude the formation of a communicative bond with the infant. In other instances, factors pertaining to the infant may serve to stifle the development of an adaptive relationship within the dyad. For example, if the infant is born prematurely and the caregiver cannot spend sufficient time with the infant during the first few weeks of life because of medical intervention, the caregiver may subsequently be hesitant about initiating a relationship with the infant. Or the caregiver may be incapable of initiating a relationship because of the infant's withdrawn state. Or the caregiver may fear that the infant is too fragile for full-fledged interaction and may withhold interactional behavior as a consequence.

Moreover, if the infant is premature or of low birth weight, normative development may be slowed. With extremely immature and physically ill infants, a diffusely organized response lacking in specificity and without integrated functioning endures well into the first year of life, and this seemingly diminished level of functioning may cause the caregiver to hesitate in forging a bond with the infant. Nurturing such an infant during the first few months of life can be frustrating to a caregiver whose predictions of a responsive infant are sharply discrepant from the relatively nonresponsive infant who is brought home from the hospital. Caregivers, in other words, are often ill-equipped to deal with an infant whose immature physiological state-although temporary-makes him unlike previously conceived notions of a healthy, responsive baby. Indeed, the contrast between the fantasized infant the caregiver has envisioned and represented during the pregnancy and the premature infant actually born may be shocking and unexpected. As discussed in Chapter 3, the manner in which the caregiver resolves the discrepancy between the envisioned image of the unborn infant and the actual disposition of the infant after birth may exert a significant impact on the interaction that transpires within the dyad.

Some infants-like the infant whose mother I referred to above frustrated by irregular behavior patterns during the first few months of life which are as yet not susceptible to medical or psychological explanation. One example of such an aberrant behavior pattern is found in the colicky infant who cries uncontrollably for no apparent reason and whose caregiver becomes increasingly more agitated due to an inability to quell the discomfort. Dyads in which such an interpersonal problem exists may be especially prone to risk because during the first few months of life, when a harmonious form of interaction ordinarily develops between caregiver and infant, such pairs are instead caught in the throes of an incomprehensible tug-of-war, in which the caregiver's efforts to assuage the infant are unsuccessful. Even if the infant's crying abates by six months, there is always the possibility that the residue of frustration the caregiver experienced during the first few months of the infant's life will linger and contaminate future interaction. Such caregivers may feel that they have given birth to unpredictable infants and thus will be hesitant about representing the infant's future behavior, and about devising previewing behaviors for the infant. The caregiver may believe that the infant's uncontrollable and unpredictable behavior patterns will resurface during interaction. As a result, a sense of uncertainty may insinuate itself into the interactions between the caregiver and the infant. In turn, the infant may interpret this uncertainty as a form of insecure attachment.

The unique temperamental proclivities of the infant, as well as the caregiver, the psychological profile of the caregiver, the physiological status of the infant at birth, and finally, conditions which cause the infant to deviate from the typical behavior patterns of newborns, such as colic or excessive lethargy are all factors which pose a challenge to the caregiver who has anticipated a healthy, interactive partner with whom a mutually rewarding relationship can occur. It must be stressed, however, that infants with problems in each of the areas outlined above are still capable of responding to their caregivers in a rewarding fashion. But in these instances the caregiver will often need guidance and tutoring to recognize how to stimulate such infants appropriately and how to enhance incremental progress as the baby matures each day. Moreover, caregivers suffering from depression-whether in the form of postpartum blues or a more pervasive clinical depression-can also be taught to work through these states to achieve a more adaptive relationship with the infant.

There is yet another factor that may exert a potent influence on the formation of a reciprocal dyadic exchange during the first months of life. This factor is the caregiver's psychological status and its impact upon her capacity to stimulate the infant in an appropriate fashion. Even the most responsive and temperamentally easy infant will encounter obstacles in development if the caregiver's mood is depressed or anxious. Both of these psychological states may cause the caregiver to misconstrue infant signals, so that the infant is not provided with the kinds of stimulation he needs. If such a pattern persists, the infant may eventually abandon efforts to interact with the caregiver in a developmentally enhancing manner. Newly acquired skills, such as vocal exchange, motor coordination and facial discrimination, will not be exercised to their fullest and such infants may eventually come to display the kind to apathy described by Spitz (1944) in his study of institutionalized infants deprived of a consistent, attentive caregiver. The ability of such infants to formulate representations may also be impaired. Such infants will most likely not be exposed to sufficient contingency relationships and their predictive skills will therefore not be challenged. These infants may not strive to acquire new developmental skills, nor will they exercise maturational potential to the fullest extent, because the caregiver is providing minimal reinforcement to fuel the infant's predictive skills.

One goal of this chapter is to provide the therapist with strategies for caregivers who, for whatever reason, are incapable of forging an adaptive relationship with the infant. First, the therapist must teach the caregiver how to represent the signals from her infant. Second, once the caregiver has learned how to read the developmental cues being emitted by the infant, it is essential to use this new understanding to provide the infant sufficient exposure to predictable, contingency sequences. In other words, the caregiver be taught interventive strategies that will be most effective in encouraging her to provide the infant with optimal patterns of stimulation.

Once the caregiver has become more adept at interpreting the cues of her infant and has learned to predict and represent the infant's typical behavior patterns, the therapist will be challenged to instruct the caregiver in methods for previewing imminent development to the infant. As will be seen, in some instances caregivers will require tutoring in the basic intuitive responses that are so natural and spontaneous to other mothers. Although these skills have been labeled intuitive in earlier chapters, there are caregivers for whom appropriate eye contact, vocalizations and body contact will be almost new components of establishing a relationship. These mothers may also harbor representational deficits which impair their capacity to envision the infants when they are removed from their immediate presence and to attribute particular behaviors to them. In such cases, the therapist will need to encourage the emergence of representational skills that enable the caregiver to perceive of the infant as a continually developing and maturing personality. Eventually, as the caregiver comes to appreciate the unique status of the infant's individuality, she will be able to devise strategies designed to promote optimal growth and the full realization of developmental potential. These strategies will emerge most vividly in the form of previewing behaviors the caregiver directs to the infant.

Interpreting Developmental Signals

To understand how to treat caregivers who are impaired in their capacity to relate to their infants, it is helpful to first examine the qualities that typify adaptive caregivers. Caregivers who are adept at interpreting the developmental signals of their infants are often described as being able to provide adequate stimulation. Even from the first hours of birth, adaptive caregivers appear especially equipped to create a harmonious mood which permeates all interactions with the infant. It is as if such caregivers are, even at that early stage, so attuned to their infant's needs that they can read the cues the babies are emitting.

Papousek and Papousek (1987) have probed this capacity for adequate stimulation by subjecting isolated sequences of interaction to microanalytic examination. These researchers have focused on the ability of the caregiver to direct an adequate amount of vocal communication toward the infant, as well as on the caregiver's skill in regulating the intensity and complexity of speech, the elongated rate of articulation, and the segmenting and repetition of prose patterns. Each of these behaviors helps to foster the infant's capacity to predict how the caregiver will respond vocally to his behaviors. In addition, such caregivers are able to modulate the degree of bodily contact and tactile stimulation provided to the infant, as well as to modulate eye contact. Papousek and Papousek have commented that caregivers who displayed harmonious interludes with their infants were also capable of coordinating sequences so that visual cuing, vocal communication and tactile stimulation were interwoven into one unified response. In effect, such caregivers possess a comprehensive impression or representation of the infant's development and are able to use this representation of the infant to formulate interactive behaviors that stimulate and sustain the dyadic relationship.

Adequate stimulation, based on the regulation of these criteria, is evident when fluid interactive episodes of relatively lengthy duration are achieved. Such sequences occur gradually, eventually intensify to a level of sustained, moderated activity and then slowly abate. Significantly, the temporal demarcations between periods of adequate stimulation and periods of quiescence are smooth and fluid and appear to respond to the infant's moods. In describing this type of interaction, Papousek and Papousek have emphasized the almost rhythmic-like quality that characterizes such an exchange. The caregiver intervenes in a nonintrusive fashion, responding to the infant in a reciprocal way and finally, disengaging from the exchange slowly and in rhythm with the infant's mood.

Stern (1985) has referred to this quality as *affect attunement,* identifying its emergence at approximately nine months of age. Affect attunement, according to Stern, is a kind of harmonious mood that suffuses the interaction. It is as if the caregiver and infant are in complete emotional accord and are capable of communicating needs fully to one another without words. Although Stern has identified the full-fledged emergence of this quality at nine months, it is possible to observe the qualities that typify this kind of attuned interaction at a far earlier age as the caregiver and infant begin to forge an attachment within the first months of life.

But describing this attuned form of interaction and observing it are quite different from explaining how a particular dyadic pair manages to achieve this kind of adaptive exchange. What behaviors, in other words, constitute the foundation for attuned interaction and how do caregivers from the first weeks of the infant's life onward use these behaviors to weave an interactive, mutually predictable rapport with the infant?

Bowlby (1969) has referred to early interactive exchange that is harmonious as a *goal-corrected partnership.* As this partnership evolves, the caregiver becomes increasingly more cognizant of subtle distinctions in the messages being conveyed by the infant. I have had this notion confirmed when I asked mothers of young infants whether they could tell the difference between their infant's crying sounds. Did one type of cry mean the infant was hungry, while another cry indicated a need for a diaper change, while yet a third cry meant that the infant desired to be cuddled? Surprisingly, I was informed that these caregivers were capable of discerning subtle distinctions between infant cries, but equally as surprising, I was told that they really hadn't thought about it that way before. Thus, many of the ingredients that contribute to making the dyadic interaction predictable and harmonious may occur at a subliminal level of awareness. One method of enhancing caregiver perception and skill, then, may lie in bringing these behaviors to consciousness, so that the caregiver can use such capacities to support the infant's burgeoning developmental skills in a more intentional and adaptive fashion. In other words, helping the caregiver to become conscious of how she predicts infant response may translate into more intentionally adaptive behaviors, which help the infant formulate predictions about the way in which the caregiver responds.

What then are some of these intuitive behaviors that incrementally provide an adaptive atmosphere for interaction with the infant? As discussed in Chapter 2 researchers have identified visual cuing on the part of the caregiver as one such interactive mechanism that fosters adaptive behavior. Visual cuing occurs when caregiver and infant are positioned face-to-face and exchange a regulated form of direct eye contact. Haekel (1985) has reported that visual cuing is capable of evoking a distinct greeting response from the infant that seems to be contingent upon presentation of the caregiver's face. This greeting response has been observed in three-month-olds. Papousek and Papousek (1987) have described particular sequences of visual cuing in which the caregiver positions herself in the middle of the neonate's visual field and then strives to achieve direct eye contact. Once such contact is achieved, an exaggerated greeting response is emitted by the caregiver by way of signaling the infant. In addition, Papousek and Papousek also report that caregivers respond to motor responses of the infant-for instance, limb gestures and clenched fists-with heightened attention to the infant's eye area. As a distinct behavior, visual cuing appears to occupy a hierarchical position in the caregiver's repertoire of responses and this form of intuitive response may fuel the infant's ability to make predictions about the world around him beginning in the first weeks of life.

One study that demonstrated the significant effect visual cuing can have on dyadic interaction was conducted by Blehar, Lieberman and Ainsworth (1977). These researchers observed interactions between caregivers and their infants of six to fifteen weeks of age. It was found that caregivers who coordinated visual cuing with playful behavior had infants who were more frequently characterized as happy, as demonstrated by more joyful bouncing, smiling and vocalizing. Caregivers who engaged in visual cuing were also more skillful in terms of pacing and modifying behavioral initiations to infant signals. Finally, Blehar et al. commented that those infants who experienced the most predictable interactions with caregivers were capable of differentiating their behavior significantly when confronted by a stranger, suggesting that in such infants an awareness of the distinct identity of the caregiver emerges early. This awareness is then used by the infant to compare the caregiver with others and to represent predictable sequences of behavior that may be anticipated from interaction with the caregiver. Field (1978) has stressed that the caregiver's ability to engage the infant visually during the first few months of life exerts a dramatic impact on whether interaction in the dyad will be harmonious and rhythmic. According to this researcher, if the caregiver fails to use visual cuing to elicit a state of alertness in the infant, a disturbed or asynchronic exchange can eventually evolve, a finding that has been confirmed by Brazelton, Koslowski and Main (1974).

The significance of adaptive maternal visual behavior was highlighted in a study conducted by Termine and Izard (1988), who examined infant responsiveness to maternal expressions of sadness and joy. The study involved nine-month-old infants whose mothers expressed sadness or joy through both facial expressions and vocalizations. After a brief induction period, mothers were instructed to display one of these emotions during an infant play period. Infant emotional expression and play behavior was analyzed, as was the amount of time the infant spent looking at the caregiver. It was found that infants expressed more joyful emotion and looked for longer periods at mothers during the maternal joy condition, while displaying more sadness, anger and gaze aversion during the maternal sadness condition. In addition, play behavior increased during the period that caregivers exhibited a joyful expression, but decreased when caregivers manifested a sad expression. The researchers noted that their findings suggest that infants are acutely aware of the emotional expression caregivers display visually and that they use this emotional display to respond accordingly.

From this study, we may infer that infants who are exposed to adequate visual cuing may be aware of their caregivers' mood and may pick up negative emotion which can dampen their desire to continue the interaction. This study, as well as the work of Papousek and Papousek, suggests that those caregivers who are not engaging in an adequate degree of visual stimulation need to be encouraged to initiate this kind of behavior with their infants. Not only will the infant be likely to benefit from the positive emotion generally conveyed during episodes of visual cuing, but the infant may also be prevented from experiencing the negative emotional signals that have been associated with a lack of visual stimulation.

Another component of harmonious interaction that contributes to the optimal stimulation of the newborn is vocal communication. Although the caregiver emits vocalizations almost immediately after birth, a distinctive pattern can be identified at approximately six to eight weeks of age. When focusing on vocalization during dyadic exchange with infants, researchers have particularly commented on changes in voice pitch, alterations in contour, quality of voice, the communication of negative emotions and vocal matching to the infant's repertoire. Each of these behaviors is designed to enhance the infant's predictive abilities and, further, to preview conversational dialogue for the infant.

In characterizing vocal communication, Papousek and Papousek (1987) have differentiated two forms of utterance. Initially, the caregiver verbalizes a reference that is in keeping with the interactional context. Most commonly, this reference is in the form of a question or answering statement. Thus, while maintaining eye contact with the infant the caregiver might comment, "Mommy's here." Almost immediately the comment will be followed by an utterance in the form of nonsense speech which incorporates melodic contours, rhythmicity, tempo, pausing and the dimensions of voice pitch and quality. As an example, one sequence might sound like, "Yo, yo, yo . . . ho, ho, ho . . . " Often the caregiver will coordinate the articulation of elongated vowels with simultaneous stroking of the infant's face and enhanced facial expression. During such exercises the caregiver recognizes the need to translate meaningful language into a predictable communicative sequence that the infant can relate to and use to formulate an internal representation of the interaction. Field (1978) has reported that during interaction in the first months of life maternal speech is characteristically slower and more exaggerated than normal adult speech, while the range of pitch is expanded. Fergusen (1964) concurs with this view, stating that maternal "baby talk" is typified by fluctuations in the range of loudness, contour of pitch, rhythms and stress with vowel durations being prominently elongated.

Another barometer of the success of caregiver-infant interaction is found in the *regulation of laughter* the baby engages in during the first few months of life, according to Sroufe and Wunsch (1972). These researchers conducted a series of observational studies with more than 150 infants during the first year of life. As a result of the study, they concluded that laughter has a positive effect on caregiver-infant interaction by imbuing the exchange with pleasurable emotion that motivates further dyadic communication. The researchers reported that when the infants cried they pulled back and turned away from the stimulus, whereas when laughter occurred the baby maintained orientation toward the agent, reached for the object, and sought to reproduce the situation. The researchers concluded by observing that laughter was a seminal milestone of adaptive interaction during the first year of life. Not only does the achievement of this milestone enhance emotional growth and expression between caregiver and infant, but it is also apt to promote previewing exercises. This occurs because the infant will strive to elicit a response from the caregiver that is contingent, and hence, pleasurable.

It is important to note that just as researchers have discerned different patterns of visual cuing among mothers who are depressed or are simulating depression, so too are the vocalizations of depressed caregivers different from those of caregivers who are not depressed. This finding has been confirmed by Bettes (1988) who investigated the motherese speech patterns of depressed mothers interacting with their three- to four- month old infants.

Bettes examined thirty-six mothers and infants during interactive sequences when the caregiver was verbalizing to the infant. These interactions where recorded and records of pitch contours and relative intensity were produced for two-minute interaction sequences. Analysis of these sequences revealed that depressed mothers failed to modify their behavior according to the behavior of the infant. These mothers were significantly slower in responding to an infant vocalization and had more variable utterances and pauses in their speech than nondepressed caregivers who engaged in baby talk episodes with their infants. Moreover, depressed caregivers were less likely to utilize the exaggerated intonation contours that are characteristic of motherese.

All of the phenomena encountered in the verbal speech of the depressed mothers differed markedly from speech characteristics of nondepressed mothers. For example, it has been reported maternal utterances to infants are generally regularly spaced (Beebe, Gertsman, Carson, Dolins, Zigman, Rosensweig, Faughey and Korman, 1979) with short pauses and utterances (Stern, Beebe, Jaffe and Bennett, 1977). In general, conversational pauses between infant vocalizations and maternal response tend to be of extremely short duration, lasting usually for less than a second (Roth, 1987). Bloom (1979) has suggested that this brief interval is necessary for the infant to detect the relationship between his behavior and that of the adult. Finally, with respect to the sound of motherese, among nondepressed mothers utterances are intonally simplified and exaggerated in both pitch range and duration, according to Fernald (1983). In one study that involved a non-depressed mother and her newborn, Fernald and Simon (1984) found that the majority of the mother's utterances directed at her newborn were intoned with one of five varieties of expanded contour, including rising, falling, level, U-shaped and complex. Stern et al. (1983) have confirmed that expanded contours are prevalent in maternal speech to four month old infants.

According to Bettes, because maternal motherese patterns differ among depressed women, infants will be receiving a different kind of verbal stimulation. For example, depressed mothers fail to adjust their vocal behavior in response to infant cue, suggesting that such mothers are not imposing any structure on their vocal behavior. The relatively long time it takes a depressed mother to respond to the infant indicates that such infants are at a disadvantage in their attempts to converse with their caregivers and their speech may be perceived as noncontingent. Finally, depressed mothers fail to exaggerate their speech patterns and, therefore, a lower degree of affective variety is being conveyed to the infant. In other words, depressed mothers fail to use vocal episodes to share a positive emotional experience with their infants, to establish a contingent pattern of responsiveness through emotional exchange and to consolidate the interactional relationship. As a consequence, depressed mothers may deprive their infants of these early developmental lessons.

These findings were confirmed in studies conducted by Cohn, Matias, Tronick, Connell and Lyons-Ruth (1986) and Breznitz and Sherman (1987). The Cohn et al. study examined the face-to-face interactions of depressed mothers and their infants. The researchers were particularly interested in the communication of affect between mothers and their infants and its relationship to socioemotional and cognitive development, because it was felt that face-to-face interactions were a primary vehicle whereby personality disorder was transmitted from parent to infant. The study involved thirteen depressed mothers and their six- to seven-month-old infants. The researchers found that during face-to-face interactions these mothers were extremely variable in the level of engagement exhibited toward the infant, as well as in their intrusiveness with the baby. Contingent responsiveness tended to be lacking among these mothers, as did a high level of positive affect that is generally encountered among nondepressed caregivers. In the Breznitz and Sherman study, the speech patterns of fourteen depressed and eighteen nondepressed mothers during conversations with their three-year-old children were assessed. As with the other studies referred to, this investigation found that depressed mothers tended to vocalize less frequently and respond less often to their children's vocal cues. In stressful situations, however, such as waiting for a doctor's visit, depressed mothers significantly increased their speech output, although adaptive mothers did not. This impaired form of vocal communication may deprive the infant of the experience of contingency. Breznitz and Sherman expressed the view that failure to expose the infant and young child to sufficient contingency impaired both cognitive and affective developmental potential.

Caregiver and infant vocalization patterns may also be related to prenatal factors or factors outside of the dyadic relationship. For example, Lester and Dreher (1989) investigated the effects of marijuana use during pregnancy on the newborn's cry. The study involved a group of pregnant women who were recruited from three rural communities in Jamaica. The pregnant women were interviewed as part of a larger ethnographic medical study of marijuana use in these communities. Included in the investigation were twenty marijuana users and twenty nonusers who were followed from the beginning of their pregnancy through delivery. The researchers were particularly interested in evaluating the acoustic characteristics of the cries of these infants.

All of the infants were born in the hospital at term. There was one lowbirth weight infant in both the smoker and nonsmoker groups. Apgar scores were reported at greater than seven for all of the infants, although the reliability of these scores was questionable. Infant crying was recorded and analyzed at home on the fourth or fifth day after birth. The infant was placed in a supine position with the microphone held fifteen centimeters from the infant's mouth. Standard newborn reflexes were used in order to elicit the cry. The first ten seconds of the cry were used for acoustic analysis.

The result of the study indicated that infants whose mothers smoked marijuana during pregnancy had a lower average first response to their cries, which may be due to a malformation of the infant's respiratory tract. In general, the cries of these infants were also of a higher pitch than the cries of infants whose mothers had not smoked marijuana. Although the researchers did not indicate precisely how this different infant cry might affect caregiver behavior, they hypothesized that the cry would have an effect on the infant's developmental course. It may be suggested, for example, that if the caregiver perceives of the infant's cry as being abnormal or "sickly" she will respond to the infant in a different manner than if she believes the cry is healthy and adaptive. As a consequence, caregiver vocalizations to the infant, as well as other intuitive behaviors, will be affected not only by factors inherent to the caregiver herself, but also by factors emanating from the infant, such as the quality of the infant's cry.

Another mode of behavior that provides information about whether the caregiver is providing adequate stimulation for the infant involves body contact. Body contact actually encompasses a wide range of behaviors that include holding and cuddling the infant when he is in a quiescent state, rocking the baby to sleep, stroking the infant to assuage discomfort and providing an adequate degree of tactile contact during feeding episodes. All behaviors whereby the caregiver establishes physical contact with the infant are included in this category.

A distinctive pattern of holding behavior has been observed in dyads where the interaction is spontaneous, fluid and reciprocal. For example, Main and Weston (1982) report that within such dyads mothers display tender and gentle gestures when picking up the infant. Typically in these dyads, the caregiver picks up the infant gently, placing it in arms that are positioned so as to create a natural cradle that supports the child's head and entire body. This molded posture facilitates face-to-face contact and enables the caregiver to engage effectively in visual cuing and vocal communication. According to Main and Weston, infants held in this position were touched, caressed and rocked frequently, while the infant displayed a pleasurable response to these gestures as demonstrated by transition to a quiescent state or by gurgling contently. Once again, each of these forms of stimulation creates a predictable interlude for the infant, that may be used to formulate representations about predictable behavior.

In distinction to these dyads, Main and Weston also described dyadic pairs in which the caregiver seemed ill-equipped at providing pleasurable holding experiences for the infant. Such mothers often displayed a stiff and inert posture, held the infant in a mechanical fashion and neglected to display the cradling gestures essential for promoting adaptive face-to-face exchange. Caregivers in this category failed to attribute any special significance to the infant's facial expression and often appeared oblivious to the fact that the baby's neck needed support during periods of holding. In fact, it was not unusual for such caregivers to express a physical dislike and occasional repulsion at the idea of bodily contact with the infant. As a result, body contact was minimal, and was generally limited to such routine tasks as diapering and feeding. Clearly, caregivers who manifested behaviors of this nature were not providing their infants with adequate stimulation to evoke the full range of predictive skills needed for developmental achievement and it would not be unusual to expect that such infants displayed lags in development as the months of infancy progressed.

Disturbed body contact with infants has also been reported by Fleming, Flett, Ruble and Shaul (1988), who investigated the physical behaviors of postpartum- depressed mothers in contrast to healthy mothers who experienced no postpartum depressive episodes. These researchers found that, relative to nondepressed mothers, depressed mothers exhibited fewer affectionate behaviors toward their infants. For example, these mothers tended to engage in significantly lower levels of unconditional positive regard, displayed less continuity of rocking behavior and touched their babies less frequently than did their nondepressed counterparts. Diminished or impaired body contact towards their infants and verbalizations were also less frequent. In general, then, depressed mothers did not respond to the infant in a coordinated fashion that attempted to integrate skills and provide the infant with a sense that responsiveness was contingent upon infant behavior.

Other groups of investigators have observed patterns of maternal and infant imitation during play episodes in order to deduce whether the infant was experiencing adequate stimulation from the caregiver. One research team, Moran, Krupka, Tutton, and Symons (1987), focused on the actual performance of imitation by infants and their mothers during episodes of face-to-face play. Three-minute episodes of play between twenty mothers and their thirteen- to sixteen-week-old infants were videotaped. Instances of mouth openings, lip movements, tongue protrusions, smiling and vocalizations by both partners were coded. Sequential analysis disclosed specific patterns of imitation that were characteristic of both members of the dyad. For example, nondepressed mothers contingently imitated behavior initiated by their infants and were more likely to display similar imitations during action in the same category as their infants. This style of interaction suggests that predictive capacities are being fostered in the infant. Infants, on the other hand, did not show immediate imitative responses, but did attend to caregiver behavior and, when the behavior was repeated, showed an increased likelihood of imitating a particular sequence. The researchers concluded that imitation by the caregiver is a pervasive characteristic of early intervention and plays a vital role in the acquisition of social and emotional skills. Moreover, such imitative sequences must be initiated by the caregiver and encouraged with intuitive responses like facial expression and positive vocalization.

Moran et al.'s study was conducted with adaptive caregivers, who had received normal or above average scores on personality inventories. These caregivers displayed imitative behaviors in a spontaneous, rhythmic fashion, such that the behaviors were woven into regular patterns of interaction. It appeared, in other words, that adaptive caregivers used imitation behaviors to elicit a predictable infant response in an intuitive way. The infant was not pressured to imitate the caregiver immediately, nor did the caregivers appear perturbed when it took some time for the infant to acclimate to a new behavior. Instead, caregivers appeared content to repeat behaviors in a gentle and rhythmic fashion, patiently giving the infant an opportunity to respond. Since this study suggests the type of behavior that is typical in adaptive caregivers, clinicians should also be alert to a different type of imitation behavior that may signal a maladaptive interaction. For example, an absence of caregiver-initiated imitation during observation may signal that the caregiver is not providing the infant with adequate stimulation. At the opposite end of the spectrum, another type of caregiver may be overly anxious in forcing the infant to respond. Infants with caregivers displaying this behavior may engage in avoidance manifestations in order to protect themselves from the distress that accompanies overstimulation. The key here is the degree to which the caregiver is able to provide the infant with contingent stimulation to which the infant responds in a positive fashion.

Feeding competence is a final behavior that rounds out the caregiver's repertoire during the first years of life. Feeding competence represents perhaps one of the most intimate ways in which a caregiver establishes contact with the newborn. Not only do manifestations of this type fulfill a fundamental physiological need, but they also create the infant's first impressions of a contingent, cause-and-effect relationship with the external world, as well as with a supportive, consistent nurturing figure. It is from the contours of such contingencies that infant predictions about future interaction emerge. The discomfort experienced by hunger is generally expressed by the infant through the vocalization of a cry to which the caregiver responds by providing milk. If consistent, feeding behavior may come to signify a crucial internal working model of how the environment responds to the infant. Eventually, other more complex associations will be made, leading to categories of contingent association that are gradually represented by the infant on an interior panorama. With time, the infant converts these representations into behavioral sequences designed to predict a desired response to the caregiver. For these reasons, feeding competence is a noteworthy mode of adaptation, because it heralds an adaptive behavior from which other behavioral milestones evolve. Interestingly enough, Fleming et al. (1988) found that depressed mothers begin bottle-feeding their infants at a significantly earlier age than adaptive mothers.

The caregiver's competence while engaging in this behavior may be equally as significant because it demonstrates the mood or social attitude the infant will come to anticipate in future interactions. As a consequence, caregiver feeding competence has validity as a proliferative model for future exchanges within the dyad.

Although one method for gauging the caregiver's feeding competence is by engaging in direct observation of these sequences, Price (1983) has devised a more formalized scale for assessing the level of caregiver sensitivity during these episodes, referred to as the AMIS (Assessment of Mother-Infant Sensitivity) scale. The scale contains twenty-five items, each with a possible score of one to five points, with higher points indicating greater sensitivity. Fifteen of the items evaluate maternal behaviors, seven evaluate infant behaviors, and three evaluate dyadic behavior. The items in the scale can be grouped into three broad classes of behavior, including holding/handling, social/affective, and feeding/caregiving. Ratings are based on fifteen to thirty minute observations.

Specifically, the maternal items on the scale include the spatial distance the caregiver maintains during feeding episodes, the holding style, the predominant maternal mood or affect exhibited, the tone and content of maternal verbalization, the degree of maternal visual behavior, maternal modulation of distress periods, maternal stimulation of the infant, maternal response to the infant's changing level of activity, burping style, frequency of feeding stimulation and maternal response to infant satiation. Items on the infant scale include predominant infant state and affect, infant vocalization and distress, infant visual behavior and posture, and infant response to stimulation at the point of satiation. Finally, the AMIS measure of dyadic interaction evaluates synchrony of response to pleasurable affect, initiation of feeding and termination of the feeding episode. In sum, the scale devised by Price captures all of the primary intuitive behaviors discussed earlier that instill positive affect and contingent responsiveness in the dyadic relationship.

Each of these dimensions provides the clinician with guidelines for assessing the degree of harmony that is occurring during any discrete feeding episode. Moreover, feeding episodes serve as miniature paradigms of interactive patterns that are likely to promote predictive skills in the infant and to suggest the course of future development. For example, a caregiver who forces the nipple into the infant's mouth despite signs of protest or who withdraws the bottle when the infant is still displaying a sucking reflex, is likely to be oblivious to infant cues in other situations beyond basic feeding episodes. Because feeding episodes capture a wide variety of caregiver behaviors and reflect the degree to which the caregiver responds contingently to the infant, they serve as valuable models the clinician can use to diagnose the degree predictive and contingent sequences are interwoven into the caregiver-infant exchange.

Landry, Chapieski and Schmidt (1986) have proposed yet another way of interpreting the quality of caregiver-infant interaction and evaluating whether the caregiver is offering an appropriate level of stimulation for the infant. These researchers focused on the relationship between maternal attention-directing strategies during play interactions with twelve-month-olds and infant response level. The researchers sought to determine whether such attention-directing strategies differed among caregivers with full term infants, as opposed to caregivers with preterm infants. The key strategies investigated included the maintenance of the infant's attention via verbal and nonverbal techniques designed to capture interest and an evaluation of behaviors designed to assess levels of contingency within the dyad.

The results of the study indicated that maternal attention-directing strategies did indeed differ across full-term and preterm groups. Mothers of full-term infants tended to rely more on verbal cues, rather than body gestures to direct the attention of their infants than did the caregivers of preterm infants. The differences in verbal behavior were related to severity of medical complications associated with prematurity. In addition, these caregivers engaged in attention-directing behaviors more frequently. For example, caregivers of preterm infants tended to direct their infants' attention more often than mothers of full-term infants. This finding is in accord with the investigations of other researchers, such as Field (1980), who found that the caregivers of preterms were more stimulating, and perhaps overly stimulating, in early interactions. According to Brazelton, Parker and Zuckerman (1976) one explanation for the increased levels of stimulation provided by these mothers may be their efforts to compensate for what they perceive to be a lower degree of responsiveness in their infants. This study indicates that the mothers of preterm infants and other infants born with physical impairments may respond in a manner similar to that of a depressed mother with respect to initiating interaction. Although the etiology of this impaired response is different, the outcome, in terms of behavior directed to the infant, is the same. Such caregivers may believe that their infants are somehow "damaged" and therefore less capable than healthy infants of engaging in active, adaptive interaction. The caregivers of these infants may also harbor resentment that the infant was born less than "perfect" and may direct this hostility to the infant by failing to engage in adequate stimulation.

Chapieski and Schmidt reported that there was a group of infants in their sample who interacted minimally with toys. The mothers of these infants seemed to direct their attention more frequently in an attempt to heighten the infant's interaction. This increased level of stimulation engaged in by caregivers of preterm infants did not, however, seem to adversely affect the infants response to the toys. In fact, the researchers suggested that the more active behavior of the preterm mothers may represent an adaptive method of compensating for their infants' temporary lag in developmental skills due to prematurity and may prepare the infant for the challenges of future development by offering predictive models.

Given this finding, it becomes essential for therapists treating dyads to obtain an accurate clinical portrait of the pregnancy and immediate postpartum period. If the infant was, in fact, premature, then a slightly hyperactive mother who repeatedly tries to stimulate the infant may be displaying a natural response. In contrast, a frenetic attitude toward stimulation may be inappropriate for a full-term infant and may signify that the caregiver is out of synchrony with the infant's rhythm of interaction and cannot predict the direction of the infant's development.

Previewing Strategies Designed to Achieve Optimal Stimulation of the Infant

From the above discussion several factors are apparent. First, we know that in adaptive dyads where exchange is characterized by attunement, both caregiver and infant seem to have deciphered each other's signals so that each can respond to the other appropriately with an adequate level of stimulation. Such appropriate responses are comprised of adequate doses of visual cuing, vocal communication, holding behavior, tactile stimulation and feeding competence. Similarly, we also know that certain factors operate insidiously to preclude predictable interactions from oc-curing within the dyad. Among these factors are: (1) an infant tempera-ment that is either misunderstood or mismatched with respect to the care-giver's temperament; (2) a physiological condition on the part of the infant, such as prematurity, that prevents the infant's initial responses from fulfilling caregiver predictions; or (3) an idiopathic condition like colic that is of unknown origin and causes frustration in the caregiver, who feels unable to preview to this "unpredictable" child. In addition, the caregiver's own psychological status may function as an impediment to harmonious dyadic exchange. Most frequently, this can occur if the caregiver has a history of clinical depression or suffers a bout of postpar-tum depression, or if the caregiver is prone to anxiety or obsessive-com-pulsive behavior.

Confronted with this group of caregiver and infant impediments that may preclude contingent and predictable development, how can clini-cians tutor caregivers to adopt modes of interactive behavior that will promote adaptive exchange? Several practical answers are provided by Thoman and Browder (1987). These researchers have strived to teach caregivers how to integrate adaptive and predictive skills during the daily problem periods of interaction. As a general rule, Thoman and Browder advise caregivers not to try too many tactics too quickly, but rather to proceed calmly from one strategy to another, without being afraid to adopt a new technique if one method doesn't work.

To alleviate an episode of crying, for example, these researchers first recommend that the infant be picked up fairly quickly. This advice finds substantiation in a study done by Bell and Ainsworth (1972), who discov-ered that infants whose cries were ignored early in life tended to cry more often and more persistently at one year. By six months of age in these cases an expected cycle had been established between these caregivers and infants, with the infants crying so much that the caregivers felt dis-couraged about responding at all. In sharp contrast, the caregivers who responded most rapidly to their babies' cries had infants who cried the least at one year and who used other forms of communication-such as gestures and happy coos-to attract their caregivers' attention. These stud-ies indicate how vital it is to establish effective interventive strategies early, before debilitating patterns become ingrained.

Thoman and Browder also advise carrying and rocking a crying infant or treating the infant to a series of rhythmic sounds in order to alleviate the crying episode. Other techniques include providing the infant with a pacifier. Although the value of pacifier has been debated, it has been found that premature infants given pacifiers were ready to take a bottle sooner and were able to leave the hospital four days before premature infants who weren't given any extra opportunity for sucking. Another revealing finding of this study was that extra sucking helped colicky two-day-olds calm down-if the pacifier was offered when the infant indicated he wanted to engage in sucking behavior. Signals an infant may use to indicate that he wants more sucking include putting his hands to his mouth, sucking on his tongue, fist or fingers, whimpering, rooting or yawning. It is especially important to emphasize to caregivers that each infant uses his own cues, so that a caregiver first has to observe the infant carefully to learn the unique signals he is emitting. Unless such signals are understood, the caregiver will be unable to predict the direction of the infant's development and incapable of devising previewing behaviors.

Yet another technique that functions both to quell a crying infant and to assist the caregiver in becoming attuned to methods of stimulating the infant, is massage. According to Thoman and Browder, the special way a caregiver touches the infant during massage can enhance intimacy and a shared feeling of reciprocity. In addition, although massage may relax even a wailing infant, this strategy usually works best to prevent crying rather than to stop it. If the infant has a typical cry time during the day, for example, the caregiver is advised to try a massage approximately one hour beforehand. When massaging the infant, Thoman and Browder suggest that a bottle of baby oil be placed in a pan of warm water until the oil feels warm but not hot to the touch. The infant is then undressed and placed on a firm, but not too hard surface, such as a bed or changing table. The caregiver can moisten her hands with the oil and then begin the massage. It is important to rub gently, but to use enough pressure so as not to tickle. As the caregiver begins to massage, she will see how the infant responds to touch and which ways of touching are preferred. A good massage generally lasts for ten to fifteen minutes, although caregivers are advised to watch the infant to be sure he is envincing signs of pleasurable affect. A massage also presents the caregiver with an outstanding opportunity to observe the scope of the infant's developmental status, in order to later devise previewing behaviors geared to enhancing maturation.

Another interventive strategy that is often effective in facilitating the evolution of a mutually stimulating relationship between caregiver and infant involves a teaching-modeling intervention that is designed to provide caregivers with didactic lessons for optimizing interaction. This technique was used by Poley-Strobel and Beckmann (1987) who examined a sample of twenty black, primiparous, low-income caregivers. These caregivers had experienced uneventful pregnancies, labor, delivery and postpartum periods and all infants were healthy, full-term, singletons who were bottle-fed. Caregivers in the experimental group received a teaching session in which the investigator discussed caregiver behaviors which elicited adaptive interactive behaviors and promoted the skills of the infant. State control, response to stress, motor processes and interactive process were discussed. After intervention, it was found that statistically significant differences existed between the experimental group of mothers and a control group of mothers.

In this study, the Brazelton Neonatal Behavioral Assessment Scale (Brazelton, 1973) was used to evaluate the infant's ability to emit certain cues in response to specific stimuli. Assessments were made the morning of discharge from the hospital when the infant was near forty-eight hours of age. Data from the assessment were converted into a scoring system and standard scoring systems were used for three dimensions, including interactive processes, motor processes and organizational processes, such as state control. In addition to modeling the Brazelton Neonatal Scale, the researchers also selected one feeding session to observe an episode of reciprocity between caregiver and infant. During this feeding, reciprocity was measured using the Assessment of Mother-Infant Sensitivity (the "AMIS") devised by Price (1983). This instrument assesses both maternal and infant behaviors, and evaluates dialogues during a feeding. Fifteen items relating to maternal behaviors are assessed and comprise the maternal cluster, while seven items evaluate infant behaviors and comprise the infant cluster. Finally, three dyadic behaviors are considered to assess overall interaction.

As a result of these interventions, the researchers found significant differences in the control and experimental groups with respect to the maternal and interactive clusters of the AMIS. Because this intervention as well as the demonstration of the Brazelton Neonatal Assessment may have been relevant to subsequent displays of maternal sensitivity and responsiveness, the assessments were able to differentiate among the groups. The researchers felt that by demonstrating and modeling the interactive behavior of the infant, the intervention was designed to reveal the infant's predictive capabilities to the mother and to motivate her to try similar interactive behaviors with her infant designed to enhance predictive skills.

Among mothers who are suffering from postpartum depression or clinical depression, however, such techniques may not be sufficient to instill patterns of contingent response within the dyad. For these mothers a variety of techniques is recommended. First, the therapist may wish to show the mother videotapes of adaptive interaction, particularly emphasizing those intuitive behaviors that are likely to lead to an adaptive response, such as visual cuing, vocal cuing and appropriate body contact. The therapist should also take the lead in discussing how these behaviors tend to result in a positive outcome. For example, it should be explained that while the infant cannot speak, he is capable of understanding affective messages that may be conveyed through facial expressions, particular types of vocalization and physical stroking sensations. These caregivers should also be told about the role of contingent stimulation in enhancing the infant's cognitive awareness of the world around him and in promoting adaptive development. Thus, if exposed to contingencies, the infant will be more likely to develop representations and expectations about how the world operates. As a result, the infant's own responses to the world will become more predictable, both to himself and to the caregiver. As the infant becomes more predictable, so too will the caregiver be able to elicit a greater degree of positive responses. This form of caregiver control will reach a pinnacle during previewing exercises.

Once this sequence has been explained to the caregiver both verbally and through some sort of visual presentation such as videotape, the therapist should demonstrate some of these interactions with the infant in the caregiver's presence. Visual cuing, vocal behavior and appropriate holding gestures are relatively easy to model, but the therapist should also strive to point out the subtle changes in the infant's expression, vocalizations responsiveness level upon being exposed to these behaviors so that the caregiver understands the significance of these behaviors in fueling interaction.

Following this kind of demonstration, the therapist should discuss some more abstract principles with the caregiver, such as how the infant comes to evolve representations of interactive sequences and to subsequently use these representations to predict a caregiver response. The therapist should next convey that the infant will develop skills that will heighten the degree of communication within the dyad and that such development may be anticipated and predicted by the caregiver. Finally, the therapist should introduce the caregiver to the concept of previewing as a special way to encourage the infant's burgeoning developmental skills and further enhance the dyadic relationship. Initially, the therapist can engage in previewing behaviors with the infant, with the caregiver observing the interaction. Eventually, however, the caregiver should be encouraged to devise her own previewing exercises that can be performed during sessions. Once the caregiver has mastered the essentials of previewing, the therapist should ask the caregiver to use previewing in the home and to periodically report on how this technique has resulted in a better relationship with the infant.

Finally, researchers such as Susman and Katz (1988) have pointed out that postpartum depression is not the only psychophysiological aftermath of pregnancy that may exert a particularly detrimental effect on future interaction. In addition, some mothers may experience depression with the advent of the weaning process. According to Susman and Katy, the depression that attends weaning may be due to the same endocrinological factors that trigger postpartum depression in some women. As a result, caregivers who are anticipating weaning their infants should be encouraged to discuss their feeling and to communicate any onset of depressive affect. If depression should occur, the therapist should be available to help the caregiver work through the episode and should also ensure that whatever deprivations of stimulation the infant is exposed to are compensated for through the interventions of the other parent or family members.

Previewing instruction may also be used with another population of new mothers. Lutzker, Lutzker, Braunling-McMorrow and Eddleman (1987) have observed that new caregivers, particularly those who are young, are often oblivious to the unique developmental abilities of their newborns. However, a perinatal coaching class can teach such mothers to be more responsive to infant cues. Often a simple prompting procedure paired with an infant response is an effective strategy for motivating such mothers to engage in more enhanced interactions with their infants.

Based on these previous findings, Lutzer et al. instituted a program that relied heavily on the teaching of contingent behavioral response in a group of young mothers with infants ranging from three to six months. Caregivers were encouraged to further develop the interactive skills they had already demonstrated with the infant. For example, the caregiver was asked to describe one play behavior she enjoyed engaging in with the infant. If the mother responded that she liked playing peek-a-boo with the baby, then this behavior was used as a prompting procedure. As a result, contingency experiences were reinforced for both caregiver and infant. This technique is beneficial for caregivers who display some degree of skill with their infants, but who would benefit from some additional therapy and encouragement.

During training sessions, this prompting procedure was then studied with respect to infant interaction, and it was explained to the caregivers that such prompting could be used to generate an awareness of contingency in their infants. By engaging in a particular behavior that she found pleasurable, the mother was able to elicit a positive infant response and further contingent activities were demonstrated; the dyad to engaged in predictable sequences of interaction. Eventually the caregiver became adept at recognizing and initiating contingent responses on her own with the child. This study demonstrates the significance of stressing positive interaction for the caregiver and striving to help the caregiver integrate such adaptive sequences into her daily routine.

Becker (1987) examined a variety of other factors that may impact on early caregiver-infant interaction and proposed some interventive strategies for promoting adaptive exchange. According to Becker, adolescent and adult single mothers may be especially prone to developing maladaptive behavior patterns with their infants. These adolescent mothers are also good candidates for training in previewing techniques. Among such mothers developmental expectations may already be low, according to Bee, Barnard, Eyres, Gray, Hammond, Spietz, Snyder and Clark (1982), who demonstrated that the expectations of adolescent caregivers were lower than those of appropriately matched adult mothers. Becker's study confirmed that adolescent motherhood involves a risk to the infant beyond factors such as prematurity or medical complications at birth. Since these adolescents do not report higher levels of stress than their adult counterparts, Becker contends that the risk can most probably be related to psychological immaturity. The correlation found between maternal age and some of the parenting measures Becker discovered further suggests that the risks associated with immaturity do not suddenly vanish at the conclusion of adolescence and that optimal obstetric age was not necessarily synonymous with the optimal parenting age.

Becker reported, however, that while adolescent mothers were as cognizant of most of their newborns' interactive behaviors as were adult mothers, they were not as competent in translating their perceptions into behaviors. Nor did they possess as profound an understanding of the impact their behaviors had on the infant. Thus, the adolescents were able to recognize newborn capabilities during the immediate and direct experience of interacting with their infants, but were less accurate in predicting and previewing developmental competencies relating to the future of their infants' maturation.

According to Becker, situational factors such as single marital status may be more important sources of stress during pregnancy than age. In summarizing the findings of the study, Becker observed that the effectiveness of intervention to optimize the caregiving environment of infants of adolescent and adult single mothers may depend on prior assessment of the level of maturity with which the mother conceptualizes both normal infant development and the implications of developmental norms for her parenting. As described above, therapist should strive to instruct such mothers in techniques for optimizing predictive experiences, particularly because treatment can significantly enhance adaptive behavior in these caregivers.

Conclusion

Each of the studies discussed previously underscores the value of early interventive strategies for optimizing the nature of interaction within the dyad. It becomes the therapist's task to first diagnose any risk factors that harbor potential for impeding this kind of optimal development. For example, is the caregiver single or an adolescent? Was the infant premature or were there medical complications attending the birth? Does the caregiver have a history of either depression or anxiety disorder? Is the caregiver experiencing an episode of postpartum depression? Following this assessment, the therapist should observe sequences of interaction to determine whether an optimal level of stimulation is being provided to the infant. It is important here to examine such factors as the infant's temperament and the caregiver's disposition, whether medical or developmental complications existed at the birth, and whether the infant suffers from an idiosyncratic condition such as colic that tends to impede interaction. Therapists should also assess the degree to which the caregiver engages in intuitive behaviors designed to enhance the dyadic interaction and promote infant predictive abilities. Once this assessment has been made, the therapist can devise the most advantageous treatment strategies for enhancing predictable and adaptive interaction. Among strategies that have been reported to be effective are infant massage, psychotherapy that focuses on alerting the caregiver to the infant's developmental signals, modeling adaptive interaction, and encouraging the caregiver to engage in representations about future infant development and play behavior. In particular, many mothers whose relationship with the infant is impaired will also benefit from instruction in previewing techniques. Such techniques strive to introduce the caregiver to the roles played by contingencies and representational thinking in the infant's unfolding development. Each of these techniques can be modeled by the therapist, who then instructs the caregiver on how to initiate such behaviors with her infant.

CHAPTER 10

Strategies for Enhancing Previewing

Introduction

Earlier chapters provided a blueprint of the optimal patterns encountered during adaptive dyadic interaction. Such patterns of interaction tend to promote the infant's predictive capacities and are imbued with previewing behaviors manifested by the caregiver. But what can be done to remedy a caregiver-infant relationship in which these previewing behaviors are absent or appear only sporadically? What techniques can be used to isolate sources of discord that impair the caregiver's capacity for engaging in adaptive previewing within the dyad? How can the therapist best ascertain the cause of an absence of previewing behaviors and what treatment strategies are most effective in alleviating difficulty and reasserting previewing patterns during interaction? Lastly, do particular situations lead to the curtailment of previewing behaviors, thereby exerting a detrimental impact on early interaction between caregiver and infant?

A review of the data on therapeutic strategies used for treating caregivers and infants reveals that therapists have incorporated a wide variety of techniques, ranging from traditional psychoanalytically oriented interventions to innovative treatments designed to modify instances of early maladaptive interaction within the dyad. These newer therapeutic models are impressive for their innovative qualities although this degree of creativity is not so unexpected when we consider the possibilities suggested by intervention within a dyadic relationship. Paradigms for dyadic treatment have enabled therapists to select which aspect of the interaction should be highlighted for treatment. Treatment strategies can focus on altering maladaptive behavior patterns demonstrated by each or both members of the dyad. Because treatment will ineviatably involve in-depth observations of the dyadic interactions, the therapist can immediately begin viewing normative and deviant developmental patterns along with descriptive reports of the caregiver, even during the first session. This model also allows the therapist to isolate patterns of interaction that are devoid of previewing behaviors.

This chapter reviews treatment strategies used for modifying problematic dyadic interaction that hinders or impedes the emergence of previewing patterns during the first two years of life. Several suggestions are made with respect to how these techniques can be used to fullest advantage and how several techniques previously relegated to other areas of psychotherapy can be adapted for dyadic treatment.

To orient the reader, I refer continually to the previewing behaviors outlined in earlier chapters. These behaviors track the developmental changes of both the caregiver and the infant, and may be used in several ways. First, a knowledge of the previewing behaviors (including such precursory manifestations as contingency stimulation) and the chronological point at which they are expected to emerge during infant development enable researchers to diagnose deviations from optimal patterns and to isolate more precisely which dyadic member is fueling the interaction dysfunctionally. Second, because previewing behaviors embody discrete forms of optimal development, they provide therapists with clearly delineated treatment goals. Finally, the fact that the adaptive behaviors are actually hierarchically organized (in that early forms of optimal interaction *proliferate* and *differentiate* into more sophisticated forms of exchange) enables the therapist to identify specific flaws or deficits in function. For example, if the dyad is presented for treatment when the infant is eight months of age, the therapist will look for signs of social referencing and affect attunement during sequences of interaction. Assuming that evidence of an attuned orchestration of responses is either absent or sporadic, the therapist can examine whether the various precursory behaviors which cumulatively result in social referencing are in evidence. For example, is the caregiver engaging in appropriate visual cuing, vocalization and bodily contact with the infant? Conversely, are factors emanating from the infant, such as temperamental proclivities and an inability to recognize contingencies, interfering with harmonious interaction?

Throughout this discussion, the key signs of adaptive interaction discussed earlier, as well as examples of previewing, are used as reference points to identify areas of vulnerability in dyad. I have chosen to present the treatment models in a sequence that moves from situations in which the dyad is at risk of dysfunctional interaction to situations in which the etiology of disorder and maladaptation are more disguised. This order of presentation is selected because it is certainly easier to diagnose and treat maladaptive patterns when a variable that is antithetical to harmonious interaction-such as a developmental disability, a birth defect or a history of maternal depression-is introduced. As the etiology of the failed interaction becomes less apparent, more sophisticated diagnostic strategies and more complex treatment is often warranted, leading the therapist to continually refine and compare interaction with the models of previewing in adaptive dyads. Moreover, the therapist is encouraged to use his or her knowledge of previewing when formulating a diagnosis.

Treatment Techniques

The Developmentally Disabled Child

Historically, the birth of a child has been of paramount symbolic significance for the parents involved. It is no accident that an impending birth is referred to as a "blessed event," a phrase which captures the collective awe each of us experiences with the advent of new life in the world. Although we are able to grasp the cognitive dimensions of conception and in utero maturation, the emergence of an entirely new being retains an aura of mystery.

No individual experiences this sense of wonder more personally and intimately than the infant's mother who, for nine months, has undergone a budding relationship with the creature developing inside of her. By another curious twist of language, we commonly refer to the pregnant woman as an "expectant mother." This phrase is significant because it implies not merely that the mother is predicting the physical presence of a newborn baby, but also that a cognitive and emotional preconception of the personality of the infant has begun to form in her imagination. Indeed, as mentioned in Chapter 1, such expectations represent the initial form of previewing engaged in by the caregiver.

Since these maternal representations attain a high degree of potency immediately prior to birth, it is not unusual to predict that if the infant is born prematurely or with any type of obvious defect, the mother may experience an extreme discrepancy between what Horan (1982) calls "the fantasy child" who was imagined before birth and the actual child. Several researchers have pointed out that extreme discrepancy between an anticipated outcome and an actual outcome is experienced as a disrupted contingency, which, in turn, creates the impression of helplessness in an uncontrollable universe. These feelings of helplessness tend to expand to other areas of function and may result in a full-fledged depressive mood (Landry and Chapieski, 1989; Cohen, Velez, Brook and Smith, 1989).

Expectant mothers may also be prone to depression upon the birth of a *premature* or *handicapped* infant for several other reasons. It must be emphasized that pregnancy is a physiological state of relatively lengthy duration and that most expectant mothers are advised to enter a program of regular prenatal care. During this period, the potential mother will likely alter many behaviors and progressively modify her customary work routine. Expectant mothers will also be advised to relinquish such habits as smoking and drinking alcohol and may undergo such medical procedures as amniocentesis and sonograms. In essence, the mother engages in these activities to promote the birth of a healthy infant. The numerous changes and procedures undergone by expectant mothers are designed to ensure a positive outcome, and in the mother's mind, these behaviors may even serve to create the healthy outcome. Upon the birth of a premature or disabled infant, the effect of these reinforcing behaviors is rapidly and automatically challenged and contradicted, and the mother may experience the trauma and shock of extreme discrepancy. In addition, the mother's predictive fantasies about the child may be shattered. The infant is less than the "perfect baby" that has been previewed by the caregiver in her anticipatory reveries. As a result, the caregiver's disappointment may be translated into interactional behaviors that impair the infant's predictive abilities and hinder the evolution of an adaptive dyadic relationship.

The nature of this discrepancy will be obvious to the caregiver. Because the status of the infant is apparent to the parents, the medical personnel and virtually anyone who enters the neonatal intensive care unit, the caregiver is almost forced to immediately confront the fact that she has given birth to a high-risk or impaired infant. There is no transitional period for her to become accustomed to her violated predictions or to reflect on the possibility that the infant's problems may have been caused by factors beyond her control. Such mothers are also deprived of the experience of caring for the neonate, because the infant is placed in a special neonatal unit away from the parents. Shattered predictions are, therefore, twofold. Not only is the mother confronted with a live infant whose tenuous physical status contradicts her notions of the perfect child, but she must also cope with the disappointment of not being able to interact intimately with the infant, and to forge the anticipated interactional bond within the first few days of life.

Mothers in this situation are primed for feelings of depression and deprivation. Several researchers have addressed the issues of how interventive strategies can be used to assist the mother in surmounting these debilitating emotions and preparing for the establishment of a subsequent harmonious dyadic interaction. In addition, the therapist should attempt to help the caregiver realign her expectations and formulate new, more realistic predictions about the infant that can eventually be used to devise previewing behaviors appropriate to the infant's developmental status.

Kennell and Klaus (1982) have suggested an approach that integrates the mother in the infant's recuperative process. This technique may be referred to as therapeutic participation by the mother. By encouraging her involvement, Kennell and Klaus report, the negative emotions that often surround the birth of a premature or disabled infant can be alleviated somewhat, thus averting the impact of caregiver depression and laying the foundation for the evolution of an adaptive relationship. By fostering early maternal involvement despite the infant's precarious medical status, the mother is also provided with the gratification derived from early interaction, thereby alleviating some of the feelings of early deprivation upon learning that her infant was born with a disability. Early nurturing behaviors foster positive expectations and will also avoid the possibility that the mother is forced into a subservient position, both dependent and resentful of the assistance of medical personnel. Prugh, Staub, Sands, Kirschbaum and Lenihan (1953), advocates of such interventive strategies for the mothers of premature infants, feel that early interaction of this type diminishes the experience of "emotional lag," defined as the alienation virtually all new mothers experience during early relationships with the infant. This emotional lag can be especially exacerbated in the case of mothers with disabled infants.

To facilitate the caregiver's active and early participation, Kennell and Klaus recommend that neonatal nurseries be open to parents, that they receive specific instruction on how to assist in the care of the infant and then be permitted to administer this care themselves, and that they be instructed in methods of creating reciprocal interactions with the infant. Such techniques help acquaint the caregiver with the infant's developmental status. As soon as medically feasible, the mother should be encouraged to breastfeed the infant and should by provided with a "nesting area" in which intimate bonding can occur in a private and soothing environment. These interventions, designed to make the mother an immediate and primary participant in the infant's care, will generally have a positive effect on the infant. For example, Kennell and Klaus have reported that premature infants who are touched, rocked and fondled daily by caregivers in the intensive-care ward experience fewer episodes of apnea. It has also been found that when caregivers interact with premature infants prior to any instruction, they tend to be hyperactive, as if to compensate for an observable nonresponsiveness and hypoactivity on the part of the infants. After some didactic coaching, however, caregivers are generally able to calm themselves and engage in more rhythmic sequences that promote the infant's predictive capacities. This form of rhythmic response suggests the caregiver is attuned to the infant's native responsive proclivities.

Klaus and Kennell (1982) have summarized a two-step approach to participatory intervention that will most likely promote adaptive interactions. First, the mother should be integrated into the format of infant care as an *active participant*. During this phase of intervention, she should be encouraged to observe the infant and to express any concerns or voice any queries. Demonstrations of contingent stimulation should also occur at this point, to reinforce for the mother that she plays the primary role in the infant's development and that this role will not be usurped by medical personnel. The goal of these active interventive strategies is to help the mother alter her prior expectations of the child. Active-participation treatment strategies facilitate the mother's gradual acceptance of the infant's limitations and despite his impairments, the infant's capabilities of learning new skills, of interacting with his mother and of asserting mastery over the environment. Ultimately, the therapist should reinforce the notion that, although the infant is impaired, he is capable of developmental achievement which can be facilitated if the caregiver engages in sufficient previewing behaviors. This restructuring of the preconceived notion of the infant into the formulation of a new, more realistic acceptance of infant capacity is the second goal of active-participation strategies.

If the child is born with a permanent disability or even if the infant's only impairment is prematurity, interactional patterns will likely be affected during the entire period of infancy and often well into childhood. Several researchers have addressed the issue of how intervention strategies focused on the active participation of the caregiver can be integrated into infant care beyond the crisis period immediately following the birth. Strom, Rees, Slaughter and Wurster (1980) examined a group of dyads in which the infants were intellectually handicapped. The median infant age was 5.8 months, however the population included children as old as eleven years. The researchers administered a Parent-as-Teacher inventory to assess child-rearing predictions and found that among those caregivers whose expectations were low due to the intellectual impairment of the infant, intervention designed to encourage parents to participate actively in the child's development was helpful in creating an interaction based on more adaptive predictions within the dyad and in counteracting the feelings of depression and helplessness expressed by many of these parents. In particular, such parents can benefit from representational exercises that focus on the caregiver's ability to predict imminent development for the infant.

Piper (1982) recommends that the parents of disabled children be included in the decisions involving their infants. If this approach is not adopted both the caregivers and the professionals involved may view the parents as incompetent partners in the care of the infant, incapable of anticipating and preparing the infant for developmental achievement. This attitude can contaminate future interactions between medical personnel and parents, inadvertently instilling feelings of incompetence and helplessness in the parents which are inevitably transferred to the infant by failing to expose the infant to previewing exercises. To counter this debilitating cycle, Piper advises that parents be encouraged from the outset to identify developmental changes and patterns for the health-care workers, with the mother becoming the pivotal figure who interprets infant needs and capacities and conveys information to medical personnel. In this fashion, the mother's function as the infant's primary interactional partner is reinforced.

Brazelton (1984) has suggested that one effective method of participatory intervention with such caregivers is to perform the Brazelton Neonatal Assessment Scale (Brazelton, 1973) in the mother's presence. The intricacies of the assessment enable her to observe directly a diverse range of responses and to gauge the flexibility of adjustment to environmental stimuli apparent even in infants with disabilities. Brazelton notes that mothers are particularly sensitive to the teaching implications of the assessment and seem energized, after observing a testing session, to transfer some of these modes of interaction to their own relationships with their infants. By witnessing such an assessment, caregivers become convinced that the infant is capable of developmental achievement and become enthusiastic about engaging in behaviors designed to enhance such development. Manipulative play that encourages responsiveness when initiated early and continued through infancy is another effective method for channeling dyadic interaction toward adaptative maturation.

Thomas, Phemister, and Richardson (1980), for example, compared the effects of manipulative play in handicapped children with the effects of such play in normal infants. Although the developmentally handicapped children were older than the normal infants, the groups were matched with respect to developmental stage, and it was found that stimulation and manipulative play were effective in eliciting contingent interaction. Moreover, the mere presence of the caregiver fostered the children's manipulative play, even though the parent did not participate in the play. Several inferences can be drawn from this study. First, although developmentally impaired children exhibit modes of adaptation according to a delayed timetable, they nevertheless manifest these behaviors in the same sequence as normal infants. Second, caregiver presence and encouragement appears to be as vital for developmentally disabled children as for normals. Thus it becomes crucial for the parents of such infants to be instructed in methods of representing and previewing adaptive development.

Haskett and Holler (1978) reported similar results when they instituted a program of sensory reinforcement and contingency awareness among profoundly retarded children aged nine to seventeen. In this study, children were taught a contingency relationship between a light and a music stimulus. It was found that allowing the children to learn how to control stimulation enhanced responsiveness. Denhoff (1981) has labeled strategies using this orientation as enrichment programs and has noted that early intervention of this type serves to reinforce contingent interaction between caregiver and infant, encouraging interaction that stimulates previewing capacities and enabling parents to resolve ambiguous predictions with respect to developmentally disabled infants and children.

When designing sensory enrichment programs for infants with developmental disabilities, researchers can also use the manifestations inherent in previewing behaviors. During the first months of life, dyads should be observed to ascertain evidence of adequate visual cuing, such as direct eye contact, regulation of the caregiver's distance during face-to-face contact, and greeting contingent to visual contact, vocal communication, including a variety of melodic contours, rhythmicity, tempo and voice pitch, holding behavior and feeding competence. In cases where caregivers are not providing these forms of stimulation for the infant, therapists can employ a variety of strategies. For example, the therapist can videotape the interaction for the caregiver and play back the tape in slow motion, permitting the caregiver to assimilate and appreciate the nuances of behavior inherent in all interactive sequences, and in particular to observe how infant responsiveness is heightened when certain behaviors are exhibited. Parents can then be assisted in altering their own cues to elicit heightened, more adaptive responses from the infant. Or the therapist may initially demonstrate inte: action with the infant and request that the caregiver attempt to duplicate or model the interaction. In all such cases, the caregiver should feel that the infant will benefit developmentally if she takes the lead in predicting responses and providing an atmosphere conducive to previewing.

In relying on any of these techniques, it is vital that the therapist keep in mind some of the significant factors that serve to enhance dyadic exchange. First, parents of developmentally disabled infants may be acutely sensitive to the fact that their infant is delayed or impaired in manifesting developmental skills. They may resent a therapist who seeks to guide them because the prospect of treatment renews feelings of inadequacy. In their view the message becomes "not only did I give birth to an inadequate infant," but "I am also an inadequate parent." Since these sensitivities can be potent, the therapist must not usurp the parent's role. Instead, the therapist's role should remain that of a didactic helper who will instruct the caregiver to rechannel her own skills toward realistically accepting the infant and devising predictive sequences of interaction that are appropriate to the infant's developmental status. Therapy, in other words, should strive for the caregiver's optimal interaction with the infant.

In the case of a developmentally disabled or premature infant, a more formidable obstacle to harmonious interaction within the dyad may be posed by the mother's complex psychological response upon learning that the infant has developmental problems. Kennell and Klaus have outlined the stages most caregivers undergo in adjusting to the relationship with a disabled infant. Initially, they note, the mother experiences a form of anticipatory grief as a consequence of the severing of the fantasy womb relationship with the infant. As explained in Chapter 1, all new mothers undergo the transition from relating to the infant envisioned during the pregnancy to relating to real infant who has been born, resolving the discrepancy between the fantasized child and the actual baby. This transition may even be one cause for postpartum depression encountered in many mothers who have given birth to healthy infants. The transition for mothers of premature or developmentally disabled infants may be particularly difficult to master, however, because such parents are confronted with the reality of an infant whose behaviors do not conform to any expected patterns. In addition to mastering their anticipatory grief, they must overcome feelings of maternal failure upon giving birth to an infant who is not average or typical, as well as mastering debilitating emotions stemming from feelings of inadequacy and incompetence. Assuming that the anticipatory grief can be mastered and that the pervasive feelings of maternal failure can be overcome, the mother will then initiate a relationship with the infant based upon predictable patterns of response. For such a relationship to be effective, however, the parent must understand and appreciate the infant's special needs and growth patterns. This psychological course is often problematic for parents and, as many researchers have found, psychotherapy can be of assistance. Indeed, the caregiver may need to be tutored in methods of instilling intuitive responses that promote the infant's predictive capacities.

Cramer (1987) has elaborated upon the psychodynamic origin of feelings of incompetence in the parents of premature and developmentally disabled infants, and his theories are of value in formulating pragmatic treatment strategies. According to Cramer, several key themes emerge when parents of such infants are interviewed shortly after the birth. For example, debilitating feelings of failure indicative of a self-esteem deficit are encountered, as are the theme of insufficiency and inadequacy. It is common for such parents to associate the infant's incomplete maturation or abnormal status with a personal feeling of incompleteness. Cramer has hypothesized that during pregnancy, the embryo is perceived as part of the self, incorporated into the mother's own narcissism and body image. If the pregnancy is full-term, the mother will ultimately be equipped to tolerate the anatomic separation attendant to giving birth.

However, when the infant is born prematurely, there is an abrupt severing, almost an eviction, of the infant from the caregiver's body. A similar feeling of disruption may be present when the infant is born with a disability. In the latter instance, the caregiver may feel that if the pregnancy had endured for a longer period, the infant's development would have been "completed." These feelings result from the fact that the transition from "fetus" as a narcissistic aspect of the self to "infant" as a separate, autonomous entity has not occurred, and as a consequence, the infant-whether premature or impaired-is viewed as still being a part of the mother's internal organs and internal "self." Individual psychotherapy geared to assist the caregiver in experiencing the natural occurrence of the infant's autonomy is one remedy for correcting this misconception. Such caregivers may experience emotional reactions that resemble disrupted contingencies. To repair these feelings, the therapist must work with the caregiver to reestablish positive feelings about the infant's developmental future and to persuade the caregiver that the infant is a separate and autonomous being, though one who will need her supportive interventions.

Klaus and Kennell, have outlined a similar progressive psychology in mothers who have given birth to infants with congenital malformations or defects. Such parents undergo a series of five anticipated stages: shock, denial, emotional response (sadness, anger, anxiety), a period of equilibrium during which the emotional repercussions abate, and reorganization signifying a realistic acceptance of the infant's status. These researchers note that the final stage of reorganization requires that parents mourn for the loss of the idealized, imaginary child who existed prior to the birth. They should be given the time and emotional support necessary to resolve these feelings naturally. Horan (1982) concurs in this view, observing that parents, especially mothers, of infants born with a defect often dwell on attaching a cause to the infant's disability. Such parents tend to view themselves despairingly twice as frequently as they express satisfaction with themselves. It is not uncommon for them to attribute the cause of their infant's defect to some failing or incapacity on their own part and to translate these feelings into a negative response directed at the infant. Indeed, occasionally, the infant's malformation or congenital defect does stem from a genetic or hereditary flaw linked to the parent. Nevertheless, parents can magnify the significance of a hereditary connection and become mired in overwhelming feelings of guilt and remorse. When this type of reaction occurs, a more active form of psychotherapy, designed to encourage the parent to explore and master feelings of inadequacy raised by the birth, may be warranted.

Other factors, more social in nature, may also surface following the birth of a developmentally disabled infant. Waisbren (1980) has reported that such parents tend to experience sleep difficulties, engage in marital disputes and that an increased dependence on medical personnel creates feelings of helplessness and uncertainty. Overt anger may be directed at the child or at the marital relationship because of the parents' lack of ability to cloak a pervasive sense of low self-esteem that threatens to disrupt the relationship between the parents themselves or between caregivers and infant. Because these feelings can be so intense, they can impair the forging of bond based on adaptive predictive sequences of interaction within the dyad. Coaxing the parent to master the cycle of shock, denial, anger, adaptation, and reorganization is one strategy for these cases. During the period when one of the parents is unable to function adaptively with the infant, the other parent should be encouraged to assume the role of adaptive partner who projects contingency experiences to the infant.

These studies indicate that the birth of a premature or developmentally disabled infant is often experienced as a traumatizing psychological event by the parents. Treatment goals designed to surmount the debilitating effects of this trauma and to reestablish a harmonious interaction within the dyad focus on two primary strategies. First, it must be demonstrated to caregivers that, although the infant is impaired, his capacities to respond to the environment and to initiate an exchange are still extant in varying degrees. In other words, the infant will still traverse a predictable developmental course. Using didactic techniques, the caregiver should be integrated into the team administering medical attention to the infant, should be encouraged to visit the infant and, when feasible, should be given the opportunity to breast-feed or otherwise interact with the infant in a relatively private setting.

Such interventions may not be sufficient in helping parents overcome the psychological repercussions of giving birth to a disabled or high-risk infant, however. Thus, in addition to systematic intervention geared to teaching the caregiver how to minister to the needs of the infant, individual psychotherapy may also be advisable in these cases. Psychotherapy of this type should be primarily supportive, enabling the parent to undergo the naturally occurring stages of shock, denial, anger, adaptation and reorganization. If the parent appears debilitated by chronic feelings of helplessness and incompetence, a more aggressive form of psychotherapy may be advisable, which challenges the caregiver to confront the source of her feelings of incompetence and to master these feelings in order to develop an adaptive relationship with the infant. Only when the caregiver has dispelled these debilitating emotions will she be able to engage in adaptive previewing with the infant.

Caregivers of premature or developmentally disabled infants need to confront yet another challenge that has not been discussed frequently in the literature. This challenge involves the infant's developmental status and future performance. As has been demonstrated, developmentally disabled and premature infants often follow a timetable of maturational achievement that differs from the developmental schedule of a normal infant. For example, such children are likely to attain the developmental milestones as walking or talking, or even more subtle milestones such as the ability to sit up and grasp an object, at a less accelerated pace than normal.

As a result of this developmental delay, Korner (1987) has pointed out that parental predictions may be disrupted and the caregivers may be reduced to feelings of helplessness and emotional debilitation. To counter these feelings, it is recommended that the caregivers undergo counseling or other therapeutic treatment to achieve a form of cognitive mastery over events and over the status of their particular infant. Moreover, caregivers should be alerted to the fact that only when they are capable of experiencing mastery will they be able to engage in positive predictions about their infants. In general, such therapy should focus on helping the caregivers realign their notions of infant development so that they are more appropriate to their infant.

Once the caregiver's expectations have become more realistic and they have come to accept the developmental profile of their particular infant, the therapist should also strive to instill a positive attitude about the infant's developmental growth and achievement. This can be done by helping the caregivers articulate current infant developmental status and then by encouraging anticipation of a future achievement. Previewing behaviors can then be demonstrated by the therapist. In this fashion, the therapist conveys to the caregivers that, while this particular infant's development will, nonetheless, occur, and it is imperative that the caregiver actively encourage the infant's efforts.

For caregivers who are especially depressed about the potential developmental delays of their infant, therapists may adopt several of the strategies used by Salzman (1984) in his insight-oriented therapy. The key to patient progress, according to Salzman, is found in a process of enlightenment, whereby the patient comes to focus upon his or her potential for accomplishment, rather that on past failures. Ultimately, it is this feeling of accomplishment that will be conveyed to the infant through previewing behavior. With caregivers of developmentally disabled infants it becomes especially important to focus upon the potential for achievement of that particular child, because the opportunity for comparisons with normal children is obviously great. Therefore, from the outset of treatment therapists may need to play an active role in focusing attention on the infant and his potential, while simultaneously diverting attention away from notions about development that the caregivers may harbor. To this end, Weakland, Fisch, Watzlawick, and Bodin (1981) recommend focusing on present observable behavior present, rather than on flights of fancy or on regret over what might have been. Therapists treating such caregivers may also need to interact more with the infant and to model behavior in order to elicit a response that will demonstrate to the caregivers that the infant is capable of functioning as an interactive partner. Eventually, through an abundance of previewing and interactive behavior with the infant, the majority of caregivers become sufficiently motivated to begin assuming their proper role as apprentice to the infant's development.

Post Partum Depression

One of the most debilitating experiences for both the neonate and the caregiver is the onset of postpartum depression. Postpartum depression is a particularly insidious disorder, because it threatens to undermine the establishment of an adaptive relationship between caregiver and infant during the first weeks, and sometimes months of life.

Several researchers have highlighted this time as a critical period, during which the infant's initial experience with the external world occurs. If there is no supportive caregiver present to minister adaptively to the infant's needs and to provide an appropriate amount of stimulation for the infant, the infant may represent the external environment as chaotic, disorganized and uncontrollable. In addition, this sense of uncontrollability may also be generalized to the developmental changes occurring within the infant's body, which the infant may also perceive as being uncontrollable and incapable of being mastered.

Such perceptions can wreak havoc on the future course of development. As has been highlighted in previous chapters, it is vital that the infant be exposed to a sufficient degree of contingency stimulation in the form of the caregiver's intuitive manifestations early in life in order for adaptive predictive capacities to begin functioning. As has been discussed in earlier chapters, the caregiver's use of intuitive behaviors motivates the infant to begin recognizing contingencies and discrepancies in his environment. During the first six months of life, an awareness of these phenomena enables the infant to evolve an incipient communication network with the caregiver, whereby the infant's essential needs for food, physical stimulation and soothing are conveyed. Perhaps the first such contingency experience occurs when the infant cries for food and the caregiver responds by offering the breast or bottle. The infant's need for stimulation is attended to when the caregiver engages in direct eye contact and vocalizations, while the need to be soothed is responded to by the provision of appropriate maternal holding behaviors and stroking gestures. The attentive caregiver, ever cognizant of the infant's behavioral manifestations, is essential if adaptive development is to emerge during the first three months of life.

Once the infant has developed contingency and discrepancy awareness, and has learned to integrate his perceptions amodally, he most likely begins representing the experiences he has undergone. As explained in earlier chapters, representation here refers to the capacity to envision and retain a particular sequence of interaction that has occurred in the past. The infant will be most likely to represent those sequences which have been repeated consistently by the caregiver and from such representations, predictions about the future emerge. In other words, certain representations will be used by the infant to derive forecasts about how the caregiver will be likely to interact in the future. The infant relies upon these predictions to create his own repertoire of responses designed to elicit a particular caregiver behavior.

Moreover, as has been noted in several chapters, the caregiver will use the behavioral cues and manifestations exhibited by the infant to represent imminent developmental achievement. From these representations, she will devise previewing exercises designed to acquaint the infant with what the full-fledged experience of the impending developmental milestone will be like. These exercises will be integrated into normal daily interaction and the caregiver will gradually curtail the previewing exercise when she senses that the infant is ready to return to his current developmental status.

As can be seen from the above description, during the first year of life the caregiver plays a seminal role in shaping the course of the infant's development through intuitive behaviors, overall responsiveness to the infant's needs and previewing behaviors. If the caregiver is suffering from postpartum depression, however, it is unlikely that she will be able to provide this support and as a result, the infant may experience developmental delay. This delay is caused by the fact that the infant may come to experience the world as uncontrollable and beyond mastery. Moreover, with no interactional partner, the infant will lack the motivation to engage in any form of significant exploration and may lapse into the kinds of withdrawn state that has been described by Spitz in his study of institutionalized infants.

Psychotherapeutic Techniques for Treating Depression

In the event that such postpartum depression does occur, the therapist's first task is to identify some surrogate figure-whether the father or another relative-to provide responsive care for the infant. This step is vital. Although the caregiver may recover her capacities within a short period of time, postpartum depression remains a somewhat unpredictable disorder. While the caregiver may eventually be able to resume normal interactive activities with the infant, the infant should not be deprived of a supportive other who responds to his needs, even if it is only for a few weeks. This is because the first few weeks and months are viewed by numerous researchers as a critical period during which the infant is particularly sensitive to the environment and especially in need of a supportive other to whom he can bond.

After the infant's immediate needs are cared for in this fashion, the therapist should focus on treating the caregiver. Depending upon the degree of depression the caregiver is manifesting, the therapist may use such techniques as modeling, representational exercises, previewing and using videotapes to depict how various intuitive behaviors may be integrated into the interaction with the infant. Caregivers who are seriously depressed may benefit most from modeling and videotaping techniques, because they can use their imitative skills to mirror adaptive behavior. However, it is only by engaging in representational and previewing exercises that the full awareness of the infant's burgeoning developmental course will be attained. Helping such caregivers engage in these exercises can be a lengthy and painstaking process. Nevertheless, it signifies what appears to be the best approach to surmounting depression and establishing an adaptive rapport with the infant.

Conclusion

Although the representational and previewing exercises discussed in this and other chapters can benefit virtually all mother-infant dyads, these techniques are of particular value for the therapist treating a caregiver who has given birth to a developmentally disabled or premature infant or a caregiver who experiences an episode of postpartum depression after the birth. These techniques can be used along with more conventional forms of treatment including modeling, videotape techniques and insight-oriented psychotherapy.

Therapists must recognize, however, that such caregivers often require unique kinds of treatment. For example, mothers who give birth to premature or developmentally disabled infants may experience a discrepancy between the ideal, fantasy infant who predominated during antenatal reveries and the actual infant. In such cases, the caregiver needs to be made aware of how her infant is unique and how development will proceed. It may be necessary for such caregivers to expiate their guilt over the loss of the ideal, fantasy infant in order to move on to an acceptance of the infant as he actually is. For depressed mothers, the therapist's emphasis should be on instilling representations of adaptive development. Helping the caregiver recognize the crucial role she plays in her infant's life may be a slow and painstaking process which the therapist can facilitate by reinforcing developmental trends and highlighting the intuitive manifestations that dominate previewing exercises.

Glossary

Auxiliary Coordination: The physical and psychological support the caregiver provides the infant during episodes of interaction, and in particular, during previewing episodes when the infant is introduced to an imminent developmental change. The caregiver offers auxiliary coordination by helping the infant coordinate developmental precursors into full-blown developmental milestones.

Caregiver: A consistent "other," often the mother, who serves as the infant's primary interactive partner during the first years of life.

Contingency Awareness: The cognizance that a stimulus and response are connected in a cause-and-effect relationship. Infants are capable of perceiving a contingency relationship by approximately three months of age.

Discrepancy Awareness: The cognizance of the degree of similarity or disparity between stimuli. Infants are capable of perceiving gross discrepancies a few days after birth and more subtle discrepancies by approximately three months of age.

Expectancy Awareness: The emotional and cognitive recognition that a particular stimulus is likely to occur in the imminent future. Infants are capable of representing expectancy awareness by approximately three months of age.

Intuition: Refers to the caregiver's behavioral manifestations that are ostensibly spontaneous, like reflexes, and simultaneously demonstrate an awareness of subtle behavioral cues. Such caregiver manifestations as visual cuing, vocal cuing and appropriate holding gestures are examples of intuitive behavior.

Milestones: Developmental events that signify the consolidation of a cluster of precursory tendencies into one coherent and identifiable skill. Some examples of developmental milestones include crawling, walking and talking.

Multimodal Perception: The capacity to integrate or synthesize sensations captured from diverse sensory pathways, such as sight, hearing, tactile perception, and smell, by discriminating the invariant elements of a stimulus so that a coherent representation of an object or experience can be established.

Precursors: Developmental manifestations that suggest a full-fledged milestone is on the verge of being consolidated. Sensitive caregivers are attuned to the emergence of the precursory manifestations of the infant and respond supportively in order for the infant to coordinate function.

Play: Refers to behaviors engaged in by the caregiver and infant, that enable the infant to experiment with developmental skills in an atmosphere distinctive for its pleasurable affect.

Predictive Capacities: The ability to anticipate upcoming interactions with the environment and upcoming somatic changes.

Previewing: A self-perpetuating dyadic process during which the caregiver envisions imminent developmental trends, translates such trends into behavior designed to introduce the infant to the experience of what a future developmental milestone will be like and what the implications of such changes are for future interactions with the caregiver. During the end of a previewing episode, the caregiver gradually returns the infant to the developmental level exhibited prior to the onset of the previewing activity.

Developmental Psychopathology: The study of the continuity and discontinuity of dyadic processes that motivate the members of the dyad to reinforce maladaptive interactions.

Representation: A reflective state during which perceptions of the current and future interactions become accessible to thought processes through the images perceived in the environment or encountered in the past. Representation involves the retention of visual images on the stage of active consciousness.

References

Acredolo, L. and Goodwyn, S. (1988). Symbolic gesturing in normal infants. *Child Development, 59,* 450–466.

Ahrens, R. (1954). Beitrag zur Entwicklung des Physiognomie und Mimiker-kennens. *Zeitscrift fur experimentelle und angewandte Psychologie, 2,* 412–454.

Ainsworth, M.D.S., and Bell, S.M. (1969). Some contemporary patterns in the feeding situation. In A. Ambrose (Ed.), "Stimulation in early infancy." London: Academic.

Ainsworth, M. D. S., and Bell, S. M. (1979). Attachment, exploration, and seperation: Illustrated by the behavior of one-year-olds in a Strange Situation. *Child Development, 41,* 49–67.

Ainsworth, M.D.S., Bell, S.M., and Stayton, D. (1974). Infant-mother attachment and social development. In M.P. Richards (Ed.), "The introduction of the child into a social world." London: Cambridge University Press.

Ainsworth, M.D.S., and Wittig, B. (1969). Attachment and exploratory behavior of one-year-olds in a strange situation. In B.M. Foss (Ed.), "Determinants of infant behavior, IV." London: Metheun.

Allen, T.W., Walker, K., Symonds, L., and Marcell, M. (1977). Intrasensory and intersensory perception of temporal sequences during infancy. *Developmental Psychology, 13,* 225–229.

Als, H. (1985). Reciprocity and autonomy: Parenting a blind infant. *Zero to Three, 5* (5), 8–10.

Altman, M. (1968). Mothers and children on psychiatric wards: II. The benefits of admitting infants with their mothers. *Hospital and Community Psychiatry, 19* (11), 356–359.

Areskog, B., Uddenberg, N., and Kjessler, B. (1981). Fear of childbirth in late pregnancy. *Gynecologic and Obstetric Investigation, 12,* 262–266.

Aslin, R.N., Pisoni, D.B., and Juscy, P.W. (1983). Auditory development and speech perception in infancy. In M.M. Haith and J.J. Campos (Eds.), "Handbook of child psychology (Vol.2)." New York: Wiley.

Assor, A., and Assor, T. (1985). Emotional involvement in marriage during the last trimester of the first pregnancy: A comparison of husbands and wives. *The Journal of Psychology, 119* (3), 243–252.

Austin, J.L. (1962). "How to do things with words." Oxford: Oxford University Press.

Bahrick, L.E. (1987). Infant's intermodal perception of two levels of temporal structure in natural events. *Infant Behavior and Development, 10*, 387–416.

Bahrick, L.E. (1988). Intermodal learning in infancy: learning on the basis of two kinds of invariant relations in audible and visible events. *Child Development, 59*, 197–209.

Bahrick, L.E., and Pickens, J.N. (1988). Classification of bimodal English and Spanish language passages by infants. *Infant Behavior and Development, 11*, 277–296.

Baldwin, D.A., and Markham, E.M. (1989). Establishing word-object relations: A first step. *Child Development, 60*, 381–398.

Ballou, J.W. (1978). "The Psychology of Pregnancy." Lexington, MA: Lexington Books.

Barrera, M.E., and Maurer, D. (1981). The perception of facial expressions by the three-month-old. *Child Development, 52*, 203–206.

Bates, E., O'Connell, B. and Shore, C. (1987). Language and communication in infancy. In J.D. Osofsky (Ed.), "Handbook of infant development." 2nd edition (pp. 149–203). New York: John Wiley and Sons.

Bateson, G. and Jackson, D.D. (1964). Some varieties of pathogenic organization. In "Disorders of Communication" Vol. 42. Research publications. Association for Research in nervous and mental disease (pp. 270–283).

Bayley, N. (1969). "Bayley Scales of Infant Development." New York: Psychological Corp.

Becker, P.T. (1987). Sensitivity to infant development and behavior: a comparison of adolescent and adult single mothers. *Research in Nursing and Health, 10*, 119–127.

Bee, H.L., Barnard, K.E., Eyres, S.J., Gray, C.A., Hammond, M.A., Spietz, A.L., Snyder, C., and Clark, B. (1982). Prediction of IQ and language skill from perinatal status, child performance, family characteristics, and mother-infant interaction.

Beebe, B., Gertsman, L., Carson, B., Dolins, M., Zigman, A., Rosensweig, H., Faughey, K., and Korman, M. (1979). Rhythmic communication in the mother-infant dyad. In M. Davis (Ed.), "Interaction rhythms" (pp. 79–100). New York: Human Sciences Press.

Beebe, B., and Stern, D.N. (1977). "Engagement-Disengagement and early object experiences." New York: Plenum.

Bell, S.M. (1970). The development of the concept of object as related to infant-mother attachment. *Child Development, 36* (1–2, Serial No. 142).

Bell, S. M. and Ainsworth, M. D. (1972). Infant crying and maternal responsiveness. *Child Development, 43*, 1171–1190.

Benedek, T. (1970). The psychobiology of pregnancy. In E.J. Anthony, T. Benedek (Eds.), "Parenthood; its psychology and psychopathology" (pp. 137–151). Boston: Little, Brown.

Bernstein, L. (1967). "The contribution of the social sciences to psychotherapy." Springfield, Ill.: Thomas.

Bertenthal, B.I., and Fischer, K.W. (1978). Development of self-recognition in the infant. *Developmental Psychology, 14* (1), 44–50.

Bettes, B.A. (1988). Maternal depression and motherese: temporal and intonational features. *Child Development, 59*, 1089–1096.

Bibring, G. (1961). A study of the psychological processes in pregnancy and the earliest mother-child relationship, Parts I and II. *The Psychoanalytic Study of the Child, 16,* 9–24.

Bibring, G. (1966). Recognition of psychological stress often neglected in OB care. *Hospital Topics, 44,* 100–103.

Blehar, M.C., Lieberman, A.F., and Ainsworth, M.D.S. (1977). Early face-to-face interaction and its relation to later infant-mother attachment. *Child Development, 48,* 182–194.

Blomberg, S. (1980a). Influence of maternal distress during pregnancy on fetal development and mortality. *Acta Psychiatrica Scandinavica, 62,* 298–314.

Blomberg, S. (1980b). Influence of maternal distress during pregnancy on fetal development and mortality. *Acta Psychiatrica Scandinavica, 62,* 315–330.

Bloom, K. (1979). Evaluation of infant vocal conditioning. *Journal of Experimental Child Psychology, 27,* 60–70.

Bloom, K. (1988). Quality of adult vocalizations affects the quality of infant vocalizations. *Journal of Child Language, 15* (3), 469–480.

Bloom, K. (1989). Duration of early vocal sounds. *Infant Behavior and Development, 12,* 245–250.

Bloom, L., Beckwith, R., and Capatides, J.B. (1988). Developments in the expression of affect. *Infant Behavior and Development, 11,* 169–186.

Bloom, L. and Capatides, J.B. (1987). Expression of affect and the emergence of language. *Child Development, 58,* 1513–1522.

Bodin, A. (1972). The use of videotapes. In A. Ferber, M. Mendelsohn, and A. Napier (Eds.), "The Book of Family Therapy." New York: Science House.

Boehm, F. (1930). The feminity complex in men. *International Journal of Psycho-Analysis, 11,* 444–469.

Bogren, L.Y. (1983). Couvade. *Acta Psychiatrica Neurologica, 68,* 55–65.

Bower, T.G.R. (1974). The evolution of sensory systems. In R.B. MacLeod and H.L. Pick, Jr. (Eds.), "Perception: Essays in honor of James J. Gibson" (pp. 141–165). Ithaca, NY: Cornell University Press.

Bowlby, J. (1969). "Attachment and loss" (Vol. 1). New York: Basic Books.

Bowlby, J. (1980). "Attachment and loss: Vol. 3 Loss." New York: Basic Books.

Bowlby, J. (1982). "Attachment and loss: Vol. 3 Attachment." (2nd Ed.). New York: Basic Books.

Brazelton, T.B. (1973). "Neonatal behavioral assessment." London: Spastics International Medical Publishers.

Brazelton, T.B. (1975). Mother-infant reciprocity. In M.H. Klaus, T. Leger, and M.A. Trause (Eds.), "Maternal attachment and mothering disorders: A round table" (pp. 51–54). North Brunswick, NJ: Johnson and Johnson Baby Products.

Brazelton, T.B. (1978). The remarkable talents of the newborn. *Birth and Family Journal, 5,* 4–10.

Brazelton, T.B. (1984). "Neonatal Behavioral Assessment Scale (2nd Ed)." Philadephia: Lippincott.

Brazelton, T.B., Koslowski, B., and Main, M. (1974). The origins of reciprocity: the early mother-infant interaction. In M. Lewis and L. Rosenblum (Eds.), "The effect of the infant on its caregiver." New York: Wiley.

Brazelton, T.B., Parker, W.B., Zuckerman, B. (1976). "Importance of behavioral assessment of the neonate." Chicago, Ill: Year Book Medical Pub.

Brazelton, T.B., and Yogman, M.W. (Eds.). (1986). "Affective Development in Infancy." New Jersey: Ablex.

Brazelton, T.B., Yogman, M.W., Als, H., and Tronick, E. (1979). The infant as a focus for family reciprocity. In M. Lewis and L.A. Rosenblum (Eds.), "The Child and its Family." New York: Plenum Press.

Bretherton, I. (1987). New perspectives on attachment relations: security, communication, and internal working models. In J.D. Osofsky (Ed.), "Handbook of Infant Development" (2nd Ed.). New York: Wiley.

Bretherton, I., and Bates, E. (1979). The emergence of intentional communication. In I. Uzgiris (Ed.), *New Directions for Child Development, 4*, 81–100.

Breznitz, Z. and Sherman, T. (1987). Speech patterning of natural discourse of well and depressed mothers and their young children. *Child Development, 58*, 395–400.

Brownell, C.A. (1988). Combinatorial skills: converging developments over the second year. *Child Development, 59*, 675–685.

Bruner, J.S. (1973). Organization of early skilled action. *Child Development, 44*, 1–11.

Bruner, J.S. (1974). The organization of early skilled action. In M.P.M. Richards (Ed.), "The interaction of a child into a social world." Cambridge: Cambridge university Press.

Bruner, J.S. (1983). The acquisition of pragmatic commitments. In R.M. Golinkoff (Ed.), "The transition from prelinguistic to linguistic communication" (pp. 27–42). Hillsdale, NJ: Erlbaum.

Burham, D.L. (1970). Varieties of reality reconstruction in schizophrenia. In R. Cancro (Ed.) "The schizophrenic reactions." New York: Brunner Mazel.

Bushnell, E.W. (1981). The ontogeny of intermodal relations: Vision and touch in infancy. In R.W. Walk and H.L. Pick (Eds.), "Intersensory perception and sensory integration" (pp. 5–36). New York: Plenum.

Campos, J.J., Campos, R.G., and Barrett, K.C. (1989). Emergent themes in the study of emotional development and emotion regulation. *Developmental Psychology, 25* (3), 394–402.

Campos, J.J., Hiatt, S., Ramsey, D., Henderson, C., and Svejda, M. (1978). The emergence of fear of heights. In M. Lewis and L. Rosenblum (Eds.), "The development of affect." New York: Plenum.

Campos, J.J. and Stenberg, C. (1981). Perception, appraisal and emotion: The onset of social referencing. In M. Lamb and L. Sherrod (Eds.), "Infant, social cognition." (pp. 273–314). Hillsdale, NJ: Erlbaum.

Caplan, G. (1959). "Concepts of mental health and consultation: Their application in public health social work" (DHEW Publication No. 373). Washington, DC: U.S. Government Printing Office.

Caron, A., Caron, R., Caldwell, R., and Weiss, S. (1973). Infant perception of the structural properties of the face. *Developmental Psychology, 9*, 385–399.

Caron, R.F., Caron, A.J., and Meyers, R.S. (1982). Abstraction of invariant face expressions in infancy. *Child Development, 53*, 1008–1015.

Cernock, M.J., and Porter, R.H. (1985). Recognition of maternal axillary odors by infants. *Child Development, 56*, 1593–1598.

Clinton, J.F. (1987). Physical and emotional responses of expectant fathers throughout pregnancy and the early postpartum period. *International Journal of Nursing Studies, 24* (1), 59–68.

Cohen, P., Velez, C.N., Brook, J., and Smith, J. (1989). Mechanisms of the relation between perinatal problems, early childhood illness, and psychopathology in late childhood and adolescence. *Child Development, 60*, 701–709.

Cohn, J. F., Matias, R., Tronick, E. Z., Connell, D., Lyons-Ruth, K. (1986). Face-to-face interactions of depressed mothers and their infants. In E. Z. Tronick and T. Field (Eds.), "Maternal depression and infant disturbance" (pp. 31–45). San Francisco: Josey-Bass Inc.

Cohn, J.E., and Tronick, E.Z. (1987). Mother-infant face-to-face interaction: the sequence of dyadic states at 3, 6, and 9 months. *Developmental Psychology, 23* (1), 68–77.

Coley, S.B., and James, B.E. (1976). Delivery: A trauma for fathers? *Family Coordinator, 25,* 359–363.

Condon, W.S., and Sander, L.W. (1974a). Neonate movement is synchronized with adult speech: interactional participation and language acquisition. *Science, 183* (120), 99–101.

Condon, W.S., and Sander, L.W. (1974b). Synchrony demonstrated between movements of the neonate and adult speech. *Child Development, 45* (2), 456–462.

Cramer, B.G. (1987). Objective and subjective aspects of parent-infant relations: an attempt at correlation between infant studies and clinical work. In J.D. Osofsky (Ed.), "Handbook of Infant Development" (2nd ed.). New York: Wiley.

Culp, R.E., Appelbaum, M.I., Osofsky, J.D., and Levy, J.A. (1988). Adolescent and older mothers: comparison between prenatal maternal variables and newborn interaction measures. *Infant Behavior and Development, 11,* 353–362.

De Gramont, P. (1987). Language and the self. *Contemporary Psychoanalysis, 23,* 77–121.

Decarie, T.G. (1978). Affect development and cognition in a Piagetian context. In M. Lewis and L.A. Rosenblum (Eds.), "The Development of Affect." (pp. 183–204). New York: Plenum.

DeCasper, A.J., and Carstens, A.A. (1981). Contingencies of stimulation: effects of learning and emotion in neonates. *Infant Behavior and Development, 4,* 19–35.

DeCasper, A.J., and Fifer, W.P. (1980). Of human bonding: New borns prefer their mother's voices. *Science, 208,* 1174–1176.

DeCasper, A.J., and Spence, M.J. (1986). Prenatal maternal speech influences newborn's perception of speech sounds. *Infant Behavior and Development, 9,* 133–150.

Demos, V. (1984). Empathy and affect: Reflections on infant experience. In J. Lichtenberg, M. Borenstein and D. Silver (Eds.), "Empathy" (Vol. 2) (pp. 9–34). Hillsdale, NJ: Analytic Press.

Denhoff, E. (1981). Current status of infant stimulation or enrichment programs for children with developmental disabilities. *Pediatrics, 67,* 32–37.

Deutsch, H. (1945). "The psychology of women" (Vol. 2). New York: Grune and Stratton.

Dodd, B. (1979). Lip reading in infants: Attention to speech presented in- and out-of-synchrony. *Cognitive Psychology, 11,* 478–484.

Eilers, R.E. and Minifie, F.D. (1975). Fricative discrimination in early infancy. *Journal of Speech and Hearing Research, 18* (1), 158–167.

Eimas, P. (1985). The perception of speech in early infancy. *Scientific American, 252* (1), 46–61.

Emde, R. N. (1984). The affective self: Continuities and transformations from infancy. In J. D. Call, E. Galenson, and R. L. Tyson (Eds.), "Frontiers in child development: Vol. 2." (pp. 38–54). New York: Basic Books.

Emde, R.N., Gaensbauer, T., and Harmon, R. (1976). Emotional expression in infancy: a biobehavioral study. *Psychological Issues Monograph Series, 10* (1), 37.

Emde, R.N., Kligman, D.H., Reich, J.H., and Wade, T. (1978). Emotional expression in infancy. 1. Initial studies of social signalling and an emergent model. In. M. Lewis and L. Rosenblum (Eds.), "The Development of Affect." Plenum: New York.

Emde, R.N., and Sorce, J.F. (1983). The rewards of infancy: Emotional availability and maternal referencing. In J.D. Call, E. Galenson, and R.L. Tyson (Eds.), "Frontiers of infant psychiatry" (pp. 17–30). New York: Basic Books.

Entwisle, D.R., and Doering, S.G. (1981). "The first birth." Baltimore: Johns Hopkins University Press.

Erikson, E.H. (1963). "Childhood and society." New York: Norton.

Farber, E.A., Vaughn, B. and Egeland, B. (1981). The relationship of prenatal maternal anxiety to infant behavior and mother-infant interaction during the 1st 6 months of life. *Early Human Development, 5* (3), 267–277.

Fenson, L., Kagan, J., Kearsley, R.B., and Zelazo, P.R. (1976). The developmental progression of manipulative play in the first two years. *Child Development, 47,* 232–236.

Ferguson, C.A. (1964). Baby talk in six languages. *American Anthropologist, 66,* 103–114.

Fernald, A. (1983). The perceptual and affective salience of mothers' speech to infants. In L. Feagens (Ed.), "The origins and growth of communication" (pp. 5–29). New Brunswick, NJ: Ablex.

Fernald, A. and Kuhl, P. (1987). Acoustic determinants of infant preference for motherese speech. *Infant Behavior and Development, 10,* 279–293.

Fernald, A., and Simon, T. (1984). Expanded intonation contours in mother's speech to newborns. *Developmental Psychology, 20,* 104–113.

Field, T. (1978). The three Rs of infant-adult interactions: Rhythms, repertoires, and responsivity. *Journal of Pediatric Psychology, 3* (3), 131–136.

Field, T. (1980). Preschool play: Effects of teacher/child ratios and organization of classroom space. *Child Study Journal, 10,* 191–205.

Field, T., Cohen, D., Garcia, R., and Greenberg, R. (1984). Mother-stranger face discrimination by the newborn. *Infant Behavior and Development, 7,* 19–25.

Field, T., Goldstein, S., Vega-Lahr, N., and Porter, K. (1986). Changes in imitative behavior during early infancy. *Infant Behavior and Development, 9,* 415–421.

Field, T. M., Woodson, R., Greenberg, R., and Cohen, D. (1982). Discrimination and imitation of facial expressions by neonates. *Science, 218,* 179–182.

Fitts, W.H. (1965). "Tennessee self-concept scale." Nashville: Counselor Recordings and Tests.

Fleming, A. S., Ruble, D. N., Flett, G. L., and Shaul, D. L. (1988). Postpartum adjustment in first-time mothers: Relations between mood, maternal attitudes, and mother-infant interactions. *Developmental Psychology, 24,* 71–81.

Fogel, A. (1980). The effect of brief separations on 2-month-old infants. *Infant Behavior and Development, 3,* 315–330.

Freeman, T. (1951). Pregnancy as a precipitant of mental illness in men. *British Journal of Medical Psychology, 24,* 49–54.

Fuchs, A.R., and Fuchs, F. (1984). Endicrinology of term and preterm labor. In F. Fuchs and P.G. Stubblefield (Eds.), "Preterm birth: Causes, prevention, and management" (pp. 39–63). New York: Macmillan.

Gaffney, K.F. (1986). Maternal-fetal attachment in relation to self-concept and anxiety. *Maternal-Child Nursing Journal, 15* (2), 91–101.

Gerzi, S., and Berman, E. (1981). Emotional reactions of expectant fathers to their wives' first pregnancy. *British Journal of Medical Psychology, 54,* 259–265.

Gibson, E.J. (1969). "Principles of perceptual learning and development." New York: Appleton-Century-Crofts.

Goldberg, P. (1989). Actively seeking the holding environment. *Contemporary Psychoanalysis, 25* (3), 448–476.

Goldman, B.D., and Ross, H.S. (1978). Social skills in action: an analysis of early peer games. In J. Glick and K.A. Clarke-Stewart (Eds.), "The development of social understanding" (pp. 177–212). New York: Gardner Press.

Greenberg, N.H. (1971). A comparison of infant-mother interactional behavior in infants with atypical behavior and normal infants. In J. Hellmuth (Ed.), "Exceptional infant"(Vol. 2). New York: Brunner/Mazel.

Grieser, D., and Kuhl, P.K. (1989). Categorization of speech by infants; Support for speech-sound prototypes. *Developmental Psychology, 25* (4), 577–588.

Gunnar, M.R., and Stone, C. (1984). The effects of positive maternal affect on infant responses to pleasant, ambiguous, and fear-provoking toys. *Child Development, 55,* 1231–1236.

Haekel, M. (1985). Greeting behavior in three-month-old infants during mother-infant interaction. Presentation at the Eighth Biennial Meetings of the International Society for the Study of Behavioral Development, Tours, France. Abstracted in *Cahiers de psychologie cognitive, 5,* 275–276.

Haith, M.M., Bergman, T., and Moore, M.J. (1977). Eye contact and face scanning in early infancy. *Science, 198,* 853–855.

Haith, M.M., Hazan, C., and Goodman, G.S. (1988). Expectation and anticipation of dynamic visual events by 3.5-month-old babies. *Child Development, 59,* 467–479.

Harding, C.G. (1982). Development of the intention to communicate. *Human Development, 25* (2), 140–151.

Harding, C.G., and Golinkoff, R.M. (1979). The origins of intentional vocalizations in prelinguistic infants. *Child Development, 50,* 33–40.

Haskett, J., and Holler, W.D. (1978). Sensory reinforcement and contingency awareness of profoundly retarded chidren. *American Journal of Mental Deficiency, 83* (1), 60–68.

Haviland, J.M., and Lelwica, M. (1987). The induced affect response: Ten-week-old infants' responses to three emotion expressions. *Developmental Psychology, 23* (1), 97–104.

Hayes, A., and Elliott, T. (1979). "Gaze and vocalization in mother-infant dyads: conversation or coincidence?" Paper presented at the biennial meeting of the *Society for Research in Child Development*, San Francisco.

Heinicke, C., Diskin, S., Ramsey-Klee, D., and Given, K. (1983). Prebirth characteristics and family development in the first year of life. *Child Development, 54,* 194–208.

Hodapp, R.M., Goldfield, E.C., and Boyatzis, C.J. (1984). The use and effectiveness of maternal scaffolding in mother-infant games. *Child Development, 55,* 772–781.

Hoffman, M.L. (1975). Developmental synthesis of affect and cognition and its implications for altruistic motivation. *Developmental Psychology, 11,* 607–622.

Hoffman, M.L. (1984). Interaction of affect and cognition in empathy. In C.E. Izard, J. Kagan, and R.B. Zajonc (Eds.), "Emotions, cognition and behavior" (pp. 103–131). Cambridge, England: Cambridge University Press.

Hopkins, B., and van Wulfften Palthe, T. (1985). Staring in infancy. *Early Human Development, 12,* 261–267.

Horan, M.L. (1982). Parental reaction to the birth of an infant with a defect: an attributional approach. *Advances in Nursing Science, 5* (1), 57–68.

Hornik, R., and Gunnar, M. R. (1988). A descriptive analysis of infant social referencing. *Child Development, 59,* 626–634.

Hornik, R., Risenhoover, N., and Gunnar, M. (1987). The effects of maternal positive, neutral, and negative affective communications on infant responses to new toys. *Child Development, 58,* 937–944.

Hughes, M. (1987). The relationship between symbolic and manipulative (object) play. In D. Gorlitz and J. F. Wohlwill (Eds.), "Curiosity, imagination, and play" (pp. 247–257). Hillsdale, NJ: Erlbaum.

Isabella, R.A., Belsky, J., and von Eye, A. (1989). Origins of infant-mother attachment: An examination of interactional synchrony during the infant's first year. *Developmental Psychology, 25* (1), 12–21.

Istvan, J. (1986). Stress, anxiety, and birth outcomes: A critical review. *Psychological Bulletin, 100* (3), 331–348.

Jaffe, D. S. (1968). The masculine envy of woman's procreative functions. *Journal of the American Psychoanalytic Association, 16,* 521–548.

Jaffe, J., Stern, D.N., and Peery, J.C. (1973). Conversational coupling of gaze behavior in prelinguistic human development. *Journal Psycholinguist Research, 2,* 321–330.

Jarvis, W. (1962). Some effects of prenancy and childbirth on men. *Journal of the American Psychoanalytic Association, 10,* 689–700.

Kaye, K. (1982). Construction of the person. In K. Kaye (Ed.) "The mental and social life of babies: How parents create persons." Chicago: University of Chicago Press.

Kaye, K. and Fogel, A. (1980). The temporal structure of face-to-face communication between mothers and infants. *Developmental Psychology, 16,* 454–464.

Keller, H., and Scholmerich, A. (1987). Infant vocalizations and parental reactions during the first 4 months of life. *Developmental Psychology, 23* (1), 62–67.

Kennell, J.H., and Klaus, M.H. (1982). Caring for the parents of premature or sick infants. In "Parent-Infant Bonding" (2nd Ed.). St. Louis: The C.V. Mosby Company.

Klaus, M. and Kennell, J. (1982). Interventions in the premature nursery-impact in development. *Pediatric Clinics of North America, 29* (5), 1263–1273.

Klinnert, M.D., Campos, J.J., Sorce, J.F., Emde, R.N., and Svejda, M. (1983). Emotions as behavior regulators: Social referencing in infancy. In R. Plutchik and H. Kellerman (Eds.), "Emotions in early development." New York: Academic Press.

Koopmans-van-Beinum, F.J., and van der Stelt, B. (1985). Early stages in the development of speech movements. In B. Lindblom and R. Zetterstrom (Eds.), "Precursors of early speech." Basingstrake, Hampshire: MacMillan.

Kopp, C.B. (1989). Regulation of distress and negative emotions: A developmental view. *Developmental Psychology, 25* (3), 343–354.

Korner, A.F. (1987). Preventive intervention with high-risk newborns: theoretical, conceptual, and methodological perspectives. In J.D. Osofsky (Ed.), "Handbook of Infant Development." New York: Wiley.

Korner, A.F., Gabby, T., and Kraemer, H.C. (1980). Relation between prenatal maternal blood pressure and infant irritability. *Early Human Development, 4,* 9–18.

Kuhl, P., and Meltzoff, A. (1982). The bimodal perception of speech in infancy. *Science, 218,* 1138–41.

Kuhl, P., and Meltzoff, A. (1984). The intermodal representation of speech in infants. *Infant Behavior and Development, 7,* 361–381.

Kumar, R., Robson, K.M., and Smith, A.M.R. (1984). Development of a self-administered questionnaire to measure maternal adjustment and maternal attitudes during pregnancy and after delivery. *Journal of Psychosomatic Research, 28* (1), 43–51.

Kurzweil, S.R. (1988). Recognition of mother from multisensory interactions in early infancy. *Infant Behavior and Development, 11,* 235–243.

Lacan, J. (1977). "Ecrits." New York: W.W. Norton and Co.

Lacan, J. (1982). "Ecrits." New York: W.W. Norton and Co.

Landry, S.H., and Chapieski, M.L. (1989). Joint attention and infant toy exploration: Effects of Down Syndrome and prematurity. *Child Development, 60,* 103–118.

Landry, S.H., Chapieski, M.L., and Schmidt, M. (1986). Effects of maternal attention-directing strategies on preterms response to toys. *Infant Behavior and Development, 9* (3), 257–269.

Lawson, K.R. (1980). Spatial and temporal congruity and auditory-visual integration in infants. *Developmental Psychology, 16,* 185–192.

Lederman, E., Lederman, R. P., Work, B. A., Jr., and McCann, D. S. (1981). Maternal psychological and physiological correlates of fetal-newborn health status. *American Journal of Obstetrics and Gynecology, 139,* 956–958.

Lederman, R.P. (1986). Maternal anxiety in pregnancy: Relationship to fetal and newborn health status. *Annual Review of Nursing Research, 4,* 3–19.

Lederman, R.P., Lederman, E., Work, Jr., B.A., and McCann, D.S. (1979). Relationship of psychological factors in pregnancy to progress in labor. *Nursing Research, 28,* 94–97.

Legerstee, M., Pomerleau, A., Malcuit, G., and Feider, H. (1987). The development of infants' responses to people and a doll: Implications for research in communication. *Infant Behavior and Development, 10,* 81–95.

Leifer, M. (1980). "Psychological effects of motherhood: A study of first pregnancy." New York: Praeger.

Lester, B. M. and Dreher, M. (1989). Effects of marijuana use during pregnancy on newborn cry. *Child Development, 60,* 765–771.

Levy, J.M., and McGhee, R.K. (1975). Childbirth as a crisis: A test of Janis' theory of communication and stress resolution. *Journal of Personality and Social Psychology, 31,* 171–179.

Lewis, M., and Feiring, C. (1989). Infant, mother, and mother-infant interaction behavior and subsequent attachment. *Child Development, 60,* 831–837.

Lewis, M., Wolan-Sullivan, M., and Brooks-Gunn, J. (1985). Emotional behavior during the learning of a contingency in early infancy. *British Journal of Developmental Psychology, 3,* 307–316.

Lieberman, P. (1970). Towards a unified phonetic theory. *Linguistic Inquiry, 1,* 307–322.

Lieberman, P. (1973). On the evolution of human language: A unified view. *Cognition, 2,* 59–94.

Little, R.E. (1977). Moderate alcohol use during pregnancy and decreased infant weight. *American Journal of Public Health, 67,* 1154–1156.

Lounsburg, M. L. (1979). Acoustic properties of and maternal reactions to infant cries as a function of infant temperament. *Dissertation Abstracts International, 39* (9-B), 4585–4586.

Lowe, M. (1975). Trends in the development of representational play in infants from one to three years-an observational study. *Journal of Child Psychology and Psychiatry and Allied Disciplines, 16,* 33–47.

Lutzker, S.Z., Lutzker, J.R., Braunling-McMorrow, D., and Eddleman, J. (1987). Prompting to increase mother-baby stimulation with single mothers. *Journal of Child and Adolescent Behavior, 4* (1), 3–12.

Lyons-Ruth, K. (1977). Bimodal perception in infancy: Response to auditory-visual incongruity. *Child Development, 46,* 820–827.

MacKain, K., Studdert-Kennedy, M., Spieker, S., and Stern, D. (1983). Infant intermodal speech perception is a left-hemisphere function. *Science, 219,* 1347–1349.

Mahler, M.S., Pine, F., and Bergman, A. (1975). "The psychological birth of the human infant." New York: Basic Books.

Main, M., Kaplan, K., and Cassidy, J. (1985). Security in infancy, childhood and adulthood. A move to the level of representation. In I. Bretherton and E. Waters (Eds.), "Growing points of attachment theory and research." *Monographs of the Society for Research in Child Development, 50* (1–2, Serial No. 209), 66–104.

Main, M., and Weston, D. (1982). Avoidance of the attachment figure in infancy: Descriptions and interpretations. In C.M. Parkes and J. Stevenson-Hinde (Eds.), The place of attachment in human behavior. New York: Basic Books.

Marlatt, G.A. (1983). Stress as a determinant of excessive drinking and relapse. In L. A. Pohorecky and J. Brick (Eds.), "Stress and alcohol use" (pp. 279–294). New York: Elsevier.

Mast, V.K., Fagen, J.W., Rovee-Collier, C.K., and Sullivan, M.V. (1980). Immediate and longterm memory for reinforcement context: The development of learned expectancies in early infancy. *Childhood Development, 51,* 700–707.

McCall, R.B. and Kagan, J. (1967). Stimulus-schema discrepancy and attention in the infant. *Journal of Experimental Child Psychology, 5,* 381–390.

McCall, R.B., and Kagan, J. (1970). Individual differences in the infant's distribution of attention to stimulus discrepancy. *Developmental Psychology, 2* (1), 90–98.

McCall, R.B., and McGee, P.E. (1977). The discrepency hypothesis of attention and affect in infants. In I.C. Uzgiris and F. Weizmann (Eds)., "The Structuring of Experience" (pp. 179–210). New York: Plenum Press.

McCarthy, D. (1972). "Manual for the McCarthy scales of children's abilities." New York: Psychological Corporation.

McNeil, T.F., and Wiegerink, R. (1971). Behavioral patterns and pregnancy and birth complication histories in psychologically disturbed children. *Journal of Nervous and Mental Disease, 152,* 315–323.

McNeil, T.F., Wiegerink, R., and Dozier, J.E. (1970). Pregnancy and birth complications in the births of seriously, moderately, and mildly behaviorally disturbed children. *Journal of Nervous and Mental Disease, 151,* 24–34.

Mebert, C.J., and Kalinowski, M.F. (1986). Parent's expectations and perceptions of infant temperament: "Pregnancy Status" differences. *Infant Behavior and Development, 9,* 321–334.

Mehra, B., and Pines, D. (1972). Study of promiscuous girls under the auspices of the Centre for Adolescent Research. Unpublished.

Meltzoff, A. N. (1981). Imitation, intermodal coo-ordination, and representation in early infancy. In G. Butterworth (Ed.), " Infancy and epistemology" (pp. 85–114). Brighton, England: Harvester Press.

Meltzoff, A. N. (1988). Infant imitation after a 1-week delay: long-term memory for novel acts and multiple stimuli. *Developmental Psychology, 24* (4), 470–476.

Meltzoff, A.N. and Borton, R.W. (1979). Intermodal matching by human neonates. *Nature, 282* (22), 403–404.

Meltzoff, A.N., and Moore, M.K. (1977). Imitation of facial and manual gestures by human neonates. *Science, 24,* 75–78.

Meltzoff, A.N., and Moore M.K. (1983a). Newborn infants imitate adult facial gestures. *Child Development, 31,* 78–84.

Meltzoff, A.N., and Moore, M.K. (1983b). The origins of imitation on infancy: Paradigm, phenomena, and theories. In L.P. Lipsett (Ed.), "Advances in Infancy" (Vol. 2.) (pp. 265–301). Norwood, NJ: Ablex Publishing Company.

Mendelson, M.J. and Ferland, M.B. (1982). Auditory-visual transfer in four-month-old infants. *Child Development, 53,* 1022–1027.

Menn, L., and Boyce, S. (1982). Fundamental frequency and discource structure. *Language and Speech, 25,* 341–383.

Messer, D. J. (1978). The integration of mothers' referential speech with joint play. *Child Development, 49* (3), 781–787.

Messer, D.J., McCarthy, M.E., McQuiston, S., MacTurk, R.H., Yarrow, L.J., and Vietze, P.M. (1986). Relation between mastery behavior in infancy and competence in early childhood. *Developmental Psychology, 22* (3), 366–372.

Messer, D.J., and Vietze, P.M. (1988). Does mutual influence occur during mother-infant social gaze? *Infant Behavior and Development, 11,* 97–110.

Moran, G., Krupka, A., Tutton, A., and Symons, D. (1987). Patterns of maternal and infant imitation during play. *Infant Behavior and Development, 10,* 477–491.

Muller, J.P., and Richardson, W.J. (1982). "Lacan and language: A reader's guide to Ecrits." New York: International Universities Press.

Mundy, P., Sigman, M., Kasari, C., and Yirmiya, N. (1988). Nonverbal communication skills in down syndrome children. *Child Development, 59,* 235–249.

Mura, E.L. (1974). Perinatal differences: A comparison of child psychiatric patients and their siblings. *Psychiatric Quarterly, 48,* 239–255.

Murray, L. and Trevarthan, C. (1986). The infant's role in mother-infant communications. *Journal of Child Language, 13* (1), 15–29.

Nelson, C.A. (1985). The perception and recognition of facial expressions in infancy. In T.M. Field and N.A. Fox (Eds.), "Social perception in infants" (pp. 101–125). Norwood, NJ: Ablex.

Nelson, C.A. (1987). The recognition of facial expressions in the first two years of life: Mechanisms of development. *Child Development, 58,* 889–909.

Nelson, C.A., and Dolgin, K. (1985). The generalized discrimination of facial expressions by 7-month-old infants. *Child Development, 56,* 58–61.

Nelson, C.A., and Horowitz, F.D. (1983). The perception of facial expressions and stimulus motion by 2- and 5-month-old infants using holographic stimuli. *Child Development, 54,* 868–877.

Nelson, C.A., and Ludemann, P. (1987). The categorical representation of facial expressions by 4- and 7-month-old infants. Manuscript submitted for publication.

Nilsson, A., Almgren, P.E., Kohler, E.M., and Kohler, L. (1973). Enuresis: The importance of maternal attitudes and personality. A prospective study of pregnant women and a follow-up of their children. *Acta Psychiatrica Scandinavica, 49,* 114–130.

Oller, D.K. and Eilers, R.E. (1988). The role of audition in infant babbling. *Child Development, 59,* 441–449.

Ottinger, D.R., and Simmons, J.E. (1964). Behavior of human neonates and prenatal maternal anxiety. *Psychological Reports, 14,* 391–394.

Papousek, H., and Papousek, M. (1975). Cognitive aspects of preverbal social interaction between human infants and adults. In M. O'Connor (Ed.), "Parent-infant interaction" (pp. 241–269). Amsterdam: Elsevier.

Papousek, H., and Papousek, M. (1977). Mothering and the cognitive headstart: Psychobiological consideration. In H.R. Schaffer (Ed.), "Studies in mother-infant interactions." (pp. 63–85). London: Academic.

Papousek, H., and Papousek, M. (1987). Intuitive parenting: A dialectic counterpart to the infant's integrative competence. In J.D. Osofsky (Ed.), "Handbook of Infant Development" (2nd edition). New York: Wiley.

Papousek, M., Papousek, H., and Harris, B.J. (1987). The way to the origins of play. In D. Gorlitz and J.F. Wohlwill (Eds.), "Curiosity, imagination, and play." Hillsdale, NJ: Erlbaum.

Parke, R.D., and Sawin, D.B. (1975). Infant characteristics and behavior as elictors of maternal and paternal responsibility in the newborn period. Paper presented at the biennial meeting of the *Society for Research in Child Development,* Denver.

Pawlby, S.F. (1977). Imitative interaction. In H.R. Schaffer (Ed.), Studies in mother-infant interaction" (pp. 203–224). New York: Academic Press.

Pederson, F.A. (1975). Mother, father and infant as an interactive system. Paper presented at the *Annual Convention of the American Psychological Association,* Chicago.

Piaget, J. (1951). "Play, dreams, and imitation in childhood." London: Heinemann.

Piaget, J. (1952). "The origins of intelligence in children." New York: International Universities Press.

Piaget, J. (1953). "The origins of intelligence in the child." London: Routledge.

Piaget, J., and Inhelder, B. (1956). "The child's conception of space." London: Routledge.

Pines, D. (1972). Pregnancy and motherhood: interaction between fantasy and reality. *British Journal of Medical Psychology, 45,* 333–343.

Piper, M.P. (1982). A parent's perspective: Prevention or crisis intervention? *Developmental and Behavioral Pediatrics, 3* (4), 236–238.

Pohlman, E.W. (1968). Changes from rejection to acceptance of pregnancy. *Social Science and Medicine, 2,* 337–340.

Poley-Strobel, B.A., and Beckmann, C.A. (1987). The effects of a teaching-modeling intervention of early mother-infant reciprocity. *Infant Behavior and Development, 10,* 476–476.

Price, G.M. (1983). Sensitivity in mother-infant interactions: The AMIS scale. *Infant Behavior and Development, 6,* 353–360.

Prugh, D.G., Staub, E.M., Sands, H.H., Kirschbaum, R.M., and Lenihan, E.A. (1953). A study of the emotional reactions of children and families to hospitalization and illness. *American Journal of Orthopsychiatry, 23,* 70–106.

Raphael-Leff, J. (1986). Facilitators and regulators: Conscious and unconscious processes in pregnancy and early motherhood. *British Journal of Medical Psychology, 59,* 43–55.

Rapoport, R. (1963). Normal crises: family structure and mental health. *Family Process, 2,* 68–80.

Reissland, N. (1988). Neonatal imitation in the first hour of life: observations in rural Nepal. *Developmental Psychology, 24,* 464–469.

Robson, K. (1967). The role of eye-to-eye contact in maternal-infant attachment. *Journal of Child Psychology of Psychiatry and Allied Disciplines, 8,* 13–25.

Rose, G.T. (1961). Pregenital aspects of pregnancy fantasies. *International Journal of Psycho-Analysis, 42,* 544–549.

Rose, S.A., and Ruff, H.A. (1987). Cross-modal abilities in human infants. In J.D. Osofsky (Ed.), "Handbook of Infant Behavior and Development" (pp. 318–362). New York: Wiley.

Ross, H.S. (1982). The establishment of social games among toddlers. *Developmental Psychology, 18,* 509–518.

Ross, H.S. and Lollis, S.P. (1987). Communication within infant social games. *Developmental Psychology, 23* (2), 241–248.

Roth, P. (1987). "Longitudinal study of maternal verbal interaction styles." Paper presented at the biennial meeting of the *Society for Research in Child Development,* Baltimore, MD.

Rovee-Collier, C.K., and Fagan, C.W. (1981). The retrieval of memory in early infancy. In L.P. Lipsett (Ed.), "Advances in infancy research" (Vol. 1). Norwood, NJ: Ablex.

Rubin, R. (1975). Maternal tasks of pregnancy. *Maternal-Child Nursing Journal, 4* (3), 143–153.

Rubin, R. (1977). Binding-in in the postpartum period. *Maternal-Child Nursing Journal, 6* (2), 67–75.

Ruddy, M.G., and Bornstein, M.H. (1982). Cognitive correlates of infant attention and maternal stimulation over the first year of life. *Child Development, 53,* 183–188.

Rutter, D.R., and Durkin, K. (1987). Turn-taking in mother-infant interaction: An examination of vocalizations and gaze. *Developmental Psychology, 23* (1), 54–61.

Ryan, T.A. (1970). "Intentional behavior: an approach to human motivation." NY: Ronald.

Salzman, L. (1984). Change and the therapeutic process. In J.M. Myers (Ed.), "Cures by Psychotherapy: What effects change?" New York: Praeger.

Shainess, N. (1968). Abortion. Social, psychiatric, and psychoanalytic perspectives. *New York State Journal of Medicine, 68* (23), 3070–3073.

Shereshefsky, P.M., and Yarrow, L.J. (Eds.) (1970). "Psychological aspects of a first pregnancy and early postnatal adaptation." New York: Raven Press.

Snow, C.E. (1977). Mothers' speech research: From input to interaction. In C.E. Snow and C.A. Ferguson (Eds.), "Talking to children: Language input and acquisition." Cambridge, England: Cambridge University Press.

Sorce, J.F., Emde, R.N., Campos, J., and Klinnert, M.D. (1985). Maternal emotional signaling: Its effect on the visual cliff behavior of one-year-olds. *Developmental Psychology, 21* (1), 195–200.

Sosa, R., Kennell, J., Klaus, M., Robertson, S., and Urrutia, J. (1980). The effect of a supportive companion on perinatal problems, length of labor, and mother-infant interaction. *New England Journal of Medicine, 303,* 597–600.

Spelke, E.S. (1979). Perceiving bimodally specified events in infancy. *Developmental Psychology, 15,* 626–636.

Spelke, E.S. (1981). The infant's acquisition of knowledge of bimodally specified events. *Journal of Experimental Child Psychology, 31,* 279–299.

Spelke, E.S., Born, W.S., and Chu, F. (1983). Perception of moving, sounding objects by four-month-old infants. *Perceptions, 12,* 719–732.

Spence, D.P. (1982). "Narrative truth and historical truth: meaning and interpretation in psychoanalysis." New York: W.W. Norton and Company.

Spence, M. J. and DeCasper, A. J. (1987). Prenatal experience with low-frequency maternal-voice sounds influence neonatal perception of maternal voice samples. *Infant behavior and Development, 10,* 133–142.

Spielberger, C., Gorsuch, R., and Lushene, R. (1970). "STAI Manual." Palo Alto, CA: Consulting Psychologists Press.

Spitz, R.A. (1944). Psychosomatic principles and methods and their clinical application. *Medical Clinics of North America, 28,* 553–564.

Spitz, R.A. (1945). Hospitalism. An inquiry into the genesis of psychiatric conditions in early childhood. *Psychoanalytic Study of the Child, 1,* 53–74.

Spitz, R.A. (1946). Anaclitic depression. *Psychoanalytic Study of the Child, 2,* 113–117.

Spitz, R.A. (1953). "Science and human behavior." New York: Macmillan.

Sroufe, L.A., and Wunsch, J.P. (1972). The development of laughter in the first year of life. *Child Development, 43,* 1326–1344.

Standley, K., Soule, A.B., and Copans, S.A. (1979). Dimensions of prenatal anxiety and their influence of pregnancy outcome. *American Journal of Obstetrics and Gynecology, 135,* 22–26.

Standley, K., Soule, A.B., Copans, S.A., and Klein, R.P. (1978). Multidimensional sources of infant temperament. *Genetic Psychology Monographs, 98,* 203–231.

Stern, D.N. (1974). Mother and infant at play: The dyadic interaction involving facial, vocal, and gaze behaviors. In M. Lewis and L.A. Rosenblum (Eds.), "The effect of the infant on its caretaker," Vol. 1. New York: Wiley.

Stern, D.N. (1979). Play and learning in the first year: new insights. *Pediatric Nursing, 5* (5), Suppl. B-G.

Stern, D.N. (1985). "The interpersonal world of the infant: A view from psychoanalysis and developmental psychology." New York: Basic Books.

Stern, D.N., and Gibbon, J. (1978). Temporal expectancies of social behaviors in mother-infant play. In E. Thoman (Ed.), "Origins of the infant's social responsiveness" (pp. 409–429). New York: Erlbaum Press.

Stern, D.N., and Gibbon, J. (1980). Temporal expectancies of social behaviors in mother-infant play. In E. Thoman (Ed.), "Origins of the Infant: Social Responsiveness." New York: Erlbaum.

Stern, D.N., Spieker, S., Barnett, R.K., and MacKain, D. (1983). The prosody of maternal speech: Infant age and context related changes. *Journal of Child Language, 10,* 1–15.

Stevenson, M.B., Ver Hoeve, J.N., Roach, M.A., and Leavitt, L.A. (1986). The beginning of conversation: early patterns of mother-infant vocal responsiveness. *Infant Behavior and Development, 9* (4), 423–440.

Strang, V.R., and Sullivan, P.L. (1984). Body image attitudes during pregnancy and the postpartum period. *Journal of Obstetric, Gynecologic, and Neonatal Nursing, 14* (4), 332–337.

Strom, R., Rees, R., Slaughter, H., and Wurster, S. (1980). Role expectations of parents of intellectually handicapped children. *Exceptional Children, 47* (2), 144–147.

Susman, V. L., and Katz, J. L (1988). Weaning and depression: another postpartum complication. *American Journal of Psychiatry, 145* (4), 498–501.

Tamis-LeMonda, C.S., and Bornstein, M.H. (1989). Habituation and maternal encouragement of attention in infancy as predictors of toddler language, play, and representational competence. *Child Development, 60,* 738–751.

Taylor, M., and Gelman, S.A. (1989). Incorporating new words into the lexicon: Preliminary evidence for language hierarchies in two-year-old children. *Child Development, 60,* 625–636.

Tennen, H., Affleck, G., and Gershman, K. (1986). Self-blame among parents of infants with perinatal complications: The role of self-protective motives. *Journal of Personality and Social Psychology, 50* (4), 690–696.

Termine, I., and Izard, C.E. (1988). Infant's responses to their mother's expressions of joy and sadness. *Developmental Psychology, 24* (2), 223–229.

Theut, S.K., Pedersen, F.A., Zaslow, M.J., and Rabinovich, B.A. (1988). *Journal of the American Academy of Child and Adolescent Psychiatry, 27* (3), 289–292.

Thoman, E.B., and Browder, S. (1987). "Born dancing." New York: Harper and Row.

Thomas, A. and Chess, S. (1986). "Temperament in clinical practice." NY: Guilford.

Thomas, G.V., Phemister, M.R., and Richardson, A.M. (1980). Some conditions affecting manipulative play with objects in severely mentally handicapped children.

Trad, P. V. (1986). "Infant depression: Paradigms and Paradoxes." New York: Springer-Verlag.

Trad, P. V. (1987). "Infant and childhood depression: Developmental factors." New York: Wiley.

Trad, P. V. (1989a). "The preschool child: Assessment, Diagnosis, and Treatment." New York: Wiley.

Trad, P. V. (1989b). Self-mutilation in a new mother: a strategy for separating from her infant. *American Journal of Psychotherapy, 43*, 414–425.

Trevarthen, C. (1979). Communication and cooperation in early infancy: a description of primary intersubjectivity. In M. Bullowa (Ed.), "Before speech: The beginning of interpersonal communication." Cambridge: Cambridge University Press.

Trevarthen, C. (1980). The foundations of intersubjectivity: Development of interpersonal and cooperative understanding in infants. In D.R. Olson (Ed.), "The social foundations of language and thought: Essays in honor of Jerome S. Bruner" (pp. 316–342). New York: W.W. Norton and Company.

Trevarthen, C. (1985). Facial expressions of emotion in mother-infant interaction. *Human Neurobiology, 4*, 21–32.

Trevarthen, C., and Hubley, P. (1979). Secondary intersubjectivity: Confidence, confiding, and acts of meaning in the first year. In A. Lock (Ed.), "Action, gesture, and symbol" (pp. 183–229). London: Academic.

Tronick, E.Z., and Cohn, J.F. (1989). Infant-mother face-to-face interaction: Age and gender differences in coordination and the occurrence of miscoordination. *Child Development, 60*, 85–92.

Tronick, E.Z., Cohn, J., and Shea, E. (1986). The transfer of affect between mothers and infants. In T.B. Brazelton and M.W. Yogman (Eds.), "Affective development in infancy." Norwood, NJ: Ablex Publishing.

Uzigris, I., and Hunt, J, McV. (1975). "Assessment in infancy: Ordinal scales of psychological development." Urbana, IL: University of Illinois Press.

Van der Zanden, J.W. (1981). "Human development." New York: Knopf.

Vygotsky, L.S. (1962). Thought and language (E. Haufmann and G. Vakaer, Eds. and Trans.). Cambridge, MA: M.I.T. Press.

Vygotsky, L.S. (1978). "Mind in society: The development of higher psychological processes." (M. Cole, V. John-Steiner, S. Scribner, and E. Souberman, Eds.), Cambridge, MA: Harvard University Press.

Waisbren, S.E. (1980). Parents' reactions after the birth of a developmentally disabled child. *American Journal of Mental Disorders, 4*, 345–351.

Walden, T.A., and Ogan, T.A. (1988). The development of social referencing. *Child Development, 59*, 1230–1240.

Walker, A.S. (1982). Intermodal perception of expressive behaviors by human infants. *Journal of Experimental Child Psychology, 33*, 514–535.

Walsh, W.H. (1958). Plain and significant narrative in history. *Journal of Philosophy, 55*, 479–484.

Watson, J.S. (1966). The development of and generalization of "contingency awareness" in early infancy. *Merrill Palmer Quarterly, 12*, 123–125.

Watson, J.S. (1972). Smiling, cooing and "the game." *Merrill Palmer Quarterly, 18*, 323–339.

Watson, J.S. (1977). Perception of contingency as a determinant of social responsiveness. In E.B. Thoman (Ed.) Origins of the infant's social responsiveness (pp. 33–63). New Jersey: Erlbaum.

Watson, J.S., and Ramey, C.T. (1972). Smiling, cooing, and "the game." *Merrill Palmer Quarterly, 18*, 323–339.

Watzlawick, P., Beavin, J., and Jackson, D. (1967). "Pragmatics of Human Communication." New York: Norton.

Weakland, J.H., Fisch, R., Watzlawick, P., and Bodin, A.M. (1981). Brief therapy. In R. J. Green and J. L. Framo (Eds.), "Family Therapy: Major Contributions." New York: International Universities Press.

Werner, E., Simonian, K., Bierman, J.M., and French, F.E. (1967). Cumulative effect of perinatal complications and deprived environment on physical, intellectual, and social development of preschool children. *Pediatrics, 39,* 490–505.

Werner, H., and Kaplan, B. (1963). "Symbol formation." New York: Wiley.

Winnicott, D.W. (1965). "The maturational processes and the facilitating environment." New York: International Universities Press.

Winnicott, D.W. (1971). "Playing and Reality." London: Penguin Books.

Witelson, S. F. (1987). Neurobiological aspects of language in children. *Child Development, 58,* 653–688.

Woodson, R.H., Jones, N.G., da Costa-Woodson, E., Pollock, S., and Evans, M. (1979). Fetal mediators of the relationships between increased pregnancy and labour blood pressure and newborn irritability. *Early Human Development, 3,* 127–139.

Yarrow, L.J. (1967). The development of focused relationships during infancy. In J. Hellmuth (Ed.), "Exceptional Infant" (Vol. 1). Seattle: Special Child Publications.

Young-Browne, G., Rosenfeld, H.M., and Horowitz, F.E. (1977). Infant discrimination of facial expressions. *Child Development, 48,* 555–562.

Zelazo, P.R., and Kearsley, R.B. (1980). The emergence of functional play in infants: Evidence for a major cognitive transition. *Journal of Applied Developmental Psychology, 1,* 95–117.

Author Index

Subject Index